1.08

2008

Standards for **Ambulatory Care**

SAC

Accreditation Policies

Standards

Elements of Performance

Scoring

DISCARDED
GEORGE WASHINGTON UNIVERSITY
PAUL HIMMELFARB HEALTH SCIENCES LIBRARY
2300 EYE STREET N. W
WASHINGTON, D.C. 20037

AF784587

The Joint Commission
Accreditation
Ambulatory Care

http://www.jointcommission.org

Joint Commission Mission

The mission of The Joint Commission is to continuously improve the safety and quality of care provided to the public through the provision of health care accreditation and related services that support performance improvement in health care organizations.

© 2008 by The Joint Commission on Accreditation of Healthcare Organizations

Joint Commission Resources, Inc. (JCR), a not-for-profit affiliate of the Joint Commission, has been designated by the Joint Commission to publish publications and multimedia products. JCR reproduces and distributes these materials under license from the Joint Commission.

JCR educational programs and publications support, but are separate from, the accreditation activities of the Joint Commission. Attendees at JCR educational programs and purchasers of JCR publications receive no special consideration or treatment in, or confidential information about, the accreditation process.

All rights reserved. No part of this publication may be reproduced in any form or by any means without written permission from the publisher.

Printed in the U.S.A. 5 4 3 2 1

Requests for permission to make copies of any part of this work should be mailed to
Permissions Editor
Department of Publications
Joint Commission Resources
One Renaissance Boulevard
Oakbrook Terrace, Illinois 60181
permissions@jcrinc.com

ISBN: 978-1-59940-135-5
ISSN: 1096-455X

For more information about the Joint Commission, please visit http://www.jointcommission.org.

REF
RA
974
.S98
2008

Contents

How to Use This Book

The "How to Use This Book" chapter is designed to help ambulatory care organizations understand both the purpose and the content of this book. This chapter highlights new and updated initiatives about the evolving accreditation process and orients readers to the structure of this book.

The *Standards for Ambulatory Care* (*SAC*) is designed to facilitate an ambulatory care organization's continuous operational improvement, as well as the self-assessment of its performance against Joint Commission ambulatory care standards. The *SAC* includes all the information an ambulatory care organization needs for continuous operational improvement: standards, rationales, elements of performance (EPs), scoring, National Patient Safety Goals, decision rules, and accreditation policies and procedures. The standards are provided in a user-friendly format that fosters a better understanding of each standard, its rationale (when applicable), and its EPs. Additional chapters that support ongoing accreditation efforts provide guidance on how to use the standards-related information found throughout the book.

What Is the Purpose of the Book?

The *SAC* is designed to provide ambulatory care organizations with information about the accreditation process. The *SAC* includes more than the latest standards and compliance information; it also includes material that supports an ambulatory care organization's continuous operational improvement and its accreditation efforts.

The *SAC* also provides a better understanding of the connection between safety- and quality-focused standards and day-to-day activities and the accreditation process. In essence, the book is a one-stop resource for ambulatory care accreditation and continuous standards compliance.

What Does This Book Include?

Changes to the *SAC* are made in response to suggestions from accredited ambulatory care organizations and relate to important issues that clearly support high-quality care, treatment, and services.

"The Accreditation Process" (ACC) chapter explains The Joint Commission's accreditation process. This chapter includes a description of the components of the accreditation process, sample time lines, and the decision categories and decision rules for ambulatory care organizations. The chapter provides current information on types of surveys and accreditation policies and procedures relevant to all health care organizations. The Joint Commission's Information Accuracy and Truthfulness Policy and its Public Information Policy are also explained. Updated information about the accreditation and appeals procedures with specific links to the "Accreditation Participation Requirements" (APR) chapter are provided to facilitate an understanding of the policies that appear in both chapters.

HB

The "Sentinel Events" (SE) chapter contains background information on the Joint Commission's Sentinel Event Policy, including the definition of a sentinel event, the goals of the policy, which adverse events constitute sentinel events, sentinel event–related standards, definitions of what occurrences are reviewable under the policy, and the various activities that surround the policy.

The "National Patient Safety Goals" (NPSG) chapter details the Joint Commission's current National Patient Safety Goals for ambulatory care organizations.

"Accreditation Participation Requirements" (APRs) addresses the ongoing requirements for continued participation in the accreditation process and includes requirements related to the integration of the Periodic Performance Review (PPR) into the accreditation process. These requirements are scorable during an organization's on-site survey.

The central portion of the book is divided into two sections—Patient-Focused Functions and Organization Functions. The two sections contain the nine functional chapters of the safety- and quality-focused standards, rationales, EPs, and scoring that apply to ambulatory care organizations.

Section 1 includes patient functions directly related to the provision of care, treatment, and services. Patient-focused standards appear in the following four functional chapters:
1. "Ethics, Rights, and Responsibilities" (RI)
2. "Provision of Care, Treatment, and Services" (PC)
3. "Medication Management" (MM)
4. "Surveillance, Prevention, and Control of Infection" (IC)

Section 2 contains organization functions that, although not directly experienced by the patient, are vital to the ambulatory care organization's ability to provide high-quality care, treatment, and services. Organization standards appear in the following five functional chapters:
1. "Improving Organization Performance" (PI)
2. "Leadership" (LD)
3. "Management of the Environment of Care" (EC)
4. "Management of Human Resources" (HR)
5. "Management of Information" (IM)

Functions include the processes and activities common to all health care organizations that cut across and are performed in all areas of an ambulatory care organization. The standards in the nine functional chapters have been adapted to ambulatory care organizations and focus on processes, activities, and outcomes related to both the patient and the ambulatory care organization itself.

The Glossary (GL) provides definitions of many terms used throughout the book.

A comprehensive Index (IX) appears at the end of the book.

What Do the Functional Chapters Include?

One goal of the Joint Commission accreditation decision initiative is to ensure and enhance the relevance of the Joint Commission standards to critical patient safety and health care quality issues.

The standards are displayed in the following format:

- Each chapter has an Overview that provides background and explanatory information
- **Standards** are statements that define the performance expectations and/or structures or processes that must be in place for an ambulatory care organization to provide safe, high-quality care, treatment, and services. An ambulatory care organization's compliance with a standard is either "compliant" or "not compliant". Accreditation decisions are based on simple counts of the standards that are determined to be "not compliant."
- A **rationale** is background, justification, or additional information about a standard. A rationale is included for those standards needing additional text describing the purpose of the standard. In some cases, the rationale for a standard is self-evident. Therefore, not every standard has a written rationale. A rationale is *not* scored.
- **Elements of performance** (EPs) are statements that detail the specific performance expectations and/or structures or processes that must be in place in order for an organization to provide high-quality care, treatment, and services. EPs are scored and determine an ambulatory care organization's overall compliance with a standard. EPs are evaluated by the following scale:

0	Insufficient compliance
1	Partial compliance
2	Satisfactory compliance
NA	Not applicable

  Some EPs have a Measure of Success (MOS) associated with them, which is indicated by an MOS icon—Ⓜ—next to the EP. An MOS needs to be developed for certain EPs when a standard is judged to be out of compliance through the on-site survey. An MOS is defined as a quantifiable measure, usually related to an audit, that can be used to determine whether an action has been effective and is being sustained.*
- Scoring helps you determine your compliance with the requirements in the functional chapters. Two components are scored for all EPs: (1) compliance with the actual requirement itself; and (2) compliance with the track record for that requirement. Scoring has been simplified from past editions of the book, and track record achievements, which have always been part of the scoring, have been appropriately modified. The functional chapters in this book have been designed to help you assess your compliance with the EPs. To do so, take the steps described below (*see* pages 4–8).

---

* For more information about MOS, *see* "The Accreditation Process" (ACC) chapter in this book.

Note: *Some standards and EPs in the* SAC *do not apply to ambulatory care organizations; these standards and EPs are marked "not applicable" and the related text is not included. Your ambulatory care organization does not have to comply with standards and EPs marked "not applicable."*

In addition, some standards and EPs that do apply to ambulatory care organizations might not apply to the specific care, treatment, and services that your individual ambulatory care organization provides. Although these standards and EPs are included in the book, you are not expected to comply with them. If you are unsure about the standards or EPs that apply to your ambulatory care organization, please contact the Joint Commission's Standards Interpretation Group at 630/792-5900.

Step 1: Score Your Compliance with Each Element of Performance

Before you can determine your compliance with the standards, you must score your compliance with each EP. First look at the EP scoring criterion category listed immediately preceding the scoring scale in the margin next to the EP. There are three scoring criterion categories: A, B, and C (described below). Please note that for each EP scoring criterion category, your ambulatory care organization must meet the performance requirement itself and the track record achievements (*see* page 6).

Category A

These EPs relate to the presence or absence of the requirement(s) and are scored either yes (2) or no (0); however, score 1 for partial compliance is also possible based on track record achievements (*see* page 6).

If a category A EP has multiple components designated by bullets, your ambulatory care organization must be compliant with all the bullets to receive a score of 2. If your ambulatory care organization does not meet one or more requirements in the bullets, you will receive a score of 0.

Category B

Category B EPs are scored in two steps:

1. As with category A EPs, category B EPs relate to the presence or absence of the requirement(s). If your ambulatory care organization does not meet the requirement(s), the EP is scored 0; there is no need to assess your compliance with the principles of good process design (*see* below).
2. If your ambulatory care organization does meet the requirement(s), but there is concern about the quality or comprehensiveness of the effort, then and only then should you assess the qualitative aspect of the EP. That is, review the applicable principles of good process design and ask how the principles were applied in the situation under discussion. Good process design has the following characteristics:
   - Is consistent with your ambulatory care organization's mission, values, and goals
   - Meets the needs of patients

- Reflects the use of currently accepted practices (doing the right thing, using resources responsibly, using practice guidelines)
- Incorporates current safety information and knowledge such as sentinel event data and National Patient Safety Goals
- Incorporates relevant performance improvement results

This two-part evaluation applies to both simple and bulleted category B EPs. First, the EPs are assessed to determine if the requirements are present. If the EP has multiple components designated by bullets, as with the category A EPs, your ambulatory care organization must meet the requirements in all the bulleted items to get a score of 2. If your ambulatory care organization meets none of the requirements in the bullets, it receives a score of 0. If your ambulatory care organization meets *at least one, but not all,* of the bulleted requirements, it will receive a score of 1 for the EPs.

Use the following rules to determine your EP score:

- Your EP score is 0 if your ambulatory care organization does not meet the requirement(s); you do not need to assess your compliance with the preceding applicable principles of good process design
- Your EP score is 1 if your ambulatory care organization does meet the requirement(s), but considered only some of the preceding applicable principles of good process design
- Your EP score is 2 if your ambulatory care organization does meet the requirement(s) and considered all the preceding principles of good process design

Your EP score is also based on consistent implementation in all applicable situations at all times (when there is not a corresponding EP to separately score implementation of the requirement). If the requirement is applied in all applicable situations, your EP score is 2 (satisfactory compliance); if the requirement is applied in fewer than all applicable situations, your EP score is 1 (partial compliance); if the requirement is not applied in any applicable situation, your EP score is 0 (insufficient compliance).

Category C

Category C EPs are scored 0, 1, or 2 based on the number of times your ambulatory care organization does not meet the EP. These EPs are frequency based and require totaling the number of occurrences (that is, results of performance or nonperformance) related to a particular EP. Each situation discovered by a surveyor(s) will be counted as a separate occurrence.

Note: *Multiple events of the same type related to a single patient and single practitioner/staff member are counted as only one occurrence.*

Use the following rules to determine your EP score:

- Your EP score is 2 if you find one or fewer occurrences of noncompliance with the EP
- Your EP score is 1 if you find two occurrences of noncompliance with the EP
- Your EP score is 0 if you find three or more occurrences of noncompliance with the EP

If an EP in the C category has multiple requirements designated by bullets, the following scoring guidelines apply:

- If there are fewer than two findings in all bullets, the EP is scored 2
- If there are three or more findings in all bullets, the EP is scored 0
- In all other combinations of findings, the EP is scored 1

Track Record Achievements for Organizations Undergoing Re-Survey

In addition to meeting the requirement(s) in each EP, regardless of category, your ambulatory care organization must also meet the following track record achievements:

Score	Re-Survey
2	12 months or more
1	6 to 11 months
0	Fewer than 6 months

Sample Sizes

If, during an on-site survey, your ambulatory care organization has been found to be not compliant with one or more standards, you must demonstrate Evidence of Standards Compliance (ESC) for each standard that is not compliant. The ESC must address compliance at the EP level. When an EP within a not compliant standard requires an MOS, your ambulatory care organization must demonstrate whether each MOS identified in the organization's ESC report was reached.

Note: *Not every EP requires an MOS. EPs that do require an MOS are clearly marked in the standards chapters in this book. Organizations are required to demonstrate achievement with an MOS only for EPs within a not compliant standard that require an MOS. Organizations do not need to demonstrate achievement with an MOS for any EP within a compliant standard.*

When demonstrating achievement with an MOS during the ESC process, your ambulatory care organization is required to use the following sample sizes, which were established because of their statistical significance, their relative simplicity in application, and their sensitivity to an ambulatory care organization's population size:

- For a population size of fewer than 30 cases,* sample 100% of available cases
- For a population size of 30 to 100 cases, sample 30 cases
- For a population size of 101 to 500 cases, sample 50 cases
- For a population size greater than 500 cases, sample 70 cases

Note: *Organizations are* encouraged, but not required, *to follow this sample size when demonstrating achievement with an MOS for an EP within a not compliant standard after conducting a full, option 1, or option 2 PPR.*

---

* *Case* refers to a single instance in which a situation related to a survey finding occurs. For example, if a survey finding was related to **pain assessment,** then a case would be any patient record. If a survey finding was related to **pain management,** a case would be any patient record for patients receiving pain management.

When conducting PPR (optional use) or demonstrating an ESC (mandatory use), use the following percentages to determine your EP score: 90% through 100% of your sample size is in compliance = score 2; 80% through 89% of your sample size is in compliance = score 1; less than 80% of your sample size is in compliance = score 0.

In addition, the following information should govern your ambulatory care organization's selection of samples:

- The appropriate sample size should be determined by the specific population related to the survey findings
- The sampling approach should involve either systematic random sampling (for example, your ambulatory care organization selects every second or third case for review) or simple random sampling (for example, your ambulatory care organization uses a series of random numbers generated by a computer to identify the cases to be reviewed)
- If your ambulatory care organization chooses not to use these sample sizes while conducting PPR options 1 or 2, you should make sure that your sample size is sufficiently large enough to ensure statistical significance
- When submitting a clarifying ESC, if your ambulatory care organization selects records as part of its sample, the records should be from a period of no more than three months before the last date of the survey
- Assessment of MOS compliance is conducted for a four-month period following the date of ESC approval. Your ambulatory care organization should select records as a part of your sample following the date of ESC approval and use the required sample sizes. MOS percentage compliance rates are derived from the average of all four months.

Step 2: Use Your EP Scores to Gauge Your Compliance with the Standards

Now that you have evaluated and scored each EP for a particular standard, use these simple rules to determine your compliance with the standard itself:

- Your ambulatory care organization is not in compliance (that is, "not compliant") with the standard if any EP is scored 0
- Otherwise, your ambulatory care organization is in compliance with a standard if 65% or more of its EPs are scored 2

The format for the functional chapters in this book separates the rationale for the standard (explanatory or educational background) and its scorable requirements (EPs). Ambulatory care organizations will know exactly what surveyors will be looking for when scoring compliance with the standards.

In addition, a standard numbering system is being used with the standards, which allows for flexibility to add standards while maintaining the current number for each standard.

A sample of a standard appears below.

Standard PI.2.10

Data are systematically aggregated and analyzed.

HB

Rationale for PI.2.10

Aggregating and analyzing data means transforming data into information. Aggregating data at points in time enables the organization to judge a particular process's stability or a particular outcome's predictability in relation to performance expectations. Accumulated data are analyzed in such a way that current performance levels, patterns, or trends can be identified.

Elements of Performance for PI.2.10

B 1. Collected data are aggregated and analyzed.

B 2. Data are aggregated at the frequency appropriate to the activity or process being studied.

B 3. Statistical tools and techniques are used to analyze and display data.

B 4. Data are analyzed and compared internally over time and externally* with other sources of information when available.

B 5. Comparative data are used to determine if there is excessive variability or unacceptable levels of performance when available.

See Table 1 (pages 9–10) for a list of information resources at the Joint Commission and Joint Commission Resources.

* **External sources** of information include recent scientific, clinical, and management literature, including sentinel event alerts, well-formulated practice guidelines or parameters, reference databases, other organizations with similar processes, and standards that are periodically reviewed and revised.

HB

Table 1. Where Should I Go If I Still Have Questions?

The following is a list of information resources at the Joint Commission and Joint Commission Resources.

The Joint Commission's **main telephone number** is **630/792-5000.** The Joint Commission's business hours are 8:30 A.M. to 5:00 P.M. central standard time, Monday through Friday.

Written correspondence should be sent to:
Joint Commission on Accreditation of Healthcare Organizations
One Renaissance Boulevard
Oakbrook Terrace, IL 60181
ATTN: ____________________
[Area Indicated (such as Account Representative or Accreditation and Certification Operations)]

The Joint Commission's **main fax number** is **630/792-5005.** If you experience difficulties in transmission, please call 630/792-5541.

Call your **account representative** at **630/792-3002** for information about ambulatory care organizations or with questions about the following:

- Request for survey for ambulatory care organizations
- Scheduling of surveys
- Survey agenda or survey process
- Status of a survey report
- Content of a survey report
- Follow-up process required for post on-site survey
- Focused surveys

Call the **Standards Interpretation Group** at **630/792-5900** for information and questions about the following:

- Interpretation of ambulatory care standards
- How to comply with ambulatory care standards
- Credentialing

The **Customer Service** telephone number is **630/792-5800.** Joint Commission customer service representatives are available from 8:00 A.M. to 5:00 P.M. central standard time, Monday through Friday. Call Joint Commission's Customer Service with questions about the following:

- General information on Joint Commission services, mission, or history
- How to apply for a survey for the first time
- Ernest A. Codman Award program and for applications
- Your organization's accreditation status or history
- Obtaining a list of accredited organizations
- Checking the current accreditation status of an organization
- Quality Reports
- Help in accessing information on The Joint Commission's Web site

The Joint Commission's **Web site** address is **http://www.jointcommission.org.** For an extensive e-mail or telephone list of contacts, click on **"Contact Us"** located near the top of the Joint Commission's home page. In general, e-mail addresses consist of the first letter of the

continued on next page

Table 1. Where Should I Go If I Still Have Questions? *(continued)*

HB

person's first name and the entire last name @jointcommission.org. In most cases, to reach the appropriate person and department by telephone, dial **630/792-** and the extension number listed.

Joint Commission Resource's **main** telephone number is **630/268-7400.** Joint Commission Resources' business hours are 8:30 A.M. to 5:00 P.M. central standard time, Monday through Friday. Visit the Web site at **http://www.jcrinc.com** for information or questions, or to order the following:

- Continuous Service Readiness
- Custom education
- Domestic consulting services
- Educational seminars
- International accreditation services
- Publications

Joint Commission Resources' **Customer Service** telephone number for publication orders and education program registration is **877/223-6866.** Customer service representatives are available from 8:00 A.M. to 8:00 P.M. central standard time, Monday through Friday. Call Customer Service for the following:

- Obtaining a free catalog for Joint Commission Resources publications or education
- Orders for Joint Commission Resources publications and registration for education seminars
- Multimedia education products
- Publications or education related to specific care programs (such as Disease Management)

Call **630/792-5120** with request for permission to reprint any Joint Commission Resources publication

Call **Joint Commission Satellite Network (JCSN)** at **800/711-6549** for information and questions about how to sign up for the series of education programs broadcast across the United States.

The Accreditation Process

Overview

This chapter combines the former "The Joint Commission Accreditation Process" (ACC) and "Accreditation Policies and Procedures" (APP) chapters. This new chapter is arranged in the order of the accreditation process and begins with general information about the accreditation process, including the application, types of surveys, the Periodic Performance Review (PPR), priority focus areas (PFAs), and clinical/service groups (CSGs). The chapter then details what organizations can expect during the accreditation survey, including the survey agenda, tracers, and scoring guidelines. Finally, the chapter includes information important to organizations after the survey, including the accreditation decision, decision rules, Evidence of Standards Compliance (ESC), and the review and appeal process.

The policies and procedures described in this chapter are relevant to all health care organizations interested in Joint Commission accreditation whether they are applying for the first time or seeking continued accreditation. You can locate the policies and procedures applicable to your organization according to where your organization is in its accreditation cycle. All organizations must follow the policies and procedures listed in this chapter to participate in (and continue to participate in) the accreditation process. Failure to follow the policies and procedures described in this chapter can result in denial or withdrawal of accreditation. Because this information is reviewed and revised as necessary on a continuous basis, all organizations are responsible for keeping track of these policies and procedures.

Note: *The "Accreditation Participation Requirements" chapter includes specific requirements for accreditation participation. The Accreditation Participation Requirements (APRs) are existing policies and are currently effective for accreditation purposes. Cross-references to the APRs are noted in the applicable sections of this chapter.*

Key Milestones in the Accreditation Process

- Each accredited organization is required to update its PPR annually.
- For initial announced surveys,* The Joint Commission will electronically provide PPR access (after the application and deposit are received at the Joint Commission), the output of the Priority Focus Process (PFP) (*see* pages 33–36 for more information), and instructions to your ambulatory care organization on how to proceed with the PPR. (Although access is granted to the electronic PPR tool, its completion is not required for ambulatory care organizations undergoing initial survey.)
- Your ambulatory care organization is encouraged to use this continuous PPR access to evaluate compliance with standards using EPs on an ongoing basis to ensure the continuous provision of safe, high-quality care (*see* the section Scor-

* Deemed status ambulatory program surveys are unannounced.

ing Compliance and Track Record Achievements on pages 56–57 for more information). For standards identified as "not compliant," your ambulatory care organization will develop a plan of action with measures of success (MOS), if required.

- The PPR process will also evaluate compliance with all applicable Accreditation Participation Requirements and National Patient Safety Goals.
- Full PPR: Your organization must annually update and transmit its PPR to the Joint Commission and, if appropriate, its plan(s) of action and relevant MOS. The plan(s) of action must address all not compliant standards areas as identified in the PPR. (*See* Table 1 on pages 34–35 for more information, and the "Accreditation Participation Requirements" chapter for the full text of the PPR and its options.)
- Organizations that select PPR option 2 or option 3 are required to undergo annual announced option 2 or option 3 surveys. Each year you may choose the full, option 1, option 2, or option 3 PPR process.
- After the annual update and transmission of your PPR, your organization may elect to participate in an optional conference call with Joint Commission staff to reach final agreement on the plan of action and MOS and/or discuss standards-related issues and receive approval of the submitted plan(s) of action and MOS.
- For organizations that selected the full PPR, option 1, or option 2, at the time of your organization's full survey, surveyors will ask to see your MOS data, which will indicate that performance has been achieved and sustained. Surveyors will use this information as a data source, similar to PFP data.
- Your accreditation decision is not affected by the results of your PPR.
- On the day of your survey, your organization will receive PFP information for its top PFAs and CSGs on its secure extranet site. (For more information on this process, please *see* the PFP component on page 33.) The surveyor(s) scheduled to conduct your survey will also receive the PFP output for your ambulatory care organization. This information will help the surveyor(s) to focus the survey process on issues that are unique to your ambulatory care organization.
- Full on-site survey occurs. The surveyor(s) will visit various services/programs using the tracer methodology. (For more information on this process, please *see* the tracer methodology component on pages 51–54.)
- After evaluating your ambulatory care organization's performance, the surveyor(s) will review the results of his or her findings. Before the closing conference, the surveyor(s) will enter his or her findings into laptop computers, thus producing an Accreditation Survey Findings Report. After the report has been rendered, the surveyor or the survey team leader will meet with your ambulatory care organization's chief executive officer (CEO) to provide him or her with a copy of the report. It is up to the CEO to decide whether the report will be distributed at the exit conference; however, the surveyor(s) will use the contents of the report during the exit conference. (For more information on this process, please *see* pages 50–51.) In special surveys (announced and unannounced), no survey report will be left on site.
- Shortly after your survey has taken place, the Joint Commission will post your Accreditation Survey Findings Report on a secure automated area of The Joint

Commission Connect™ extranet site that is password protected for each organization. If the surveyor(s) finds requirements for improvement in your organization, you have 45 days following the posting of your organization's Accreditation Survey Findings Report on the extranet to submit an ESC. During the 45-day period, your ambulatory care organization's prior accreditation decision will remain in effect.

- Clarification (optional): If your organization believes that it was in compliance with a standard identified as "Not Compliant" at the time of survey and that there was adequate evidence of compliance available to the surveyor or the survey team, you may submit evidence in a narrative format via electronic means to support that contention. All submissions of clarifying evidence must be included as part of the ESC submission. An organization may also submit detailed evidence of information that was not immediately available at the time of survey. The submission of clarifying evidence should include an explanation as to why the surveyor(s) did not have access to the information or why it was not provided to the surveyor(s) at the time of survey. Such information must be from the time of survey, not generated after the survey date. If an organization submits clarifying evidence, it may not also submit a plan of action, an evaluation method, and an MOS for that same EP.
- **On-site Validation Survey:** If, as the result of a survey, the organization meets a decision rule for Preliminary Denial of Accreditation or Conditional Accreditation, the organization will have 10 business days from the date the survey findings are posted to the extranet to submit clarifying evidence of standards compliance. If, after reviewing the clarifying evidence, it is determined that the organization continues to meet a rule of Preliminary Denial of Accreditation or Conditional Accreditation, the survey results will be submitted to the Accreditation Committee for a decision. If after reviewing the organization's clarifying evidence it is determined that the organization no longer meets the decision rule for Preliminary Denial of Accreditation or Conditional Accreditation, a Joint Commission staff member will conduct an on-site validation survey to:
    - Seek to validate the clarifying evidence submitted and determine if such information or data was available to the previous on-site survey team
    - Determine whether the organization does or does *not* meet a decision rule for Preliminary Denial of Accreditation or Conditional Accreditation

If the organization does *not* meet a rule for Preliminary Denial of Accreditation or Conditional Accreditation, it will be awarded Accreditation (if it is compliant with all standards) or it will be required to submit an ESC (if it still has requirements for improvement [RFIs]). However, if the organization does meet a decision rule for Preliminary Denial of Accreditation or Conditional Accreditation, the Joint Commission staff will recommend to the Accreditation Committee that the organization remain in Preliminary Denial of Accreditation or Conditional Accreditation. If the results of the on-site validation survey suggest that the organization falsified its clarifying evidence, a recommendation will be made to the Accreditation Committee as to whether the Information Accuracy and Truthfulness Policy should be invoked.*

---

* *See* pages 71–81 for more information on decision rules.

There will be no charge to the organization for having an on-site validation survey.

- If, at the end of the 45-day period, your ambulatory care organization successfully addresses its RFIs, it will receive an accreditation decision of "Accredited" provided you had not met a rule for Conditional Accreditation or Preliminary Denial of Accreditation. After the 45-day time frame, either the ESC report is received and approved or your organization will receive an accreditation decision of "Provisional Accreditation." Your Quality Report will be made available to the public on Joint Commission's Quality Check®.

Eligibility

Organizations Eligible for Accreditation

General Eligibility Requirements

Any health care organization may apply for Joint Commission accreditation under the standards in this book* if all the following requirements are met:

- The organization is in the United States or its territories or, if outside the United States, is operated by the U.S. government, or under a charter of the U.S. Congress
- The organization assesses and improves the quality of its services. This process includes a review of care by clinicians, when appropriate.
- The organization identifies the services it provides, indicating which services it provides directly, under contract, or through some other arrangement
- The organization provides services addressed by the Joint Commission's standards

Policies

Scope of Accreditation Surveys

General Survey Categories

The Joint Commission surveys and accredits health care organizations using standards from one or more of the following manuals:

- *Comprehensive Accreditation Manual for Ambulatory Care*
- *Comprehensive Accreditation Manual for Behavioral Health Care*
- *Comprehensive Accreditation Manual for Critical Access Hospitals*
- *Comprehensive Accreditation Manual for Home Care* (includes standards for home health, personal/support care, hospice, home medical equipment, and pharmacies)
- *Comprehensive Accreditation Manual for Hospitals: The Official Handbook*
- *Comprehensive Accreditation Manual for Laboratory and Point-of-Care Testing*
- *Comprehensive Accreditation Manual for Long Term Care*
- *Comprehensive Accreditation Manual for Office-Based Surgery Practices*

In addition to using standards, the Joint Commission also surveys organizations by using the standards, elements of performance (EPs), performance measurement data (when applicable), and APRs, including the Joint Commission National Patient Safety Goals (*see* the "National Patient Safety Goals" chapter). Used in conjunction with the standards, these items help assess an organization's performance.

---

* The Joint Commission will work with the organization to determine which standards from other accreditation books are applicable.

Tailored Survey Policy

The Joint Commission survey, assuming satisfactory compliance, provides one accreditation award for all the organization's services, programs, and related organizations. Another service, program, or related entity (that is, component), whether providing services directly or through a contractual arrangement, is included in the survey of the applicant organization under the following circumstances:

- There are Joint Commission standards applicable to the component
- The component is overseen and managed by the applicant organization through organizational and functional integration

Note: *Any service, program, or related entity that is a component of an accreditation-eligible organization may independently seek accreditation if it can meet Joint Commission survey eligibility requirements. The results of such a separate accreditation survey will still apply to the overall organization's decision in accordance with applicable decision rules.*

Organizational and functional integration refers to the degree to which the component is overseen and managed by the applicant organization. *Applicant organization* refers both to an organization seeking accreditation and to an organization that is currently accredited. A *component* is a service, program, or related entity that delivers care or services and is eligible for survey under one of the Joint Commission's accreditation programs. These include the following:

- General, acute psychiatric, pediatric, critical access, surgical specialty, long term acute care, and rehabilitation hospitals
- Home care organizations, including those that provide home health services, personal care and support services, home infusion and other pharmacy services, long term care pharmacies and infusion centers, durable medical equipment services, and hospice services
- Skilled nursing facilities, nursing homes and other long term care facilities
- Behavioral health care organizations, including those that provide mental health services, substance abuse treatment services, foster care services, and services for persons with developmental disabilities of various ages and in various organized service settings
- Ambulatory care providers, including surgery centers and office-based surgery practices, rehabilitation centers, sleep labs, imaging centers, group practices, community health centers, student health centers, and others
- Clinical laboratories

Organizational integration exists when an applicant organization's governing body, either directly or ultimately, controls budgetary and resource allocation decisions for the component or, where individual corporate entities are involved, there is greater than 50% common governing board membership for the applicant organization and on the board of the component.

Functional integration exists when the entity meets at least three of the following eight criteria:

1. The applicant organization and the component do the following:
   - Use the same process for determining membership of licensed independent practitioners in practitioner panels or medical or professional staff, and/or
   - Have a common organized medical or professional staff for the applicant organization and the component
2. The applicant organization's human resources function hires and assigns staff at the component and has the authority to do the following:
   - Terminate staff at the component
   - Transfer or rotate staff between the applicant organization and the component
   - Conduct performance appraisals of the staff who work in the component
3. The applicant organization's policies and procedures are applicable to the component, with few or no exceptions
4. The applicant organization manages significant operations of the component; that is, the component has little or no management authority or autonomy independent of the applicant organization
5. The component's patient records are integrated into the applicant organization's patient record system
6. The applicant organization applies its performance improvement program to the component and has authority to implement actions intended to improve performance at the component
7. The applicant organization bills for services provided by the component under the name of the applicant organization
8. The applicant organization and/or the component portrays to the public that the component is part of the organization through the use of common names or logos; references on letterheads, brochures, telephone-book listings, or Web sites; or representations in other published materials

A checklist to assist in determining organizational and functional integration is found on page 17.

The Joint Commission evaluates all health care services provided by the organization for which the Joint Commission has standards and makes one accreditation decision and Accreditation Survey Findings Report. An organization must be prepared to provide evidence of its compliance with each applicable standard. To gain accreditation, an organization must demonstrate overall compliance with the standards and their EPs.

Complex Organization Survey Process

The complex organization survey process is applied to organizations that are governed by the Tailored Survey Policy. The Joint Commission conducts a complex organization survey based on the services provided by the organization, as reported in its electronic application (e-App). Because a complex organization survey process involves standards in more than one of the manuals listed in this chapter, the Joint Commission provides the organization with a copy of each of the manuals to be used in the survey before it is conducted.

ACC

Checklist to Determine Organizational and Functional Integration

Organizational	Description	Check Yes or No		Comments
1. Governance	Governing body of the organization applying for accreditation controls budget and resource allocation for component	Yes	No	
2. Shared governance	If separate corporate entities, over 50% of governing body membership is shared by the organization applying for accreditation and the component	Yes	No	

Functional	Description	Check Yes or No		Comments
1. Common medical staff and/or licensed independent practitioner process	Unified process for credentialing of licensed independent practitioners	Yes	No	
2. Human resources	The organization applying for accreditation has hiring/firing/performance appraisal authority over the component's staff	Yes	No	
3. Policies and procedures	Common policies and procedures	Yes	No	
4. Management	Component is managed by the organization applying for accreditation	Yes	No	
5. Patient records	Integrated patient record system	Yes	No	
6. Performance improvement	Integrated performance improvement program, with organization authority to implement performance improvement actions at component	Yes	No	
7. Billing	Component's services are billed by applicant organization	Yes	No	

continued on next page

ACC

Checklist to Determine Organizational and Functional Integration *(continued)*

Functional	Description	Check Yes or No	Comments
8. Public	There is public portrayal of components as part of parent organization through names or logos, etc.	Yes No	

Note: Applicant organization needs minimum of one (1) "Yes" response for Organizational Integration; and three (3) "Yes" responses for Functional Integration to include components as "sites" on application.

An organization that has acquired a new component that requires a survey in an accreditation program that is new to the organization is given a 12-month grace period from the time the component is acquired before the performance of that component is factored into the organization's overall accreditation decision. The newly acquired component is usually surveyed within six months of its acquisition as an extension survey, even though the component would still be considered accredited.

Single Accreditation Award

The Joint Commission survey, assuming satisfactory compliance, provides one accreditation award for all of the organization's services, programs, and related organizations. Included in each organization's survey and accreditation decision are all services, programs, and related organizations that are organizationally and functionally integrated. If, after accreditation is rendered to an organization, the organization's structure changes whereby one or more of its services, programs, or related organizations is no longer part of the organization that was originally surveyed, the service, program, or related organization is no longer included in the organization's accreditation.

System Accreditation for Ambulatory Care Programs

System accreditation involves awarding a single accreditation decision to a "system," composed of an organization that has a corporate office or a main site, and multiple sites under the auspices of the main site. The main site has oversight of the performance of the sites in the system. Under the system accreditation approach, the corporate office or main site is visited to assess systemwide policies and functions and then a random sample of sites within the system are visited to assess the execution of the policies and the delivery of care. The sites are selected based on their size and risk levels. Selected sites undergo unannounced surveys. Extension surveys may be conducted at sites newly established as part of the system.

With system accreditation, the entire system undergoes the accreditation process during a concentrated period of time. Additionally, the entire system will be assigned a single, dedicated account representative.

Eligibility requires a minimum of four sites and a common governance structure with system management in the following areas:

- Overseeing quality of care
- Overseeing performance improvement
- Setting strategic goals and expectations
- Developing policies and monitoring execution
- Approving and monitoring site budgets
- Overseeing site managers' performance
- Credentialing/privileging licensed independent practitioners

If a system wishes to have each of its sites independently accredited in order to meet deemed status requirements, the system remains eligible for evaluation under this approach.

After surveys are completed, the system receives an accreditation certificate and a consolidated report of findings, leading to a three-year accreditation decision. Each site within the system can display a copy of the system's accreditation certificate.

For more information about System Accreditation for ambulatory care organizations, please contact Michael Kulczycki, executive director, Ambulatory Care Accreditation Program at 630/792-5290 or mkulczycki@jointcommission.org.

Contracted Services

The Joint Commission evaluates an organization's assessment of the quality of services provided under contractual arrangements. The Joint Commission reserves the right to evaluate, as part of its survey, services provided by another organization or provider. It may survey performance issues between the contracted organization and the applicant organization, regardless of the accreditation decision of the contracted organization. The Joint Commission also surveys services provided on-site under contract.

Notifying the Public About a Joint Commission Survey

Because an organization will not be able to post its survey date and, therefore, individuals cannot request to have a Public Information Interview (PII), a new APR was established. APR 8 requires an organization to demonstrate how it communicates to its public that if members of the public have any quality of care or safety concerns about an organization, they should notify the Joint Commission. The organization may notify the public by posting an accreditation certificate, posting information on its Web site and/or in patient admission brochures, or by using any other effective means of its choice.

The public includes, but is not limited to, the following:

- Patients and their families
- Patient advocates and advocacy groups

- Members of the community for whom services are provided
- Staff members

Initial Surveys

An organization that is seeking Joint Commission accreditation for the first time or that has not been unaccredited by the Joint Commission during the previous six months is eligible for an initial survey. The full scope of applicable standards is reviewed during the survey. The Joint Commission's policy for assessing and monitoring organizations new to the accreditation and certification process is as follows:

- Elimination of the requirement that organizations new to the accreditation and certification process be able to demonstrate a four-month track record of compliance with the standards at the time of the initial survey.*
- If an organization new to the accreditation or certification process demonstrates compliance with Joint Commission standards, without consideration of track record requirements, the organization will receive Accreditation or Certification, respectively.
- Organizations new to the accreditation or certification process that provide **high risk/critical services** (for example, specialty hospitals)—based on criteria yet to be determined—will be subject to a one-year follow-up survey to assess sustained compliance with the standards.
- All organizations new to the accreditation or certification process that become accredited after their initial survey will be included in a 5% "pool" of organizations undergoing a validation survey of their Evidence of Standards Compliance (ESC).
  - In October 2005, the Joint Commission's Accreditation Committee approved the progressive elimination of Random Unannounced Surveys by the end of 2008, and the introduction of a new validation survey—Random Unannounced Validation Surveys of Evidence of Standards Compliance. The latter will be conducted to validate information in organizations' ESCs and to evaluate how effectively corrective actions are sustained over time.
  - The new Random Unannounced ESC Validation Surveys will provide a timely mechanism for monitoring continued standards compliance for organizations new to the accreditation or certification process, versus using the organization's prior track record to predict future performance.

The accreditation effective date for an organization that undergoes an initial survey is the date on which an acceptable ESC was submitted, if the organization has a requirement for improvement. If there are no requirements for improvement, the effective date is the date after the last day of the survey.

For organizations receiving an initial survey that receive a Conditional Accreditation decision, the effective date will be the date of the Accreditation Committee meeting at which the decision was made, if the organization has submitted an acceptable ESC. If the organization has yet to submit an acceptable ESC that

---

* **Initial survey** An accreditation survey of a health care organization not previously accredited by the Joint Commission, or an accreditation survey of an organization performed without reference to any prior survey findings.

resolves all requirements for improvement at the time of the Accreditation Committee meeting, then the effective date for the accreditation decision is set retroactively as the date when the acceptable ESC is submitted.

Survey Postponement Policy for Initial Announced Surveys

A postponement is an organization's request to alter an already-scheduled survey date. An organization should direct a request for a postponement to its account representative. A request to postpone a survey may be granted if one or more of the following criteria are met:

1. A natural disaster or other major unforeseen event has occurred that has totally or substantially disrupted operations
2. The organization is involved in a major strike, has ceased admitting patients, and is transferring patients to other facilities or organizations
3. Patients and/or the organization is being moved to a new building on the day or days of the survey

Note: *If an organization is undergoing an unannounced survey and on the day of the survey the organization experiences one of these situations, the survey may be postponed.*

Fees for Postponements for Initial Surveys

In rare circumstances, the Joint Commission may, at its discretion, approve a request to postpone a survey for an organization not meeting any of the criteria described here. In such cases, the organization may be charged a fee to defray costs. In addition, if the initial survey is of a new program or service of a complex organization already accredited, the organization may be required to undergo an extension survey. Please contact your account representative or the Pricing Unit at 630/792-5115.

Information Accuracy and Truthfulness Policy

The accuracy and veracity of relevant information, whether actually used in the accreditation process or not, are essential to the integrity of the Joint Commission's accreditation process. Information provided at any time by the organization must be accurate and truthful. Such information may do the following:

- Be provided verbally or in writing
- Be obtained through direct observation or interview by Joint Commission surveyors
- Be derived from documents supplied by the organization to the Joint Commission, including, but not limited to, an organization's root cause analysis (RCA) in response to a sentinel event, an organization's request for accreditation, or a plan of correction submitted as part of the Conditional Accreditation process
- Involve data or documents transmitted electronically to the Joint Commission, including, but not limited to, data or documents provided as part of the e-App process

  or
- Involve an attestation that an organization has not knowingly used Joint Commission full-time, part-time, or intermittent surveyors to provide any accreditation-related consulting services after January 1, 2004. Examples of such services include, but are not limited to, the following:

- Helping an organization meet Joint Commission standards
- Helping an organization in the PPR process
- Conducting mock surveys for an organization
- Helping an organization in the ESC process

or

- Providing consultation to an organization to address PFP information

Falsification, as the term is used in the Joint Commission's Information Accuracy and Truthfulness Policy, applies to both commissions and omissions in sharing information with the Joint Commission.

Policy Requirements

The Joint Commission's Information Accuracy and Truthfulness Policy includes the following:

1. An organization must never provide the Joint Commission with falsified information relevant to the accreditation process. The Joint Commission construes any effort to do so as a violation of the organization's obligation to engage in the accreditation process in good faith.
2. *Falsification* is defined for this policy as the fabrication, in whole or in part, and through commission or omission, of any information provided by an applicant or accredited organization to the Joint Commission. This includes, but is not limited to, any redrafting, reformatting, or content deletion of documents.
3. The organization may submit additional material that summarizes or otherwise explains original information submitted to the Joint Commission. These materials must be properly identified, dated, and accompanied by the original documents.
4. The Joint Commission conducts an evaluation when it has cause to believe that an accredited organization may have provided falsified information to the Joint Commission relevant to the accreditation process. Except as otherwise authorized by the president of the Joint Commission, the evaluation includes an unannounced on-site survey. This survey uses special protocols designed to address the alleged information falsification. It assesses the degree of actual organization compliance with the standards and EPs that are the subject of the allegation, if appropriate.
5. The Joint Commission takes action to deny accreditation to an accredited organization whenever the Joint Commission is reasonably persuaded that the organization has provided falsified information.
6. The Joint Commission notifies responsible federal and state government agencies of any organization subject to such action.
7. If an organization is denied accreditation because it provided falsified information, the Joint Commission prohibits it from participating in the accreditation process for a period of one year. The president of the Joint Commission, for good cause only, may waive all or a portion of this waiting period.

Good Faith Participation in Accreditation

The Joint Commission requires each organization seeking accreditation or reaccreditation to engage in the accreditation process in good faith. The Joint Commission may deny accreditation to any organization that fails to participate in the accreditation process in good faith.

Ways of interfering with good faith participation can fall into the following categories:

- *Deceiving the Joint Commission.* Compliance with the Information Accuracy and Truthfulness Policy requires a commitment on the part of the accredited organization not to deceive the Joint Commission in any aspect of the accreditation process, such as during the completion of an application for accreditation, during the PPR process, or during a survey.
- *Deceiving the public.* An accredited organization is not acting in good faith if it misleads the public about the meaning and limitations of accreditation. Also, an accredited organization must not inaccurately suggest to the public that its accreditation award applies to any unaccredited affiliated or otherwise related activities.
- *Reprisals.* The Joint Commission invites open communication from any accredited organization's staff and recipients of care and services about any standards compliance or other issue relating to the accreditation process. An organization's good faith participation in the accreditation process is questioned if the organization does any of the following:
    - Attempts to discourage such communication—for example, by taking disciplinary steps against an employee solely because that employee provides information to the Joint Commission
    - Threatens those who communicate with the Joint Commission with a defamation lawsuit based solely on what was said to the Joint Commission
    - Allows the treatment or access to services of any individual or staff member to be adversely affected by his or her or a family member's communication with the Joint Commission
- *Standards compliance.* If an organization's conduct reflects a lack of commitment to standards compliance, issues of good faith may be raised. For example, an intentional refusal to attempt to comply with a standard could suggest a cavalier view of the accreditation process.

The good faith participation requirement applies continuously throughout the accreditation cycle.

Deemed Status Option for Medicare-Certified Ambulatory Surgical Centers

An ambulatory surgical center (ASC) that is eligible to achieve or continue Medicare certification may choose to participate in a Joint Commission accreditation survey that can be used for both Medicare certification and accreditation. An ASC that chooses to have its survey conducted by the Joint Commission will undergo a Joint Commission survey in place of a Medicare survey conducted by a state agency. Once an organization is accredited by the Joint Commission through this process, the Centers for Medicare & Medicaid Services (CMS) would determine the ASC to be in compliance with federal requirements specified in the Conditions for Coverage for ASCs. The CMS retains the authority to conduct random validation surveys and complaint investigations for Medicare-certified organizations. This option, referred to as *deemed status,* applies only to an organization that meets the Medicare definition of an ASC and is eligible for certification, as determined by the federal regulations. The CMS applies the following specific definition for ASCs eligible to receive reimbursement for facility services from Medicare:

An ambulatory surgical center means any distinct entity that operates exclusively for the purpose of providing surgical services to patients not requiring hospitalization, has an agreement with CMS to participate in Medicare as an ASC, and meets the conditions for coverage as defined by regulation. For purposes of deeming, CMS considers all applicants as Ambulatory Health Care Organizations regardless of the number of patients under anesthesia at any given time.

Joint Commission accreditation is voluntary, and seeking deemed status through Joint Commission accreditation is an option, not a requirement. An ASC interested in seeking Medicare certification through Joint Commission accreditation must declare its intention to seek deemed status by indicating such on the e-App, as well as by notifying CMS and/or the state.

Public Information Policy*

The Joint Commission is committed to making relevant and accurate information about health care organizations available to interested parties. Information regarding a health care organization's quality and safety of care helps organizations improve their services. This information may also help educate consumers and health care purchasers in making informed choices about health care. At the same time, it is important that confidentiality be maintained regarding certain information to encourage candor in the accreditation process. The Joint Commission's primary vehicles for providing this information publicly are Quality Check® and Quality Reports.

Quality Check. Quality Check is the Joint Commission's Web site for making available descriptive and performance information, as applicable, about accredited and non-accredited organizations.

To provide the public with a direct link to the Joint Commission, the accreditation certificate publicly posted in accredited organizations includes the following statement: "The Joint Commission on Accreditation of Healthcare Organizations is an independent, not-for-profit, national body that oversees the safety and quality of health care and other services provided in accredited organizations. Information about accredited organizations may be provided directly to the Joint Commission at 1-800-994-6610. Information regarding accreditation and the accreditation performance of individual organizations can be obtained through the Joint Commission's Web site."

Early Survey Policy

The sidebar on page 26 highlights Early Survey Policy Option 1 and Option 2. An organization wishing to be accredited for the first time by the Joint Commission

* This policy meets the requirements of the Health Insurance Portability and Accountability Act of 1996 (HIPAA).

may choose one of the two Early Survey Policy options described here. Under both Option 1 and Option 2, an organization is required to undergo two surveys. However, the nature of the surveys and potential outcomes differ. The first survey under Option 1 is a more limited survey, while the first survey under Option 2 is a full accreditation survey.

Early Survey Policy Option 1 (Preliminary Accreditation)

A. Eligibility. Early Survey Policy Option 1 is available to any organization that is currently not accredited, except an organization that has been denied accreditation. An organization must declare during the application process that it wishes to be surveyed under this option.

B. The First Survey. When an organization chooses Option 1, the Joint Commission conducts two on-site surveys, both of which will be announced.* The Joint Commission can conduct the first survey as early as two months before the organization begins operating, provided that the organization meets the following criteria:

- It is licensed or has a provisional license, according to applicable law and regulation
- The building in which the services will be offered or from which the services will be coordinated is identified, constructed, and equipped to support such services
- It has identified its chief executive officer (CEO) or administrator, its director of clinical or medical services, and its nurse executive, if applicable
- It has identified the date it will begin operations

Generally, the first survey uses a limited set of standards and assesses only the organization's physical facilities, policies and procedures, plans, and related structural considerations. For this reason, Early Survey Policy Option 1 has not been recognized by the CMS to meet the requirements for Medicare certification.

C. Preliminary Accreditation. The Joint Commission grants Preliminary Accreditation to an organization that is in satisfactory compliance with a subset of the standards and their EPs assessed in the first survey under Option 1. An organization that is not in satisfactory compliance must reapply and begin the accreditation process again.

The Preliminary Accreditation decision includes assignment of an additional announced survey against the full set of applicable standards within six months of the first survey. The survey assesses evidence of compliance with the standards for at least four months.

For an organization operating when the survey is conducted, the effective date for its Preliminary Accreditation decision is the day after the survey is conducted if the organization does not receive any requirements for improvement. If the organization receives at least one requirement for improvement and therefore must submit an acceptable ESC report that resolves all requirements for improvement, the effective date for Preliminary Accreditation is then set retroactively as the date of the acceptable ESC submission. For an organization not in operation, the effective date for its Preliminary Accreditation decision is the day after it begins operating if the

* Deemed status ambulatory program survey is unannounced under this option.

ACC

Early Survey Policy Options

Early Survey Policy Option 1

First Survey

- Conducted up to two months before opening
  - Licensed
  - Building identified, constructed, and equipped
  - CEO or administrator, director of clinical or medical services (medical director), and nurse executive identified
  - Identified opening date
- Limited set of standards (physical plant, policies and procedures)
- Announced*
- Outcome: Preliminary Accreditation

Second Survey

- Four months after the decision from the first survey
- Announced*
- Full survey
- Outcome: Change in Preliminary Accreditation decision to Accredited, Provisional Accreditation, Conditional Accreditation, Preliminary Denial of Accreditation, or Denial of Accreditation. The effective date of the accreditation decision is the day after the *second* survey if the organization does not receive any requirements for improvement. If the organization receives at least one requirement for improvement and, therefore, must submit an ESC that resolves all requirements for improvement, the effective date of the accreditation decision is then set retroactively as the date the successful ESC is submitted.

Early Survey Policy Option 2

First Survey

- Conducted when an organization
  - Has been in operation (licensed) at least one month
  - Has cared for at least 10 patients
  - Has at least 1 patient in active treatment at time of survey
- Full survey; no track record achievement required
- Announced*
- Outcome: Accredited, Conditional Accreditation, Preliminary Denial of Accreditation, or Denial of Accreditation

Second Survey

- Full, follow-up survey four months after the decision from the first survey
- Announced*
- Addresses track record and standards compliance issues
- Outcome: Accredited or Provisional Accreditation, Conditional Accreditation, Preliminary Denial of Accreditation, or Denial of Accreditation. The effective date of the accreditation decision is the day after the *first* survey if the organization does not receive any requirements for improvement. If the organization receives at least one requirement for improvement and, therefore, must submit an ESC that resolves all requirements for improvement, the effective date of the accreditation decision is then set retroactively as the date the successful ESC is submitted.

Note: *For all surveys, the organization will incur a fee. Contact the Joint Commission Department of Planning and Financial Affairs at 630/792-5115 for more information.*

---

* Deemed status ambulatory program survey is unannounced.

organization does not receive any requirements for improvement. If the organization receives at least one requirement for improvement and, therefore, must submit an acceptable ESC report that resolves all requirements for improvement, the effective date for Preliminary Accreditation is then set retroactively as the date of the acceptable ESC submission. If the organization is not in operation at the time of survey, the organization must confirm in writing the date it begins operating.

A Preliminary Accreditation decision remains in effect until the organization has completed a second, full survey or until the Joint Commission has withdrawn the Preliminary Accreditation. The Joint Commission may withdraw Preliminary Accreditation in the following situations:

- If an organization that was not providing services at the time of the first survey does not begin providing services when expected
- If an organization does not meet the survey eligibility criteria (*see* page 14)
- If an organization fails to accept the date of the second survey
  or
- If an organization is found to be not in satisfactory compliance with the applicable standards and their EPs

In any of these cases, the organization must begin the accreditation process again.

D. The Second Survey. The second survey under Early Survey Policy Option 1 is an announced full accreditation survey. The Joint Commission conducts this survey at the following times:

- Approximately six months after the first survey
- At least four months after the organization begins operating

Based on survey results, the organization's accreditation decision then changes to one of the following:

- Accredited
- Provisional Accreditation
- Conditional Accreditation
- Preliminary Denial of Accreditation
  or
- Denial of Accreditation

The effective date of the accreditation decision is the day after the second survey if the organization does not receive any requirements for improvement. If the organization receives at least one requirement for improvement and, therefore, must submit an acceptable ESC report that resolves all requirements for improvement, the effective date for Preliminary Accreditation is then set retroactively as the date of the acceptable ESC submission. The organization's accreditation cycle begins the day after the second survey was conducted, unless the Joint Commission reached a decision to deny accreditation. Submission of an acceptable ESC may be required based on the survey findings of the second survey under Option 1.

Early Survey Policy Option 2

A. Eligibility. Early Survey Policy Option 2 is available only to an organization that meets the following criteria:

- Has never been surveyed by the Joint Commission or has not had its Joint Commission accreditation revoked for the previous two years
- Has been in actual operation for at least one month
- Has cared for at least 10 patients by the time of the first survey, with at least 1 patient in active treatment at the time of survey
- Has not been denied participation in the Medicare program as a result of a survey conducted by or action taken by CMS or the state on behalf of CMS

B. The First Survey. When an organization chooses Early Survey Policy Option 2, the Joint Commission conducts an announced initial full accreditation survey. If the organization demonstrates satisfactory compliance with standards and their EPs in the first survey, it is granted an Accredited decision, including a requirement for a second survey. This accreditation decision reflects the preliminary nature of the assessed performance. The effective date of the accreditation decision is the day after the first survey if the organization does not receive any requirements for improvement. If the organization receives at least one requirement for improvement and, therefore, must submit an acceptable ESC that resolves all requirements for improvement, the effective date of the accreditation decision is then set retroactively as the date the ESC is submitted.

C. The Second Survey. The organization undergoes a full announced follow-up survey in four months. The full scope of applicable standards is reviewed, with particular attention paid to the issue of sustained performance since the first survey. Organizations surveyed under the Early Survey Policy Option 2 will also be required to complete an acceptable ESC after the second survey, as appropriate.

Before the Survey

This section provides information on the steps leading to a full accreditation survey. These steps include the application process; the assignment of an account representative; the PPR process; the PFP, the assignment of a survey team; policies regarding survey scheduling; postponements and delays; and continuous public involvement. In accordance with the requirements of the Health Insurance Portability and Accountability Act of 1996 (HIPAA), a health care organization and the Joint Commission must have a signed Business Associate agreement before the organization's survey can begin.

Application for Accreditation

An organization needs to complete its e-App once, and it is required to provide updates as appropriate. An electronic version of the e-App can be completed via the organization's secure extranet site. When an organization notifies the Joint Commission that it wishes to become accredited, the Joint Commission provides the organization with information explaining how to access and complete its application on its secure site on the Joint Commission extranet site. After an organization completes its application, it will remain valid until the organization no longer wishes to be Joint Commission accredited, as long as the organization completes and submits its updates to the Joint Commission. Initial applications are valid for six months.

Organizations that use the e-App are able to enter data directly in the application and submit the e-App to the Joint Commission electronically. The application provides essential information about the organization, including ownership, demographics, and types and volume of services provided.

The application does the following:

- Describes the organization seeking accreditation
- Requires the organization to provide the Joint Commission with all official records and reports of public or publicly recognized licensing (for example, state licenses), examining, reviewing, or planning bodies*
- Authorizes the Joint Commission to obtain any records and reports not possessed by the organization
- When accepted, establishes the terms of the relationship between the organization and the Joint Commission

For an organization that chooses not to complete its application via its secure site on the Joint Commission extranet site, the organization may request a printed copy of the application by contacting its account representative. An organization can find out who its account representative is by calling 630/792-3007.

Accreditation Contract

The Joint Commission has begun annual subscription billing. As a result, organizations seeking Joint Commission accreditation for the first time or re-accreditation with the Joint Commission must sign an accreditation contract. This contract is separate from the e-App.

Contracts are available for printing and approval via each organization's secure extranet site. An organization will not be scheduled for survey until a contract is in effect. Governmental organizations may enter into unique contracts with the Joint Commission in accordance with the scope of services available from the Joint Commission and the laws for contracting that bind that government entity.

An organization will not be scheduled for survey until it signs an Accreditation Contract. When this happens, the Joint Commission will proceed with the organization's survey plans unless the organization notifies the Joint Commission in writing of its intent to withdraw from accreditation and terminate the accreditation contract. Notification in writing is necessary to terminate the accreditation contract, halt survey scheduling, and avoid a final decision of Denial of Accreditation. If an organization fails to notify the Joint Commission in writing of its intent to withdraw from accreditation and terminate its accreditation contract before a scheduled unannounced survey, The Joint Commission's Decision Rules provide for a final decision of Denial of Accreditation.

Accuracy of the Application Information

The Joint Commission schedules surveys based on information provided in an organization's e-App. With the information provided, the Joint Commission determines the number of days required for a survey and the number of surveyors.

---

* *See* APR 1 on page 134 in the "Accreditation Participation Requirements" chapter.

Inaccurate or incomplete information in the e-App may necessitate an additional survey, which could delay the Joint Commission's Accreditation Decision and Accreditation Survey Findings Report. It may also cause the organization to incur additional survey charges.

Handling Changes Affecting Application Information

At any time during the accreditation process, an organization may undergo a change that modifies the information reported in its e-App. The organization must notify the Joint Commission in writing within 30 calendar days after such a change is made. Information that must be reported includes the following:

- A change in ownership
- A change in location
- A significant increase or decrease in the volume of services
- The addition of a new type of health service or site of care
- The acquisition of a new component
- The deletion of an existing health service or site of care
  or
- The deletion of an existing component

The Joint Commission may conduct an additional survey at a later date if its surveyor or survey team arrives at the organization and discovers that a change was not reported. The Joint Commission may also survey any unreported services and sites addressed by its standards. The Joint Commission makes the final accreditation decision for the organization only after surveying all or an appropriate sample of all services, programs, and sites provided by the organization for which the Joint Commission has standards. Information reported in the e-App is subject to the Joint Commission's Information Accuracy and Truthfulness Policy (*see* pages 21–22).

Forfeiture of Survey Deposit

A nonrefundable, nontransferable deposit toward accreditation fees is required for initial surveys only. The Joint Commission applies the deposit to the organization's accreditation fees if a survey is conducted. An organization scheduled for an initial survey forfeits its deposit if its survey is not conducted within six months of submitting its application. The organization must then reapply and submit a new deposit to begin the accreditation process again.

An Organization's Secure Site on the Joint Commission Extranet Site

A key feature of the Joint Commission's accreditation process is increased use of technology. The use of technology better enables the Joint Commission and accredited organizations to communicate accreditation-related information in a more efficient and timely manner.

To fully use technology in the accreditation process, the Joint Commission provides each organization with a secure Web site on the Joint Commission's extranet site. Access to this site can only be accomplished through the use of the organization's password. This site permits an organization to complete its e-App and PPR electronically. In addition, shortly after an organization's survey, the organization's Accreditation Survey Findings Report and its ESC report are posted on the organization's secure extranet site.

Role of the Account Representative

The Joint Commission assigns an account representative to an organization after receiving its e-App. This person serves as the primary contact between the organization and the Joint Commission. He or she coordinates survey planning and handles policies, procedures, accreditation issues or services, and inquiries throughout the accreditation cycle. If an organization does not know who its account representative is, it can call 630/792-3007.

Survey Fees

Since January 2006, the Joint Commission has used a subscription billing system for all programs. For all accredited programs, the subscription approach involves an annual billing at a base rate and the assessment of an add-on fee to cover survey-related costs in those years in which an on-site survey is conducted. The use of an annual fee subscription approach is more consistent with the continuous nature of the Joint Commission's current accreditation process.

The nonrefundable annual fee is assessed on each accredited program and is due each January. Electronic invoices will be posted to the organization's The Joint Commission Connect™ extranet site; paper invoices will not be sent. The annual fee level for an organization is determined based on the organization's size and complexity, just as in the previous approach. The annual fee for organizations applying for accreditation for the first time will be prorated, based upon the quarter in which the application for accreditation and deposit is submitted.

In addition to annual fees, organizations are also billed an on-site survey fee after the survey has been performed. The on-site survey fee, which is designed to cover the costs of performing a survey, is due upon receipt. Other types of surveys such as conditional follow-up surveys and PPR surveys, will continue to be charged separately, after the event has occurred.

For an initial survey, an organization must send a nonrefundable deposit toward accreditation fees with its e-App.

An organization that has not paid its annual or on-site accreditation fee in full prior to issuance of the accreditation decision and report must remit the outstanding balance within 60 calendar days from receipt of the report. Failure to provide timely payment of any Joint Commission fees may result in the loss of accreditation. The Joint Commission notifies an organization with significant standards compliance problems of either a Conditional Accreditation or a Preliminary Denial of Accreditation decision as soon as possible, whether or not payment has been received.

Questions regarding fees can be directed to the Pricing Unit (pricingunit@jointcommission.org) or by calling 630/792-5115.

Periodic Performance Review

The PPR process is a key component in the more continuous accreditation process. It is designed to help organizations incorporate Joint Commission standards as part of routine operations and ongoing quality improvement efforts. An organization has access to its PPR tool on a continuous basis throughout its accreditation cycle. The PPR tool becomes available to organizations seeking accreditation for the first time after submitting their e-App and deposit. The PPR tool permits the organization to evaluate compliance with all applicable Joint Commission standards and EPs. For every not compliant standard, the organization must identify a plan of action at the EP level, identifying how it plans to come into compliance with the requirement(s). This plan must include an MOS, if applicable, for each EP within a standard that is identified as not compliant and that requires an MOS. (Not all EPs require an MOS, and an organization needs to demonstrate achievement with an MOS only for an EP that is within a not compliant standard and that requires an MOS.) The MOS is a numeric or other quantitative measure, usually related to an audit, which can help determine whether a planned action was effective and sustained.

The PPR helps your ambulatory care organization review applicable standards, APRs, and National Patient Safety Goals; assess compliance; develop and implement plans of action; and identify measures by which you will gauge your success in carrying out those plans. By participating in the PPR, your ambulatory care organization will be better able to incorporate Joint Commission standards into routine operations, which in turn will help to ensure the provision of safe, high-quality care on an ongoing basis.

The evaluation and plan of action must be completed electronically on the organization's secure extranet site and transmitted to the Joint Commission by its annual due date. Following receipt of the evaluation and plan of action, and if requested by the organization, staff from the Joint Commission's Standards Interpretation Group schedule a telephone call with the organization to discuss and agree upon an acceptable plan of action. The time line for the PPR is such that the organization should have sufficient time to implement the actions identified in the plan of action. The track record will be based on the plan of action implementation date. (The PPR submission is not required of organizations undergoing initial survey.)

An organization is required to annually submit to the Joint Commission an update to its PPR. Organizations that select option 2 or option 3 are required to undergo annual option 2 or option 3 surveys.*

Due dates for annual PPR updates will be at one-year intervals after the organization's last full survey. For example, if an ambulatory care organization had its last full survey end on January 1, 2006, its next annual PPR update would be due January 1, 2007, and the following annual PPR updates would be due January 1, 2008. If a full survey occurs before an organization's anticipated PPR update due date, the PPR due date will reset accordingly. Each accredited organization must either submit its updated PPR to the Joint Commission or select option 1, option 2, or option

* *See* pages 138–139 for the full text of the PPR and its options.

3 on an annual basis. An organization may change its selection or options as often as annually. The annual update to the PPR facilitates an ambulatory care organization's ongoing quality improvement efforts and supports a continuous accreditation process.

Table 1 on pages 34–35 outlines some of the activities in each of these options.

Plans of Action

A plan of action is a detailed description of how an ambulatory care organization plans to bring into compliance any standard identified as "not compliant" in the PPR (plans of action are not required for standards where some EPs are marked "partial compliance" but where the standard does not meet the level of "not compliant"). The plan of action should include the planned action to be taken and target implementation dates. If the EP requires an MOS when lack of compliance exists, you must also describe the MOS or how you plan to measure your successful implementation of your plans of action.

The PPR will only affect an organization's accreditation decision if the organization fails to participate in the PPR process, whether the full or one of the three options, or through the PPR process an immediate threat to life situation is identified and a special survey is conducted. If you need more information while completing your PPR, please contact your account representative at 630/792-3007.

Priority Focus Process

An important component of the Joint Commission's accreditation process is the Priority Focus Process (PFP), which guides the surveyor(s) in planning and conducting your on-site survey. This focuses survey activities on the organization-specific issues that are most relevant to safety and quality of care (referred to as *priority focus areas* [PFAs]). The PFP can be considered a process for standardizing the PFAs for review during survey. The PFP uses an automated tool, which takes available data from a variety of sources—including e-Apps for accreditation, previous survey findings, complaint data, and publicly available external data—and integrates them to identify clinical service/groups (CSGs) and PFAs for your ambulatory care organization. The PFP converts these data into information that focuses survey activities, increases consistency in the accreditation process, customizes the accreditation process to make it specific to your ambulatory care organization, and guides tracer activities (*see* page 51 for more information on the tracer methodology) and is a starting point for the survey.

Your ambulatory care organization will receive PFP information for its top PFAs and CSGs on its secure extranet site. Complex organizations that are surveyed under more than one accreditation program will receive program-specific PFP information and organization-level PFP information that is a summary of all programs' data and information.

ACC

Table 1. PPR Options

Full PPR

- Organization uses the automated PPR tool to assess and score compliance with EPs for each applicable standard
- Organization creates a plan of action* addressing each EP scored partial or insufficient compliance within any standards found not compliant
- Organization identifies an MOS, if required, for each EP scored partial or insufficient compliance within any standards scored not compliant
- Organization submits PPR to Joint Commission annually
- Organization may elect to participate in a conference call with Joint Commission staff to discuss plan(s) of action, MOS, and other standards-related issues of their choosing. If a conference call is not requested, the data will be reviewed by Joint Commission staff. Should they determine a conference call is needed, your organization will be contacted to schedule a call.
- Because the Joint Commission may request a conference call even if an organization does not request one, all organizations submitting the full PPR or option 2 second submission with not compliant standards need to enter their conference call "avoid dates" when they submit their PPR. "Avoid dates" are dates on which the organization prefers that the conference call not be scheduled.
- Joint Commission staff reviews and approves plan(s) of action during conference call
- Surveyors review any required MOS at full survey

Option 1

- Organization uses PPR tool to annually affirm that, for substantive reasons, legal counsel advises the organization not to participate in the full PPR and instead complete a PPR and plan of action and identify appropriate MOS
- Organizations can use the PPR tool to score compliance and can print and view standards and EPs to conduct its assessment on paper. These data are not submitted to the Joint Commission.
- Organization affirms that it has completed an assessment of its compliance with applicable EPs and developed plans of action and MOS, as necessary, but does not submit data to Joint Commission
- Organization can submit standards-related issues in the PPR tool for telephone discussion with Joint Commission staff, if desired, and receive design approval
- Surveyors review any required MOS at full survey

Option 2

- Organization uses PPR tool to annually attest that, after careful consideration with legal counsel, it has decided not to participate in full PPR and instead intends to undergo either a limited survey, or a full-length PPR survey. The organization may choose between either the limited survey or the full-length survey. When an organization selects a full-length PPR options 2 or 3 survey, it may independently select these options without advice of legal counsel.

* A plan of action details the action(s) an organization will take to come into compliance with each standard identified as not compliant.

Table 1. PPR Options *(continued)*

- The limited survey will be approximately one-third the length of the full survey; a fee will be charged
- Organizations that choose a full-length PPR survey will also be charged a fee. The full-length PPR survey can be either announced or unannounced, depending upon the organization's request.
- Survey will be conducted using tracer methodology and PFP output; all standards are subject to review
- Surveyor leaves written report of findings with organization
- The organization must submit the tool again within 30 days of the survey. This submission addresses not compliant standards, choice of a conference call, and any other topics for discussion with Joint Commission staff.
- Organization creates a plan of action and any required MOS for each standard scored not compliant and submits data to Joint Commission via the PPR tool within 30 days of survey
- Organization may elect to participate in a conference call with Joint Commission staff to discuss the plan(s) of action and MOS. If a conference call is not requested, the data will be reviewed by Joint Commission staff. Should it determine a conference call is needed, your organization will be contacted to schedule a call.
- Joint Commission staff reviews and approves plan(s) of action during conference call
- Surveyors will review any required MOS at full survey

Option 3

- Organization uses the PPR tool to annually attest that, after careful consideration with legal counsel, it has decided not to participate in the full PPR and instead intends to undergo either a limited survey, or a full-length PPR survey. The organization may choose between either the limited survey or the full-length survey. When an organization selects a full-length PPR options 2 or 3 survey, it may independently select these options without advice of legal counsel.
- The limited survey will be approximately one-third the length of the full survey; a fee will be charged
- Organizations that choose a full-length PPR survey will also be charged a fee. The full-length PPR survey can be either announced or unannounced, depending upon the organization's request.
- Survey will be conducted using tracer methodology and PFP output; all standards are subject to review
- Unlike option 2, however, option 3 stipulates that no written report of findings will be left at the organization. The surveyor delivers an oral report of findings at the closing conference of the on-site survey.
- The organization must submit the tool again within 30 days of the survey. This submission addresses the choice of a conference call and any topics for discussion with Joint Commission staff.
- At the time of the organization's full survey, the surveyors will receive no information relating to the organization's option 3 survey findings.

From these sources, the PFP identifies PFAs for each ambulatory care organization on which surveyors will focus during the initial part of the on-site survey. Surveyors will use the PFP in the following ways:

- The surveyor(s) assigned to your ambulatory care organization will have access to your ambulatory care organization's PFP information via the surveyor extranet
- The surveyor(s) will review the PFP information for ambulatory care-specific PFAs as well as for ambulatory care-specific CSGs
- As part of the planning process, the surveyor(s) will begin to assess and plan his or her tracer activities
- During the on-site survey, the surveyor(s) will use the ambulatory care organization's active patient list to select tracer patients

As the survey progresses, the surveyor(s) may find other priority areas that need addressing and may begin to focus less on the PFP suggested list and more on what he or she is finding.

The PFP will also be used for an ambulatory care organization undergoing its initial survey. The only difference with this type of ambulatory care organization (versus an ambulatory care organization that has already gone through a survey) is in the available data inputs that feed the PFP. Ambulatory care organizations undergoing initial survey will not have previous requirements for improvement (referred to as "type I recommendations" before January 1, 2004) available to feed into the PFP. For initial surveys, the Joint Commission will only be able to feed e-App data, external data (as applicable), and Office of Quality Monitoring (OQM) data into the PFP.

After these data are transformed to become the PFP information, the process for initial surveys is no different from the process for any other type of survey. The data will be aggregated in the same manner to determine the PFAs and CSGs for the ambulatory care organization. Beginning in 2007, PFP data will be updated quarterly, as changes warrant. Organizations will receive electronic notification that a new report is available, however, updated PFP reports are only generated when there is a change to one or more of the priority focus areas (PFAs) and or clinical/service groups (CSGs) in their accredited program since the previous report.

Priority Focus Areas

PFAs are processes, systems, or structures in a health care organization that significantly impact safety and/or the quality of care provided. The list of PFAs was developed from information gathered through Joint Commission experience, published literature, and consensus. Joint Commission categorized the different processes, systems, and structures leading to improved health care in 14 PFAs. The PFAs evolved from this process of identifying common patterns that are useful in building positive health care outcomes and safe, high-quality health care.

The PFAs provide a consistent yet customized approach to providing an initial focus for the on-site survey process, and they may assist the health care organization at the time of its PPR.

The PFAs are the following:

- Assessment and Care/Services
- Communication
- Credentialed Practitioners
- Equipment Use
- Infection Control
- Information Management
- Medication Management
- Organizational Structure
- Orientation & Training
- Patient Safety
- Physical Environment
- Quality Improvement Expertise/Activities
- Rights & Ethics
- Staffing

PFAs guide the surveyor with assessing standards compliance in relation to the individual tracer activities. Outside formal conferences/interviews, much of the survey will consist of reviewing issues in the form of tracer methodology (for more information, please *see* the Tracer Methodology section on page 51). The tracer methodology incorporates the use of the PFP information, follows the care experience for individuals initially identified by CSGs, and allows the surveyor to identify performance issues that may be related to PFAs for your organization.

Definitions for the PFAs follow.

Assessment and Care/Services Assessment and Care/Services for patients comprise the execution of a series of processes including, as relevant, screening; assessment; planning care, treatment, and/or services; provision of care; ongoing reassessment of care; and discharge planning, referral for continuing care, or discontinuation of services. Assessment and Care/Services are fluid in nature to accommodate a patient's needs. Although some elements of Assessment and Care/Services may occur only once, other aspects may be repeated or revisited as the patient's needs or care delivery priorities change. Successful implementation of improvements in Assessment and Care/Services rely on the full support of leadership.

Subprocesses of Assessment and Care/Services include the following:

- Screening
- Assessment
- Reassessment
- Planning care, treatment, and services
- Provision of care, treatment, and services
- Discharge planning or discontinuation of services

Communication Communication is the process by which information is exchanged between individuals, programs/services, or organizations. Effective communication successfully permeates every aspect of a health care organization, from the provision of care to performance improvement, resulting in a marked improvement in the quality of care delivery and functioning.

Subprocesses of Communication include the following:
- Provider and/or staff–patient communication
- Patient and family education
- Staff communication and collaboration
- Information dissemination
- Multidisciplinary teamwork

Credentialed Practitioners Credentialed Practitioners are health care professionals whose qualifications to provide patient care services have been verified and assessed, resulting in the assignment of clinical responsibilities. The category varies from organization to organization and from state to state. It includes licensed independent practitioners and others who are permitted to provide patient care services under the direction of a sponsoring physician. Licensed independent practitioners are permitted by law and the health care organization to provide care and services without clinical supervision or direction within the scope of their license and consistent with individually assigned clinical responsibilities.

Equipment Use Equipment Use incorporates the selection, delivery, setup, and maintenance of equipment and supplies to meet patient and staff needs. It generally includes movable equipment, as well as management of supplies that staff members use (for example, gloves, syringes). (Equipment Use does not include fixed equipment such as built-in oxygen and gas lines and central air-conditioning systems; such items are included in the Physical Environment PFA.) Equipment Use includes planning and selecting; maintaining, testing, and inspecting; educating and providing instructions; delivery and setup; and risk prevention related to equipment and/or supplies.

Subprocesses of Equipment Use include the following:
- Selection
- Maintenance strategies
- Periodic evaluation
- Orientation and training

Infection Control Infection Control includes the surveillance/identification, prevention, and control of infections among patients, employees, physicians, and other licensed independent practitioners, contract service workers, volunteers, students, and visitors. This is a systemwide, integrated process that is applied to all programs, services, and settings.

Subprocesses of Infection Control include the following:
- Surveillance/identification
- Prevention and control
- Reporting
- Measurement

Information Management Information Management is the interdisciplinary field concerning the timely and accurate creation, collection, storage, retrieval, transmission, analysis, control, dissemination, and use of data or information, both within an organization and externally, as allowed by law and regulation. In addition to written and verbal information, supporting information technology and information services are also included in Information Management.

Subprocesses of Information Management include the following:

- Planning
- Procurement
- Implementation
- Collection
- Recording
- Protection
- Aggregation
- Interpretation
- Storage and retrieval
- Data integrity
- Information dissemination

Medication Management Medication Management encompasses the systems and processes an organization uses if an organization provides medication to individuals served by the organization. This is usually a multidisciplinary, coordinated effort of health care staff, implementing, evaluating, and constantly improving the processes of selecting, procuring, storing, ordering, transcribing, preparing, dispensing, administering (including self-administering), and monitoring the effects of medications throughout the patients' continuum of care. In addition, Medication Management involves educating patients and, as appropriate, their families, about each medication, its administration and use, and potential side effects.

Subprocesses of Medication Management include the following:

- Selection
- Procurement
- Storage
- Prescribing or ordering
- Preparing
- Dispensing
- Administration
- Monitoring

Organizational Structure The Organizational Structure is the framework for an organization to carry out its vision and mission. The implementation is accomplished through corporate bylaws and governing body policies, organization management, compliance, planning, integration and coordination, and performance improvement. Included are the organization's governance, as well as business ethics, contracted organizations, and management requirements.

Subprocesses of Organizational Structure include the following:

- Management requirements
- Corporate bylaws and governing body plans
- Organization management
- Compliance
- Planning

- Business ethics
- Contracted services

Orientation & Training Orientation is the process of educating newly hired staff in health care organizations to organizationwide, departmental, and job-specific competencies before they provide patient care, treatment, and services. "Newly hired staff" include, but are not limited to, regular staff employees, contracted staff, agency (temporary) staff, float staff, volunteer staff, students, housekeeping, and maintenance staff.

Training refers to the development and implementation of programs that foster staff development and continued learning, address skill deficiencies, and thereby help ensure staff retention. More specifically, Training entails providing opportunities for staff to develop enhanced skills related to revised processes that may have been addressed during orientation, new patient care techniques, or expanded job responsibilities. Whereas orientation is a one-time process, training is a continuous one.

Subprocesses of Orientation & Training include the following:

- Organizationwide orientation
- Program/service orientation
- Job-specific orientation
- Training and continuing or ongoing education

Patient Safety Effective Patient Safety entails proactively identifying the potential and actual risks to safety, identifying the underlying cause(s) of the potential, and making the necessary improvements to reduce risk. It also entails establishing processes to respond to sentinel events, identifying risks through root cause analysis (RCA), and making necessary improvements. This involves a systems-based approach that examines all activities within an organization that contribute to the maintenance and improvement of patient safety, such as performance improvement and risk management, to ensure that the activities work together, not independently, to improve care and safety. The systems-based approach is driven by organization leadership; anchored in the organization's mission, vision, and strategic plan; endorsed and actively supported by medical staff and nursing leadership; implemented by directors; integrated and coordinated throughout the organization's staff; and continuously re-engineered using proven, proactive performance improvement modalities. In addition, effective reduction of errors and other factors that contribute to unintended adverse outcomes in an organization requires an environment in which patients, their families, and organization staff and leaders can identify and manage actual and potential risks to safety.

Subprocesses of Patient Safety include the following:

- Planning and designing services
- Directing services
- Integrating and coordinating services
- Error reduction and prevention
- The use of *Sentinel Event Alert*
- Joint Commission's National Patient Safety Goals

- Clinical practice guidelines
- Active patient involvement in their care

Physical Environment The Physical Environment refers to a safe, accessible, functional, supportive, and effective Physical Environment for patients, staff members, workers, and other individuals by managing physical design; construction and redesign; maintenance and testing; planning and improvement; and risk prevention, defined in terms of utilities, fire protection, security, privacy, storage, and hazardous materials and waste. The Physical Environment may include the home in the case of in-home programs and foster care.

Subprocesses of Physical Environment include the following:
- Physical design
- Construction and redesign
- Maintenance and testing
- Planning and improvement
- Risk prevention

Quality Improvement Expertise/Activities Quality Improvement identifies the collaborative and interdisciplinary approach to the continuous study and improvement of the processes of providing health care services to meet the needs of consumers and others. Quality Improvement depends on understanding and revising processes on the basis of data and knowledge about the processes themselves. Quality Improvement involves identifying, measuring, implementing, monitoring, analyzing, planning, and maintaining processes to ensure they function effectively. Examples of Quality Improvement Activities include designing a new service, flowcharting a clinical process, collecting and analyzing data about performance measures or patient outcomes, comparing the organization's performance to that of other organizations, selecting areas for priority attention, and experimenting with new ways of carrying out a function.

Subprocesses of Quality Improvement Expertise/Activities include the following:
- Identifying issues and establishing priorities
- Developing measures
- Collecting data to evaluate status on outcomes, processes, or structures
- Analyzing and interpreting data
- Making and implementing recommendations
- Monitoring and sustaining performance improvement

Rights & Ethics Rights & Ethics include patient rights and organizational ethics as they pertain to patient care. Rights & Ethics addresses issues such as patient privacy, confidentiality and protection of health information, advance directives (as appropriate), organ procurement, use of restraints, informed consent for various procedures, and the right to participate in care decisions.

Subprocesses of Rights & Ethics include the following:
- Patient rights
- Organizational ethics pertaining to patient care
- Organizational responsibility

- Consideration of patient
- Care sensitivity
- Informing patients and/or family

Staffing Effective Staffing entails providing the optimal number of competent personnel with the appropriate skill mix to meet the needs of a health care organization's patients based on that organization's mission, values, and vision. As such, it involves defining competencies and expectations for all staff (the competencies of licensed independent practitioners and medical staff are addressed in the Credentialed Practitioners PFA for all accreditation programs). Staffing includes assessing those defined competencies and allocating the human resources necessary for patient safety and improved patient outcomes.

Subprocesses of Staffing include the following:
- Competency
- Skill mix
- Number of staff

Clinical/Service Groups

CSGs categorize patients and/or services into distinct populations for which data can be collected. The Joint Commission created the list of CSGs based on data gathered from e-Apps from each accreditation program and on publicly available data from external sources. The list then underwent a thorough review to make sure that all categories were actually representative of populations served or services provided by the organizations surveyed by the individual accreditation programs. Joint Commission surveyors use an ambulatory care organization's CSGs combined with other ambulatory care–specific data to get a better understanding of the ambulatory care organization's systems and the patients it serves. Tracer patients are selected according to CSGs.

The CSGs for ambulatory care organizations follow.

Clinical/Service Groups for Ambulatory Care

Surgery/Anesthesia:
- Cardiac Catheterization
- Endoscopy
- Gastroenterology Procedures
- General surgery
- In Vitro Fertilization
- Mohs Surgical Procedure
- Ophthalmology
- Oral Maxillofacial Surgery
- Orthopedic Surgery
- Plastic Surgery
- Podiatric Surgery
- Trigger Point Infections (Pain Management)
- Urologic Procedures

ACC

Medical/Dental:
- Cardiology
- Dentistry
- Dermatology
- Emergency Medicine
- Family Practice
- Gastroenterology
- General Practice
- Internal Medicine
- Neurology
- Obstetrics/Gynecology
- Occupational Health
- Oncology
- Optometry
- Orthopedic Medicine
- Otolaryngology
- Pediatric Medicine
- Pharmacy/Dispensary
- Podiatry
- Rheumatology
- Short stay/Observation/Infirmary/Recovery
- Urology
- Vascular Medicine

Diagnostic/Therapeutic Services/Other:
- Allergy
- Alternative/Complementary Care
- Audiology
- Chiropractic Medicine
- Diagnostic Imaging
- Dialysis
- Hematology
- Infusion Therapy
- Lithotripsy
- Orthotics/Prosthetics
- Pain Management
- Physical Medicine and Rehabilitation
- Pulmonary Medicine
- Radiation Oncology
- Sleep Diagnostics
- Telehealth

During the Survey

During an accreditation survey, the Joint Commission evaluates an organization's performance of functions and processes aimed at continuously improving patient outcomes. The survey process focuses on assessing performance of important patient-centered and organization functions that support the safety and quality of patient care. This assessment is accomplished through evaluating an organization's compliance with the applicable standards in this manual, based on the following:

- Tracing the care delivered to patients
- Verbal and written information provided to the Joint Commission
- On-site observations and interviews by Joint Commission surveyors
- Documents provided by the organization

The Joint Commission's accreditation process seeks to help organizations identify and correct problems and improve the safety and quality of care and services provided.

A survey is designed to be individualized to each organization, to be consistent, and to support the organization's efforts to improve performance. The Joint Commission determines the length of a survey based on information supplied in the e-App that describes the organization's size and scope of services. In addition, Joint Commission surveyors may conduct some survey activities on evenings, nights, and weekends as necessary.

The On-Site Survey

This section includes information relevant to an organization that has applied for an accreditation survey and is ready for the survey process. It provides an overview of the survey process, including use of the PFP.

The Joint Commission's accreditation process focuses on systems critical to the safety and the quality of care, treatment, and services. It represents a shift from a focus on survey preparation to a focus on continuous operational improvement by encouraging ambulatory care organizations to incorporate the standards as a guide for routine operations.

Under this accreditation process, the unannounced full survey is the on-site evaluation piece of a continuous process. (Initial surveys will continue to be announced unless required to be unannounced to meet deemed status requirements. In addition, organizations such as the Department of Defense and Bureau of Prisons and organizations providing foster care will receive advance notice of their survey date.) The accreditation process encourages organizations to embed the standards into routine operations to achieve and maintain excellent operational systems on an ongoing basis. Initiatives such as the continuous PPR (discussed on page 64) and the sharing of PFP information (discussed on pages 33–36) facilitate this.

Unannounced Surveys

The Joint Commission conducts surveys in an unannounced fashion, with the following exceptions:

- Initial surveys (that is, for organizations that are undergoing their first Joint Commission survey), including both surveys conducted under the Early Survey Policy, unless deemed status requirements specify unannounced surveys

- Situations in which it would not be logical or feasible to conduct an unannounced survey, such as with the Bureau of Prisons or the Department of Defense facilities
- Foster care (Traditional or Therapeutic)
- "Very small" organizations in certain situations (*see* Table 2 on pages 46–47, under the "Threshold" column, to understand what is meant by "very small" for each program)
- PPR option 2 and option 3 surveys (*see* pages 34–35 for more information on these options)

Between 2006 and 2008 the unannounced survey will occur in the year that the organization is due to have its triennial survey (laboratories will have their survey prior to when their current accreditation is due to expire). Subsequent unannounced surveys will occur 18 to 39 months after the organization's first unannounced survey (subsequent unannounced surveys for laboratories will occur within 24 months after its previous unannounced survey). The timing of this latter survey and all succeeding unannounced surveys will be based on pre-established criteria generated from PFP data.

With an *unannounced survey*, an accredited organization will receive *no notice* of its survey date prior to the start of the survey. In concert with the unannounced survey process, the following procedures will be implemented:

- Accredited organizations will be able to identify up to 10 days each year in which an unannounced survey should be avoided. These 10 days should not include federal holidays but may include regional events in which it may be difficult to conduct a survey during a given period. The Joint Commission will make every effort to accommodate the organization regarding avoiding these 10 days. However, the Joint Commission reserves the right to conduct a survey during an "avoid period" if the reason(s) given to avoid a survey at that time is such that a survey can be reasonably accomplished.
- An annual subscription billing model has been implemented. *See* page 31 for further details.
- Because an accredited organization will not be able to post its survey date and, therefore, individuals cannot request to have a public information interview (PII), a new APR was established. This APR requires an organization to demonstrate how it communicates to its public that if members of the public have any quality of care or safety concerns, they should notify the Joint Commission.
- On the morning of an organization's survey, the letter of introduction, the survey agendas, and the biographies and pictures of the surveyors assigned to conduct the survey will be posted to the organization's secure site on the Joint Commission extranet site.
- If an organization knows of a surveyor who works at or has worked at the organization, a competing organization, or who has had personal experience with the survey that represents a potential conflict, the organization is asked to identify the individual(s) in its e-App.

ACC

Table 2. Exemptions to Unannounced Surveys

Program	Subject	Exception	Threshold
Ambulatory Care	Initial surveys	Announced (except deemed status surveys for Medicare certification)	
	Early Survey Policy Option 1—1st survey	Announced (except for deemed status surveysfor Medicare certification)	
	Early Survey Policy Option 2—1st and 2nd surveys	Announced	
	Department of Defense facilities	5 days within certain periods of time	
	Bureau of Prisons' facilities and contracted facilities	5-day notice	
	Immigration facilities	5-day notice	
	Office-based surgery practices	5-day notice	Fewer than 1,500 annual visits
	Health care organizations that provide surgery/ anesthesia services	5-day notice	Fewer than 1,500 annual visits
	Health care organizations that provide medical/ dental services	5-day notice	Fewer than 5,000 annual visits, or less than 3 licensed independent practitioners
	Initial organizations that are using their accreditation for deemed status purposes under the Early Survey Policy Option 2	1st survey—unannounced 2nd survey—announced	

ACC

Table 2. Exemptions to Unannounced Surveys (continued)

Program	Subject	Exception	Threshold
	Organizations that provide specified diagnostic and therapeutic services* and have fewer than 3,000 annual visits or four or fewer licensed independent practitioners	5-day notice	
	Organizations that provide mobile diagnostic services	5-day notice	

* Note: This includes Allergy, Alternative/Complementary Care, Audiology, Chiropractic Medicine, Diagnostic Imaging, Dialysis, Hematology, Infusion Therapy, Lithotripsy, Orthotics/Prosthetics, Pain Management, Pulmonary Medicine, Physical Medicine, Radiation Oncology, Sleep Diagnostic, and Telehealth.

Survey Agenda

The on-site survey process shifts the focus from survey preparation to continuous operational improvement in support of safe, high-quality care, treatment, and services.

The survey agenda will include the following elements:*

Survey Planning Session. During this session, the surveyor(s) will review data and information about the ambulatory care organization, measures of success (MOS) generated from the full PPR, option 1, or option 2, and plan the survey agenda. The surveyor(s) will also select initial tracer patients. As part of the survey process, surveyors will review the organization's MOS information.

Opening Conference and Orientation to the Organization. During the opening conference, the surveyor(s) describes the structure and content of the survey to the organization, while the organization provides the surveyor(s) with information about the organization. At this time, your ambulatory care organization will briefly explain its structures, mission, vision, and relationship with the community. This provides the surveyor(s) with baseline information about the organization that can help focus subsequent survey activities.

Leadership Session. During the leadership session, surveyors discuss the following with leaders:

* Please *see* the *Survey Activity Guide*, which is available on your extranet site or your account representative if not available on the extranet site. For more detailed information on the survey process, call your Account Representative at 630/792-3007.

- Information gathering and baseline assessment of leadership-level, system issues—system standards, management oversight and direction, and other leadership responsibilities
- Leadership's approach to the PPR and methods used to address areas needing improvement
- Ongoing initiatives to improve delivery of health care
- Safety program and National Patient Safety Goals
- Oversight by governance or board
- PFP output related to CSGs and PFAs

Individual Tracers. During the individual tracer activity, the surveyor(s) will do the following:
- Follow the course of a type of care, treatment, and service provided to the patient by the ambulatory care organization
- Assess the interrelationships among disciplines and services/programs and the important functions in the care, treatment, and services provided
- Evaluate the performance of processes relevant to the care, treatment, and service needs of the patient, with particular focus on the integration and coordination of distinct but related processes
- Identify vulnerabilities in the care processes

Individual-based System Tracers. Individual-based system tracers are interactive sessions with the surveyor(s) and ambulatory care organization staff that explore the performance of important patient-related functions that cross the ambulatory care organization. The surveyor(s) and ambulatory care organization staff will address critical risk points and provide education during the individual-based system tracer sessions. The following are the individual-based system tracers:
- Data Use
- Infection Control
- Medication Management, if within the scope of the organization

As surveyors go through the individual tracers to determine standards compliance as it relates to care delivered to the selected patient, they also assess the organization's overall systems by conducting individual-based system tracers. Individual-based system tracers focus on high-risk processes across the organization.

Program-specific tracers. Program-specific tracers will be conducted if they apply to the organization being surveyed. *See* pages 51–52 for more information.

Daily Briefings. During the daily briefing session, organization staff are briefed on the previous day's survey findings and any significant patterns or trends that are becoming evident in the survey. During the daily briefing, the surveyor(s) will do the following:
- Facilitate leadership's understanding of the survey process and the findings that contribute to the accreditation decision
- Report on findings from the previous day's survey activities
- Emphasize patterns or trends of significant concern that could lead to noncompliance determinations
- Highlight any positive findings or exemplary performance

- Allow the ambulatory care organization to provide information that may have been missed during the previous survey day
- Review the agenda for the survey day ahead and make any necessary adjustments based on ambulatory care organization needs or the need for more intensive assessment of an issue

Special Issue Resolution. This session provides an opportunity for the surveyor(s) to follow up on potential findings that could not be resolved in other survey activities or address any requested PIIs.

Competence Assessment Process. This process will help the ambulatory care organization and the surveyor(s) do the following:

- Identify the competence-assessment, process-related strengths and vulnerabilities of the organization
- Begin the assessment or determine the degree of compliance with relevant standards
- Identify human resources issues requiring further exploration

Credentialing and Assigning of Clinical Responsibilities. This activity will help the organization and the surveyor(s) identify specific issues related to the following:

- Evaluation of the process the ambulatory care organization uses to collect relevant data for decisions for credentialing
- Evaluation of consistent implementation of the credentialing and assigning of clinical responsibilities process
- Evaluation of processes for the privileges
- Determination that practitioners practice within the limited scope of assigned clinical responsibilities
- Link results of peer review and focused monitoring to the credentialing process
- Identify vulnerabilities in the credentialing and assigning of clinical responsibilities

Environment of Care Session. This session will help the ambulatory care organization and the surveyor(s) do the following:

- Identify vulnerabilities and strengths in the organization's processes
- Begin to identify or determine the action(s) necessary to address any identified vulnerabilities
- Begin the assessment or determine the ambulatory care organization's actual degree of compliance with relevant standards
- Identify environment of care processes requiring further evaluation of implementation
- Identify issues requiring further exploration

***Life Safety Code*® (*LSC*) Building Tour** (as applicable). This session will help the organization and the surveyor(s) do the following:

- Identify areas of concern in the organization's processes for designing buildings to *LSC* requirements
- Identify areas of concern in the organization's processes for maintaining buildings to *LSC* requirements

- Identify areas of concern in the organization's processes for identifying and resolving *LSC* problems
- Determine the organization's degree of compliance with relevant *LSC* requirements
- Identify or determine the action(s) necessary to address any identified *LSC* problems

Clinical Leadership and Staff Discussion Session.* This group session focuses on the involvement of clinical leaders and staff in the provision of care. This activity is intended to do the following:

- Begin a dialogue with the surveyor about the quality and safety of care provided by the organization
- Address the continuum of care provided to the patients by the organization in its various clinics and locations with particular focus on the integration and coordination of processes
- Assess the interrelationships and communication between and among disciplines, departments, programs, services, or settings (as applicable) in the organization
- Provide an opportunity to confirm the surveyor's observations and/or assessment of standards-based issues
- Identify potential opportunities for organizational improvement at the organization, system, or process level
- Provide consultation and education as time permits

Governance Discussion Session.* This session focuses on the organization's governance and is intended to address the following:

- The structure and composition of the governing body
- The functioning, participation, and involvement of the governing body in the oversight and operation of the organization
- The level of communication among the board members
- The governing body's perception of its role in the organization
- The knowledge of the governing body members with respect to federal law and regulation
- The governing body's understanding of performance improvement approaches and methods and involvement in the organization's approach to performance improvement
- Pertinent Leadership standards relevant to the governing body's role in the organization

Surveyor Team Meeting. On surveys being conducted by more than one surveyor, scheduled team meetings provide an opportunity for the surveyor(s) to share information and observations, plan for upcoming survey activities, and plan for communication and coordination with the organization.

Surveyor Report Preparation. The surveyor(s) will use this time to compile, analyze, and organize the data he or she has collected throughout the survey into a report reflecting the organization's compliance with standards.

CEO Exit Briefing and Organization Exit Conference. During the CEO Exit Briefing the surveyor(s) will review the outcome of the survey, present the Accredi-

* These on-site survey activities are only applicable to Bureau of Primary Health Care–supported organizations.

tation Survey Findings Report, discuss any concerns that the CEO has with the report, and determine the need for any special arrangements for the Organization Exit Conference.

During the Organization Exit Conference the surveyor(s) will report the outcome of the survey and present the Accreditation Survey Findings Report if desired by the CEO, review the issues of standards compliance that have been identified during the survey, allow the organization a final on-site opportunity to question the survey findings or provide additional material regarding standards' compliance, and review required follow-up actions, as applicable.

Survey Team Composition

An accreditation survey may be conducted by a survey team rather than by an individual surveyor. The composition of an organization's survey team is based on the information provided in its e-App. Surveyors assess and provide education as part of the survey process.

The Survey Team Leader

If more than one surveyor is required, one of the surveyors on each organization survey team is designated as the "team leader." The team leader is responsible for integration, coordination, and communication of on-site survey activities. In addition to direct participation as an active member of the survey team, the team leader serves as the primary point of on-site contact between the organization and the Joint Commission. Among other responsibilities, the team leader leads the opening conference and the daily and exit briefings.

Tracer Methodology

The tracer methodology is the cornerstone of the Joint Commission on-site survey. The tracer methodology does the following:

- Incorporates the use of PFP information
- Follows the experience of care for a number of individuals (initially identified by CSGs) through the organization's entire health care process
- Allows the surveyor(s) to identify performance issues (that may be related to PFAs) in one or more steps of the process, or in the interfaces between processes

Program-Specific Tracers

The Joint Commission is implementing specific tracer activities in the ambulatory care program to better address the unique characteristics and relevant issues of the organizations in these programs. Table 3 on page 52 contains your program-specific tracer activities including applicability and objectives.

The goal of the program-specific tracer activity is to identify safety concerns within different levels and types of care. Program-specific tracers bring a targeted focus on important issues relevant to the following information:

- Types of services offered by the organization
- Programs being surveyed
- Organization's priority focus areas

ACC

Table 3. Program-Specific Tracer Applicability Objectives

Organization Type	Program-Specific Tracer	Applicability	Objectives
Ambulatory	Continuity of Care	Community Health Clinics/Medical Providers	• To evaluate the effectiveness of the organization's process, from prescribing a diagnostic study to patient follow-up • To identify process- and possibly system-level issues contributing to missed follow-up of diagnostic studies

Topics for the program-specific tracers were identified through a review of expert literature, research, input from the field, and subject matter expertise. Program-specific tracers evaluate program-specific issues and compliance with relevant standards that impact patient safety.

Note: *Program-specific tracers will only be conducted if they apply to the specific organization being surveyed.*

Individual Tracer Activity

The individual tracer activity is an evaluation method that is conducted during an on-site survey and is designed to "trace" the care experiences that a patient had while at the ambulatory care organization. The tracer methodology is a way to analyze an ambulatory care organization's system of providing care, treatment, and services using actual patients as the framework for assessing standards compliance. The surveyor(s) will use the following general criteria to select initial individual tracers:

- Patients in top CSGs for that organization
- Patients related to individual-based system tracer topics (*see* the Individual-Based System Tracer Activity section below), such as infection control or medication management
- Patients receiving multiple services, such as an adult diabetic who receives regular exams, medications, lab work, and services from a nutritionist and podiatrist

Patients selected for initial individual tracer activity will most likely be those identified in the ambulatory care organization's PFP information as listed in the CSGs. Based on identified CSGs, the surveyor(s) will identify individual tracers and follow specific patients through the ambulatory care organization's processes. A surveyor will not only examine the individual components of a system but will also evaluate how the components of a system interact with each other. In other words, a surveyor will look at the care, treatment, and services provided by each department/unit/program and service, as well as how departments/units/programs and services work together. The surveyor(s) may start where the patient is currently located. He or she can then move to where the patient first entered the organization's systems; an area of care provided to the patient that may be a priority for that organization; or to any areas in which the patient received care, treatment, and services. The order will vary. Along the way, the surveyor(s) will speak with the health care staff member(s) who actually provided the care to that individual tracer patient—or, if that staff member(s) is not available, will speak with another staff member(s) who provides the same type of care.

Based on the findings of the surveyor(s), he or she may select similar patients to trace. The tracer methodology permits surveyors to "pull the threads" if there is a reason to believe that an issue needs further exploration.

Individual-Based System Tracer Activity

Individual-based system tracers explore one specific system or process across the organization, focusing, when possible, on the experiences of specific patients or activities relevant to specific patients. This differs from individual tracers in that during individual tracers, the surveyor follows an individual through his or her course of care, evaluating all aspects of care as opposed to a "system." During the individual-based system tracer sessions, the surveyor(s) evaluates the system/process, including the integration of related processes and the coordination and communication among disciplines and departments in those processes.

An individual-based system tracer includes an interactive session (involving a surveyor and relevant staff members) in tracing a "system" within the organization based on information from individual tracers. Points of discussion in the interactive session include the following:

- The flow of the process across your ambulatory care organization, including identification and management of risk points, integration of key activities, and communication among staff/units involved in the process
- Strengths in the process and possible actions to be taken in areas needing improvement
- Issues requiring further exploration in other survey activities
- A baseline assessment of standards compliance
- Education by the surveyor, as appropriate

The three topics evaluated with individual-based system tracers are data use, infection control, and medication management, although the number of individual-based system tracers varies based on survey length. Despite survey length, the data use individual-based system tracer is always performed.

Data Use The data use individual-based system tracer focuses on how your ambulatory care organization collects, analyzes, interprets, and uses data to improve patient safety and care.

Infection Control The infection control individual-based system tracer explores your ambulatory care organization's infection control processes. The goals of this session are to assess your ambulatory care organization's compliance with the relevant infection control standards, identify infection control issues that require further exploration, and determine actions that may be necessary to address any identified risks and improve patient safety.

Medication Management The medication management individual-based system tracer explores your ambulatory care organization's medication management processes while focusing on subprocesses and potential risk points (such as handoff points).

The Role of Ambulatory Care Staff in Tracer Methodology

To help the surveyor(s) in the tracer methodology process, staff will be asked to provide the surveyor(s) with a list of active patients, including the patients' names, current locations in the ambulatory care organization, and diagnoses, as appropriate. The surveyor(s) may request assistance from ambulatory care organization staff for selection of appropriate tracer patients. As the surveyor(s) moves around an ambulatory care organization, he or she will ask to speak with the staff members who have been involved in the tracer patient's care, treatment, and services. If those staff members are not available, the surveyor(s) will ask to speak to another staff member who would perform the same function(s) as the member who has cared for or is caring for the tracer patient. Although it is preferable to speak with the direct caregiver, it is not mandatory because the questions that will be asked are questions that any caregiver should be able to answer in providing care to the patient being traced.

Feedback Sessions

Surveyors will communicate their observations at daily briefings, if requested to do so by the organization. If the organization has additional information that would demonstrate compliance with a standard that a surveyor has indicated may be a requirement for improvement, the organization should supply that information to the surveyor(s) as soon as possible.

Final On-Site Survey Activities

At the organization exit conference, the survey team presents survey findings and a written Accreditation Survey Findings Report. A written report is not provided at the completion of a for-cause unannounced survey.

Threat to Health or Safety

The Joint Commission may consider for accreditation purposes a surveyor's finding that some aspect of an organization's operation is having or may potentially have a serious adverse effect on patient health or safety and that immediate action must be taken.

Surveyors notify the organization's CEO and Joint Commission headquarters staff immediately if they identify any condition they believe poses a serious threat to public or patient health or safety. The president of the Joint Commission, or if the president is unavailable, his or her designee, can then issue an expedited Preliminary Denial of Accreditation decision based on such notification which includes the public posting of this decision on Quality Check. He or she promptly informs the organization's CEO and appropriate governmental authorities of this decision and the findings that led to this action. The Accreditation Committee of the Joint Commission Board of Commissioners confirms or reverses the decision at its next meeting. The Accreditation Committee may take into consideration an organization's corrective actions or responses to a serious threat situation. The organization can provide information to demonstrate that the serious threat-to-health-or-safety situation has been corrected prior to the Accreditation Committee's consideration of the Preliminary Denial of Accreditation decision.

In these situations, the corrective action is considered when a single issue leads to the adverse finding and the organization demonstrates that it did the following:

- Took immediate action to completely remedy the situation
- Prepared a thorough and credible RCA
- Adopted systems changes to prevent a future recurrence of the problem

If the organization demonstrates that it has taken corrective action, the Joint Commission will conduct an on-site survey to validate the implementation of the corrective action and that the immediate threat situation is no longer present.

The Accreditation Survey Findings Report

Following evaluation of an organization's performance of functions and processes, the surveyor (or survey team) reviews the results of integrated individual findings. Then, with the use of laptop-based decision support software, the surveyor (or survey team) produces the organization's Accreditation Survey Findings Report. The surveyor (or survey team leader) meets with the organization's CEO prior to the closing conference and provides him or her with a copy of the report. The CEO determines whether this report is distributed at the closing conference. The surveyor (or survey team) uses the report contents in making his or her closing conference presentations.

Shortly after a survey, an organization's Accreditation Survey Findings Report is posted on the organization's secure extranet site. The report includes, as appropriate, requirements for improvement and supplemental findings.

If an organization does not receive any requirements for improvement, the organization's accreditation decision is rendered at the same time that the organization's Accreditation Survey Findings Report is available, and it is effective the day after the completion of the survey. If an organization receives requirements for improvement, then the organization's accreditation decision is rendered following the submission of an acceptable ESC report. An acceptable ESC report is due within 45 calendar days following the posting of the Accreditation Survey Findings Report. The organization's accreditation decision is retroactive to the day after the last day of the survey, unless the organization is undergoing its first Joint Commission survey. In that case, the effective date for accreditation is set retroactively as the date on which an acceptable ESC that resolves all requirements for improvement is submitted. For an organization that receives a notification that it will be recommended for either Conditional Accreditation or Preliminary Denial of Accreditation, the accreditation decision is rendered by the Joint Commission's Accreditation Committee. (*See* the Evidence of Standards Compliance section on pages 78–79.)

Conducting a Public Information Interview

Because all surveys are now unannounced,* PIIs are conducted only if someone contacts the surveyor(s) during an on-site survey to request a PII and the survey schedule can accommodate the PII.

Scoring Compliance and Track Record Achievements

An accredited organization is expected to remain in continuous compliance with the standards and their EPs throughout its accreditation cycle. Standards are judged "Compliant" or "Not Compliant" based on the scoring pattern of their associated EPs. EPs are performance expectations for meeting a particular standard.

The accreditation decision will be based on a simple count of the standards that are judged not compliant. The EPs for each standard will be scored on the following scale:

0	Insufficient compliance
1	Partial compliance
2	Satisfactory compliance
NA	Not applicable

The determination as to whether an organization is compliant with a given standard is based on the scoring of that standard's EPs. An EP is a specific performance expectation related to a standard that details the specific structures or processes that must be in place for an ambulatory care organization to provide quality care, treatment, and services.

Two components are scored for each EP: (1) compliance with the requirement itself **and** (2) compliance with the track record for that requirement. (**Note:** *The track record is not applicable when assessing compliance in the PPR.*)

To determine your compliance with an EP, first look at the EP scoring category listed immediately preceding the scoring scale in the margin next to the EP. There are three scoring categories: A, B, and C. For more information on these scoring categories, please refer to the "How to Use This Book" chapter.

In addition to the requirements specifically stated in the EPs, EPs are also scored in accordance with the following track record achievements:

Score	**Re-Survey**
2	12 months
1	6 to 11 months
0	Fewer than 6 months

---

* Please *see* pages 45 and 46 for exceptions to unannounced surveys.

If during an on-site survey, your ambulatory care organization has been found to be not compliant with one or more standards, you must submit an ESC* for each standard that is not compliant. The ESC must address compliance at the EP level; when an EP within a not compliant standard requires an MOS†, your ambulatory care organization must establish an MOS compliance goal for each EP when completing the ESC.‡ Also *see* page 12 for information on submitting an optional clarification as part of the ESC for standards identified as not compliant.

See the "How to Use This Book" chapter for detailed information on sample sizes. *See* page 79 in this chapter for more information on the MOS decision rules.

After you have evaluated and scored each EP for a particular standard, use these simple rules to determine your compliance with the standard itself:

- Your ambulatory care organization is not in compliance (that is, "not compliant") with the standard if any EP is scored 0
- Your ambulatory care organization is not in compliance (that is, "not compliant") with the standard if 35% or more of its EPs are scored 1

For practical purposes, in conducting a survey, surveyors ordinarily limit their evaluation of an accredited organization's track record of compliance to 12 months for a resurvey.

Surveyors may evaluate compliance over a shorter or longer time frame, depending on circumstances encountered during the survey. For example, the required time frame for full compliance with applicable standards and EPs for new services cannot exceed the time the service has been in operation. As another example, certain activities that are conducted infrequently, such as biennial credentialing, may require evaluation over a longer interval to ensure an adequate sample size for valid assessment. For a resurvey, an organization's track record generally affects the scoring of standards as follows:

Score 0 Fewer than 6 consecutive months before survey
Score 1 6 to 11 consecutive months before survey
Score 2 12 consecutive months before survey

* **Evidence of Standards Compliance (ESC)** A report submitted by a surveyed organization within 45 days of its survey, which details the action(s) that it took to bring itself into compliance with a standard or clarifies why the organization believes that it was in compliance with the standard for which it received an RFI. An ESC must address compliance at the element of performance (EP) level and include a measure of success (MOS) (*see* definition) for all appropriate EP corrections.

† **Measure of success (MOS)** A numerical or quantifiable measure usually related to an audit that determines whether an action was effective and sustained due four months after Evidence of Standards Compliance (*see* definition) approval.

‡ **Note:** *Not every EP requires an MOS. EPs that do require an MOS are clearly marked in the standards chapters in this book. Organizations are required to demonstrate achievement with an MOS* only *for EPs within a not compliant standard that requires an MOS. Organizations* do not *need to demonstrate achievement with an MOS for any EP within a compliant standard.*

After the Survey

This section includes information relevant to an organization that has recently participated in an accreditation survey. Material includes information on the ESC process, the MOS process, the types of accreditation decisions, how to request review of Preliminary Denial of Accreditation decisions, how to appeal Denial of Accreditation decisions, and how to use and display an accreditation award.

The Evidence of Standards Compliance Process

For every requirement for improvement cited in an organization's Accreditation Survey Findings Report, the organization must submit an ESC. The ESC report is available for completion on the organization's secure extranet site at the same time that the organization's Accreditation Survey Findings Report is posted.

An acceptable ESC report must detail the action(s) that the organization took to bring itself into compliance with a standard or clarify why the organization believes that it is in compliance with the standard for which it received a requirement for improvement. An acceptable ESC must address compliance at the EP level and include an MOS, if applicable. An MOS is a numeric or quantifiable measure, usually related to an audit, which determines whether an action is effective and sustained. (*See* Measure(s) of Success Report section, page 59.)

An acceptable ESC report is due within 45 calendar days following the posting of the Accreditation Survey Findings Report. Following a successful submission of the report, the organization receives an accreditation decision. If the organization implements actions to address its requirements for improvement, the organization's accreditation decision is Accredited. If an organization's ESC report does not acceptably address its requirements for improvement, then the organization's accreditation decision is Provisional Accreditation, which can eventually lead to a Conditional Accreditation or Preliminary Denial of Accreditation decision.

Conditional Accreditation, Preliminary Denial of Accreditation, and the ESC Report

If an organization is notified that a recommendation is to be made to the Joint Commission's Accreditation Committee for either Conditional Accreditation or Preliminary Denial of Accreditation, the organization has 10 business days to provide information to clarify any of the requirements for improvement cited in its Accreditation Survey Findings Report through its ESC report.

After reviewing the organization's clarifying information and determining that the organization has no longer met the decision rule for Preliminary Denial of Accreditation or Conditional Accreditation, the Joint Commission will follow up with an on-site validation survey to do the following:

- Seek to validate the clarifying information submitted and determine if such information or data was available to the previous on-site survey team
- Determine whether the organization does or does *not* meet a decision rule for Preliminary Denial of Accreditation or Conditional Accreditation

If the organization does *not* meet a rule for Preliminary Denial of Accreditation or Conditional Accreditation, it will be awarded Accreditation (if it is compliant with all standards) or it will be required to submit an ESC (if it still has requirements for improvement). However, if the organization continues to meet a decision rule for Preliminary Denial of Accreditation or Conditional Accreditation, the Joint Commission staff will recommend to the Accreditation Committee that the organization remain in Preliminary Denial of Accreditation or Conditional Accreditation. If the results of the on-site validation survey suggest that the organization knowingly falsified its clarifying information, the staff will recommend to the Accreditation Committee that the Information Accuracy and Truthfulness Policy should apply.

Measure(s) of Success Report

If possible, an organization is required to submit an MOS report within four months of submitting an acceptable ESC report. The MOS report should demonstrate whether each MOS identified in the organization's ESC report was reached.

Accreditation Decisions

An organization's accreditation decision becomes official following submission of its acceptable ESC resolving all requirements for improvement, which is retroactive to the day after the last day of the full survey, or, in the case of Preliminary Denial of Accreditation, on the date the Accreditation Committee makes a decision. For organizations undergoing an initial survey, the accreditation decision becomes official the day of the Accreditation Committee meeting or an acceptable ESC resolving all requirements for improvement is submitted (if that occurs after the Accreditation Committee meeting). When an organization's accreditation decision becomes official, it is publicly disclosable. There are six possible accreditation decisions:

1. Accredited
2. Provisional Accreditation
3. Conditional Accreditation
4. Preliminary Denial of Accreditation
5. Denial of Accreditation
6. Preliminary Accreditation (Early Survey Policy Option 1 process only)

See Table 4 on pages 60–61 and The Accreditation Decision Process section on pages 68–69 for more information.

An organization's request to withdraw from the accreditation process after undergoing survey and before a final decision has been made does not terminate the decision-making process. The Joint Commission then issues a final accreditation decision.

Review and Appeal of Preliminary Denial of Accreditation and Denial of Accreditation Decisions

The appeal procedures are set forth in the Review and Appeal Procedures section of this chapter, on pages 86–97. Two additional procedures specific to Preliminary Denial of Accreditation and Denial of Accreditation decisions are described here.

Table 4. Joint Commission Accreditation Decisions

The Joint Commission has six accreditation decision categories. Each decision and the conditions that lead to it are described here.

ACC

Accreditation Decision Category	Conditions That Lead to This Type of Decision
Accredited	The organization is in compliance with all applicable standards at the time of the on-site survey or has successfully addressed all requirements for improvement in an ESC within 45 days following the posting of the Accreditation Survey Findings Report.
Provisional Accreditation	The organization fails to successfully address all requirements for improvement in an ESC within 45 days following the posting of the Accreditation Survey Findings Report.
Conditional Accreditation	The organization is not in substantial compliance with the applicable standards, as usually evidenced by a count of the number of standards identified as not compliant at the time of survey which is between 1½ and 3 standard deviations above the mean number of not compliant standards for organizations in that accreditation program. The organization must remedy identified problem areas through preparation and submission of an ESC and subsequently undergo an on-site, follow-up survey.
Preliminary Denial of Accreditation	There is justification to deny accreditation to the organization as usually evidenced by a count of the number of not compliant standards at the time of survey which is 3 or more standard deviations above the mean number of standards identified as not compliant for organizations in that accreditation program. The decision is subject to review and appeal prior to the determination to deny accreditation; the appeal process may also result in a decision other than Denial of Accreditation.

Table 4. Joint Commission Accreditation Decisions *(continued)*

Accreditation Decision Category	Conditions That Lead to This Type of Decision
Denial of Accreditation	The organization has been denied accreditation. All review and appeal opportunities have been exhausted.
Preliminary Accreditation	The organization demonstrates compliance with selected standards in the first of two surveys conducted under the Early Survey Policy Option 1.

When an organization receives written notice from the Joint Commission that a recommendation of Preliminary Denial of Accreditation is proposed for submission to the Accreditation Committee, the organization has 10 business days from receipt of that notification to submit to the Joint Commission an acceptable ESC report and clarifying information that demonstrates that it was, in fact, in compliance with one or more standards in question at the time of survey.

If, after Joint Commission review of any submitted materials, the Preliminary Denial of Accreditation recommendation will still be made, the organization will have five business days from receipt of this notification to submit a written response directly to the Accreditation Committee.

Weighted Decision Rules

The weighted decision rules are applied to rendering accreditation decisions in complex organizations. When a secondary component of a complex organization meets rules of Conditional Accreditation or Preliminary Denial of Accreditation as a consequence of invoking the Threat to Helath or Safety Policy or not complying with the Information Accuracy and Truthfulness Policy or an APR, that accreditation decision would apply equally to the component and the complex organization of which the component is a part.

See Table 5 on page 62 for more information on the weighted decision rules.

Award Display and Use

The Joint Commission provides each accredited organization with one certificate of accreditation per program. There is no charge for the initial certificate(s). Additional certificates may be purchased. Such requests should be sent to the certificate coordinator in the Division of Accreditation and Certification Operations at the Joint Commission.

The certificate and all copies remain the Joint Commission's property. They must be returned if either of the following situations occurs:

ACC

Table 5. Weighted Decision Rules*

Primary Program	Secondary Programs
One program in a complex organization is to be identified as "primary" (this is not a change from the previous rule).	If one of the secondary programs meets a rule for Preliminary Denial of Accreditation, the overall decision for the organization is Conditional Accreditation.
If the primary program meets a rule for Provisional Accreditation, Conditional Accreditation, or Preliminary Denial of Accreditation, the overall decision for the organization is Provisional Accreditation, Conditional Accreditation, or Preliminary Denial of Accreditation, respectively.	If one of the secondary programs meets a rule for Conditional Accreditation, the overall decision for the organization is Provisional Accreditation.
If the primary or any secondary program meets a rule for Provisional Accreditation, the overall decision for the organization is Provisional Accreditation.	If two or more of the secondary programs meet rules for Preliminary Denial of Accreditation, the overall decision for the organization is Preliminary Denial of Accreditation.
	If two or more of the secondary programs meet rules for Conditional Accreditation, the overall decision for the organization is Conditional Accreditation.
	If the primary or any secondary program meets a rule for Provisional Accreditation, the overall decision for the organization is Provisional Accreditation.

* **Note:** *Weighted decision rules are not applicable when the laboratory is the secondary program.*

- The organization is issued a new certificate, reflecting a name change
  or
- The organization's accreditation decision is changed, withdrawn, or denied for any reason

An organization accredited by the Joint Commission must be accurate in describing to the public the nature and meaning of its accreditation and its award.* When an organization receives an accreditation award, the Joint Commission sends the organization guidelines for characterizing the accreditation award.

Accreditation award certificates include language about educating patients and their families on how to contact the Joint Commission.

An organization may not engage in any false or misleading advertising of an accreditation award. Any such advertising may be grounds for the Joint Commis-

* *See* APR 11 on page 136 in the "Accreditation Participation Requirements" chapter.

sion to deny accreditation. For example, an organization may not represent its accreditation as being awarded by any of the Joint Commission's corporate members. These include the American College of Physicians, the American College of Surgeons, the American Dental Association, the American Hospital Association, and the American Medical Association. The Joint Commission has permission to reprint the seals of its corporate members on certificates of accreditation. However, these seals must not be reproduced or displayed separately from the certificate.

Any organization that materially misleads the public about any matter relating to its accreditation must undertake corrective advertising to a degree acceptable to the Joint Commission in the same medium in which the misrepresentation occurred. If an organization fails to undertake the required corrective advertising following the communication of false or misleading advertising about its accreditation decision, the organization may be subject to loss of accreditation.

The Joint Commission's logo is a registered trademark. An accredited organization may use the logo if it follows these guidelines:
- The logo must remain in the same proportional relationship as provided and should not be displayed any larger than an organization's own logo
- The logo's format cannot be changed, the name may not be separated from the symbol, and the logo must be printed in the original color
- Graphic devices such as seals, other words, or slogans cannot be added to the logo, except for the words "Accredited by"
- These guidelines apply to logo use on all print materials, Internet Web pages, and promotional items, such as coffee mugs, T-shirts, and notepads. Contact the Joint Commission Department of Communications at 630/792-5631 for questions about using the Joint Commission logo.

Additional Accreditation Activities

This section provides information that is relevant to organizations between Joint Commission surveys. Material includes the duration of an accreditation award; the process for continuing accreditation; how to notify the Joint Commission in the event of organization changes, including the opening or closing of a unit or services, addition or deletion of components, leadership changes, mergers, consolidations, and acquisitions; and unscheduled and unannounced for-cause surveys.

Reentering the Accreditation Process

For a previously accredited organization to be designated as "new," it must not have participated in the accreditation process during the previous six months. If an organization is reentering the accreditation process before six months have passed, it must demonstrate a continuing 12-month track record of compliance with the standards.

Duration of Accreditation Award

An accreditation award is continuous until the organization has its next full survey, which is usually around three years, unless accreditation is revoked for cause or as otherwise outlined in this chapter. An organization may request a full accreditation survey more frequently than when it is due to have a survey. The Joint Commission, at its discretion and in accordance with its mission, determines whether to honor the request. An organization should send such a request to its Joint Commission account representative.

Continuous Compliance

The Joint Commission expects an accredited organization to be in continuous compliance with all applicable standards and EPs. It may ask an organization to supply, in writing, information about compliance with standards. It may also survey an organization at any time with or without notice in response to complaints, media coverage, or other information that raises questions about the adequacy of patient health and safety protections (*see* Unscheduled and Unannounced For-Cause Surveys on page 67). The Joint Commission might also conduct a survey if an organization fails to respond to a request for more information.

The Joint Commission may view an organization's failure to permit a survey as the organization no longer wanting to participate in the accreditation process. In such a case, the Joint Commission begins proceedings to deny accreditation to the organization.*

Continuing Accreditation

An organization's accreditation cycle is continuous, as long as the organization does both of the following:

- Has a full, unannounced survey within 39 months of its last survey
- Continues to meet all accreditation-related requirements as required, including, but not limited to, submission of an annual PPR and an annual subscription payment

Duration of the Accreditation Decision

An organization's previous accreditation decision remains in effect until a decision is made either to accredit or to preliminarily deny accreditation to the organization.

Notifying the Joint Commission About Organizational Changes

Accreditation is neither automatically transferred nor continued if significant changes occur within an organization. When significant changes occur, the organization must notify the Joint Commission in writing not more than 30 calendar days after such change is made. The organization must also notify the Joint Commission in writing if it opens or closes any units or services. Beginning in 2006, organizations will be able to report information about changes at their organization on a continuous basis through their extranet site.

When an organization offers at least 25% of its services or programs at a new location or in a significantly altered physical plant, the organization must also fill out and submit to the Joint Commission Part 2: Basic Building Information of the Statement of Conditions™ (SOC) compliance document; Part 3E or 3F of the Statement of Fire Safety (SFS); and Part 4: Plan for Improvement, should *LSC* deficiencies be present. (For a copy of the SOC, visit the Joint Commission's Web site, at

---

* *See* APR 3 on pages 134–135 in the "Accreditation Participation Requirements" chapter.

http://www.jointcommission.org, and select Accredited Organizations, then your accreditation program, then Standards, and then Statement of Conditions.) Failure to provide timely notification to the Joint Commission of these changes may result in the organization's loss of accreditation. If completion dates for a Plan for Improvement cannot be achieved, the organization is to contact the Joint Commission's engineering staff to request an extension.

Mergers, Consolidations, and Acquisitions

In the case of a merger, a consolidation, or an acquisition, the Joint Commission may decide that the organization responsible for services must have a survey. Barring exceptional circumstances, the Joint Commission continues the accreditation of the organization undergoing the kind of changes described here until it determines whether an extension survey is necessary.

Note: *If, after accreditation is rendered to an organization, the organization's structure changes whereby one or more of its services, programs, or related organizations are no longer part of the organization that was originally surveyed, the service, program, or related organization is no longer included in the organization's accreditation.*

When an accredited organization acquires another organization and an extension survey is conducted, the survey findings resulting from the extension survey are maintained separately from, and are not reflected in, the accreditation decision of the acquiring organization for 12 months following the acquisition. After the 12-month period, any outstanding standards compliance problems in the acquired component(s) are reflected in the accreditation decision of the acquiring organization.

Extension Surveys

An extension survey is conducted at an accredited organization or at a site that is owned and operated by the organization if the accredited organization's current accreditation is not due to expire for at least nine months and when at least one of the conditions above is met. The results of an extension survey may affect the organization's accreditation decision.

An extension survey of an organization may be necessary if the organization has done any of the following:

- Instituted a new service or program for which the Joint Commission has standards
- Changed ownership and has a significant number of changes in the management and clinical staff or operating policies and procedures
- Offered at least 25% of its services at a new location or in a significantly altered physical plant
- Expanded its capacity to provide services by 25% or more, as measured by patient volume, pieces of equipment, or other relevant measures
- Provided a more intensive level of service
  or
- Merged with, consolidated with, or acquired an unaccredited site, service, or program for which there are applicable Joint Commission standards and EPs

Accreditation Status of Organizations That Cease Services After a Disaster

The Joint Commission will discontinue the accreditation of organizations that have been closed or out of service for more than six months as a result of a disaster.

The Joint Commission's complete process for determining the accreditation status of organizations that cease services following a disaster is listed below, in chronological order.

For the first 30 days after a disaster and/or the organization's decision to cease operations, the organization's original Joint Commission accreditation status will stay in effect. Once the organization resumes operation, the time frame for complying with any outstanding Joint Commission requirements (such as the PPR or ESC) will also resume. In most cases, the Joint Commission will not need to survey the affected organization to reassess its level of standards compliance. If the Joint Commission decides to conduct a survey, however, the organization's accreditation decision will be driven by the survey findings.

If the organization resumes services from 31 to 90 days after a disaster, the Joint Commission will conduct an extension survey to determine the organization's accreditation status. The circumstances surrounding the organization's closure will determine the survey's length and scope.

For organizations that resume services from 91 days up to six months after a disaster, the Joint Commission will require an environment of care on-site survey. This survey will preferably take place one to two weeks after services are resumed. It is assumed that these organizations have received clearance from the fire marshal and other local/state authorities before resuming services. In addition, the Joint Commission will conduct a second on-site survey approximately four months after services have been resumed to evaluate sustained compliance with Joint Commission standards and requirements. The track record requirement for demonstrating standards compliance will be four months.

If an organization does not resume services within six months after a disaster or the decision to cease operations, the Joint Commission will discontinue its accreditation. If the organization resumes services, it must re-apply to become accredited. In such cases, the accreditation process will involve at least two surveys. The first survey will be conducted at the organization's request, and will assess the organization's ability to provide safe patient care. The organization may qualify for an accreditation award as a result of this survey. The second survey will be conducted approximately four months later to assess sustained compliance with Joint Commission requirements. The track record requirement for demonstrating standards compliance will be four months.

The Joint Commission will continue to list all affected organizations as "Accredited" up to six months after a disaster, unless survey findings dictate otherwise.

While working with affected health care organizations in the aftermath of a catastrophic event, the Joint Commission will be sensitive to these organizations' needs and will work with responsible state and federal agencies to help re-establish the organizations' operations as well as their qualification for accreditation.

Unscheduled and Unannounced For-Cause Surveys

The Joint Commission may perform a for-cause unannounced survey when it becomes aware of potentially serious standards compliance or patient care or safety issues, or when it has other valid reasons for surveying an accredited organization.*

Note: *For-cause unannounced surveys should not be confused with regular unannounced surveys, as described on pages 44–45.*

A for-cause unannounced survey can take place at any point in an organization's accreditation cycle. No preliminary report is generated after a for-cause unannounced survey.

Note: *An organization is charged for a for-cause unannounced survey, regardless of the outcome. An organization can determine the cost of such a survey by calling the Joint Commission's Pricing Unit at 630/792-5115. However, an organization is not charged for random unannounced surveys. (For additional information on random unannounced surveys,* see *below.)*

Reasons for a for-cause unannounced survey include occurrence of any event or series of events in an accredited organization that creates either of the following significant situations:

- Concern that a continuing threat may exist to the safety or care of patients at risk or
- Indication that the organization is not or has not been in compliance with the Joint Commission's Information Accuracy and Truthfulness Policy

Such a survey can either include all the organization's services or only those areas where a serious concern may exist.

The Joint Commission may deny an organization accreditation if the organization does not allow the Joint Commission to conduct an unscheduled or unannounced survey.

Random Unannounced Surveys

A random unannounced survey is generally conducted 9 to 30 months following the accreditation date (that is, the date after the last day of the full survey). An organization receives no advance notice of a random unannounced survey. One surveyor conducts each such survey for one day. An organization is not charged for a random unannounced survey.

During a random unannounced survey, the surveyor assesses both fixed and variable components, or performance areas. Fixed components are identified each year for organizations based on the highest PFAs and selected National Patient Safety Goals. Fixed components are identified based on the degree of actual or perceived risk to the care of patients posed by noncompliance with applicable standards

---

* *See* APR 3 on page 134 in the "Accreditation Participation Requirements" chapter.

related to these elements. Fixed components for each accreditation program are published in *The Joint Commission Perspectives*® and are listed on the Joint Commission Web site. Variable components are identified through the PFP. Presurvey information run through the PFP identifies prioritized organization-specific PFAs to be evaluated. (*See* the section The Priority Focus Process on pages 33–36 for more information on presurvey information.) The surveyor may also expand the scope of a random unannounced survey based on findings at the time of that survey.

ACC

The Accreditation Decision Process

The goal of the accreditation decision and reporting approach is to move ambulatory care organizations away from focusing on achieving high scores to achieving and maintaining safe, high-quality systems of care, treatment, and services. During the decision process, there are no numerical scores, and thus no scores are disclosed to the organizations or to the public. The lack of scores facilitates shifting the focus from passing the exam to continuous operational improvement. For more information on the ambulatory care organization accreditation decision rules, *see* pages 71–81.

Key elements of the accreditation decision process include the following:

- Scoring of EPs is on the following scale: satisfactory compliance (2), partial compliance (1), insufficient compliance (0), or not applicable (NA)
- Standards are identified as compliant or not compliant based on the scoring pattern of their associated EPs
- The surveyor(s) leaves an Accreditation Survey Findings Report of findings on site (for special surveys, no report is left on site)
- The Accreditation Survey Findings Report will be posted on the ambulatory care organization's secure, password-protected extranet Web site space shortly after survey
- If requirements for improvement (RFIs) are cited, the organization has a 45-day window to submit an ESC report to address correction of the RFIs. The accreditation decision is rendered following the submission of the ESC report. For organizations receiving a Preliminary Denial of Accreditation or Conditional Accreditation decision, the decision will be effective on the day the decision is rendered. For organizations that do not receive any RFIs, the accreditation decision will be effective the day after the last day of survey.

For more information on the scoring process, *see* pages 4–7 in the "How to Use This Book" chapter.

Accreditation Decision Categories

The Joint Commission's six accreditation decision categories are as follows:*

- **Accredited**—The organization is in compliance with all standards at the time of the on-site survey or has successfully addressed all requirements for improvement in an ESC within 45 days following the posting of the Accreditation Survey Findings Report.

* Table 4 (pages 60–61) provides a description of each category and the conditions that lead to it.

- **Provisional Accreditation**—The organization fails to successfully address all requirements for improvement in an ESC within 45 days following the posting of the Accreditation Survey Findings Report.
- **Conditional Accreditation**—The organization is not in substantial compliance with the standards, as usually evidenced by a count of the number of standards identified as not compliant at the time of survey which is between 1½ and 3 standard deviations above the mean number* of not compliant standards for organizations in that accreditation program. The organization must remedy identified problem areas through preparation and submission of ESC and subsequently undergo an on-site, follow-up survey.

  Note: *These thresholds are triggers for an Accreditation Committee determination about a Conditional Accreditation decision. The Accreditation Committee considers each organization and decides whether to apply the decision rules for Conditional Accreditation based on the thresholds, or to exercise its discretion in appropriate cases and render an alternative decision on the survey.*

  The key points of reference from year to year are the standard deviations that establish the trigger points as mentioned above, not the number of actual requirements for improvement that may change over time based on field performance.
- **Preliminary Denial of Accreditation**—There is justification to deny accreditation to the organization as usually evidenced by a count of the number of not compliant standards at the time of survey which is 3 or more standard deviations above the mean number of standards identified as not compliant for organizations in that accreditation program. The decision is subject to review and appeal prior to the determination to deny accreditation; the appeal process may also result in a decision other than Denial of Accreditation.

  Note: *These thresholds are triggers for an Accreditation Committee determination about a Conditional Accreditation decision. The Accreditation Committee considers each organization and decides whether to apply the decision rules for Conditional Accreditation based on the thresholds, or to exercise its discretion in appropriate cases and render an alternative decision on the survey.*

  The key points of reference from year to year are the standard deviations that establish the trigger points as mentioned above, not the number of actual requirements for improvement which may change over time based on field performance.
- **Denial of Accreditation**—The organization has been denied accreditation. All review and appeal opportunities have been exhausted.
- **Preliminary Accreditation**—The organization demonstrates compliance with selected standards in the first of two surveys conducted under the Early Survey Policy Option 1.

Components of the Decision Process

This section provides an overview of the Joint Commission's accreditation decision process.

ACC

* The mean is based on the previous years' scoring in each program.

The surveyor(s) will leave the survey findings report with the ambulatory care organization; the survey findings will be organized by the following:

- Primary PFAs
- Standard number
- Applicable program
- Standard text
- Secondary PFA (as applicable)
- EP text
- Surveyor findings

After the on-site survey, the surveyor(s) will transmit the results described here to the Joint Commission Central Office.

Reports that contain flagged items or contain findings that under applicable accreditation rules would likely lead to a Preliminary Denial of Accreditation or Conditional Accreditation decision will be processed by Central Office staff shortly after the survey. At the time of survey, an item can be flagged for Central Office review by the surveyor(s) if there is a question about interpreting or scoring a standard. Once that review is completed, the results of the survey are then posted to the secure automated area of The Joint Commission Connect extranet site. The report includes, as appropriate, requirements for improvement and supplemental findings.

If an ambulatory care organization is in compliance with all standards at the time of the on-site survey, it will be Accredited as of the day after the last day of survey. The official Accreditation Decision Categories for 2008 are included in this chapter beginning on page 71. If the ambulatory care organization is not compliant with one or more standards at the time of survey, it is required to submit an acceptable ESC report within 45 days of the Accreditation Survey Findings Report being posted on The Joint Commission Connect extranet. As part of its ESC submission, the ambulatory care organization is required to demonstrate "correction" of not compliant standards (that is, detail the action[s] that it has taken—not just planned—to come into compliance with a standard) or "clarification" (that is, explain why the ambulatory care organization believes that it was compliant with a standard judged to be not compliant at the time of survey). The organization's acceptable ESC must address compliance at the EP level and include an MOS, if applicable, for each EP found to be partially (1) or insufficiently (0) compliant.

The acceptable ESC report is due within 45 calendar days following the posting of the Accreditation Survey Findings Report; however, the organization's accreditation decision is retroactive to the day after the last day of the survey, unless the organization is undergoing its first Joint Commission survey. In that case, the effective date for accreditation is the date on which the acceptable ESC is submitted.

The organization's ESC submission will be evaluated by Central Office staff using the same scoring guidelines used by the surveyors at the time of survey and by health care organizations when they conduct their PPR. The ESC will be considered acceptable when the ambulatory care organization has demonstrated resolution of all requirements for improvement. If the ambulatory care organization has not met a rule for Conditional Accreditation or Preliminary Denial of Accreditation and its first ESC submission is determined to be acceptable, its decision will be Accredited, and it will be required to submit the data for applicable MOS, if required, for each EP four months later.

If the ambulatory care organization has not met a rule for Conditional Accreditation or Preliminary Denial of Accreditation and it is determined that an ambulatory care organization's ESC submission is unacceptable, its accreditation decision will be Provisional Accreditation, and it will be required to submit an acceptable ESC within 30 days. If the second ESC is determined to be acceptable, the ambulatory care organization's accreditation decision will remain Provisional Accreditation until it has submitted acceptable results of the corresponding MOS four months later. If the second ESC is determined to be unacceptable, a recommendation for Conditional Accreditation will be presented to the Accreditation Committee.

Central Office staff will evaluate the MOS results, when required. If it is determined that the MOS results are acceptable, no further action will be required of the ambulatory care organization, and if the organization had a Provisional Accreditation decision, its accreditation decision will be changed to Accredited. If it is determined that an ambulatory care organization's MOS submission is unacceptable and its accreditation decision is not currently Provisional Accreditation, its accreditation decision will be changed to Provisional Accreditation; the ambulatory care organization will be required to submit a second set of MOS results in another four months. If an ambulatory care organization whose accreditation decision is Provisional Accreditation because of an unacceptable first ESC submission submits an unacceptable first MOS submission, a recommendation for Conditional Accreditation will be presented to the Accreditation Committee.

If the ambulatory care organization's first ESC submission is determined to be acceptable and the second MOS submission is determined to be acceptable, its accreditation decision will be changed to Accredited, and no further action will be required of the ambulatory care organization. If the second MOS submission is determined to be unacceptable, a recommendation for Conditional Accreditation will be presented to the Accreditation Committee. *See* Figures 1 and 2, page 72, for a time line of ESC and MOS submissions.

The organization's ESC submission and sustained implementation of it, including the MOS, are subject to review in random unannounced surveys.

A final decision letter will be posted to the ambulatory care organization's secure, password protected area of The Joint Commission Connect extranet Web site when its ESC has been reviewed and an accreditation decision has been rendered. A Quality Report will then be posted on Quality Check® on the Joint Commission's Web site.

2008 Accreditation Decision Rules for Ambulatory Care

The Joint Commission makes accreditation decisions by applying decision rules to the scored standards. Decision rules determine an accreditation decision that appropriately represents an organization's overall performance as measured by evi-

ACC

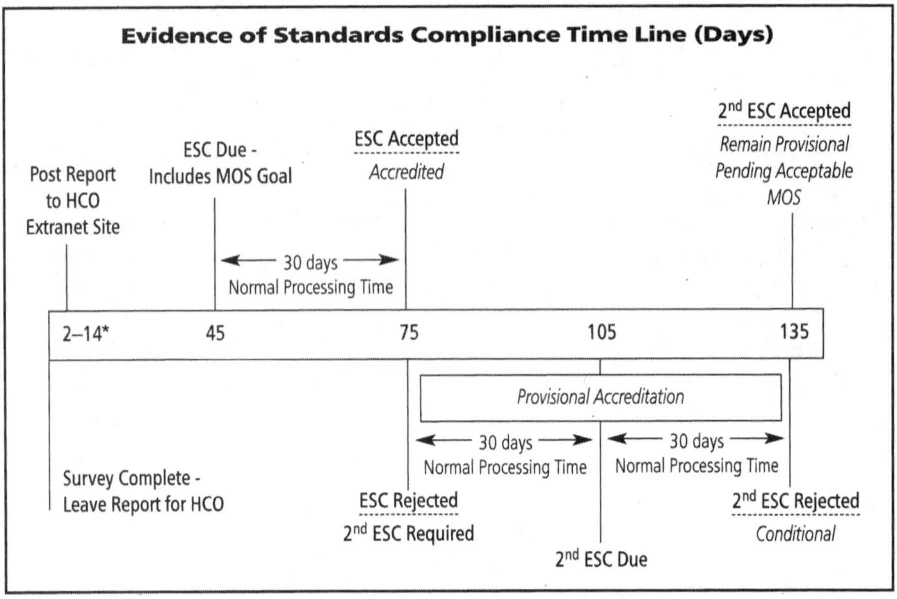

Figure 1. *This figure shows the Evidence of Standards Compliance (ESC) time line.*

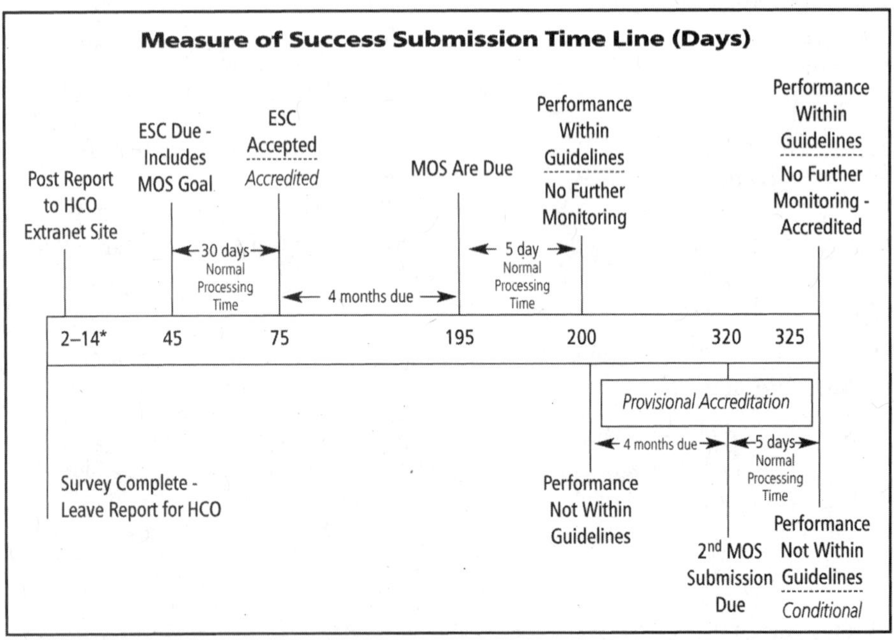

Figure 2. *This figure shows the measure of success (MOS) submission time line.*

* Those that go directly to the extranet are 2 days. If an account representative has to process it, it normally takes 14 days.

dence of compliance with the applicable standards. Decision rules are approved by the Accreditation Committee. The Committee may exercise reasonable discretion in individual cases to determine whether to vary from applicable decision rules in furtherance of the Joint Commission's mission to help enhance the quality and safety of care.

"Weighted" decision rules have been in place to limit the impact that the performance of small or secondary components of a complex organization may have on the organization's overall accreditation decision. These rules were established based on the rationale that the poor performance of a small component of a large complex organization, as determined by standards noncompliance, should not determine the accreditation decision of the entire organization. As such, the performance factors contributing to the overall accreditation decision for a complex organization were "weighted" to account for a proportional impact on overall care. The current "weighted" decision rules can be found on page 61.

The decision rules for ambulatory care follow.

Denial of Accreditation

Denial of Accreditation will be recommended when one or more of the following conditions are met:

DA01 The organization does not permit the performance of any survey by the Joint Commission. (Accreditation Participation Requirement 3)

DA02 The organization has failed to resolve a Conditional Accreditation status prior to withdrawing from the accreditation process.

DA03 The organization has failed to submit payment for survey fees or annual fees.

DA04 The organization, which was previously in Conditional Accreditation for failure to submit data and information to the Joint Commission within 61 days of the due date(s) has failed to meet all requirements for timely submission of data and information to the Joint Commission, within 91 days of the due date(s). The submissions include, but are not limited to, the Accreditation Contract, annual updates to the organization's application for Accreditation, annual PPR updates, and the electronic Statement of Conditions. (Accreditation Participation Requirement 19)

DA05 The organization, which was previously in Conditional Accreditation for failure to submit the Periodic Performance Review 61 days after the due date, has failed to submit a Periodic Performance Review, and corrective action plan as appropriate, 91 days after the due date. The organization may also be required to participate in a scheduled consultative phone call with Central Office staff as specified in the description of the full Periodic Performance Review and the Periodic Performance Review options. (Accreditation Participation Requirement 14)

Preliminary Denial of Accreditation

Preliminary Denial of Accreditation will be recommended when one or more of the following conditions are met:

PDA01 An immediate threat to patient/public health or safety exists within the organization.

PDA02 An individual who does not possess a license, registration, or certification is providing or has provided health care services in the organization that would, under applicable law or regulation, require such a license, registration, or certification and which placed the organization's patients at risk for a serious adverse outcome. (Standard HR.4.10)

PDA03 The Joint Commission is reasonably persuaded that the organization submitted falsified documents or misrepresented information in seeking to achieve or retain accreditation. Information provided by an organization and used by the Joint Commission for accreditation purposes must be accurate and truthful and may:

- Be provided verbally, in writing, or electronically
- Be obtained through direct observation or interview by Joint Commission surveyors
- Be derived from documents supplied by the organization to the Joint Commission, including, but not limited to, an organization's root cause analysis in response to a sentinel event, or an organization's application for accreditation
- Involve data or documents transmitted electronically to the Joint Commission, including, but not limited to, data or documents provided as part of the Periodic Performance Review process or the electronic application process

If accreditation is denied following implementation of this rule, the organization shall be prohibited from participating in the accreditation process for a period of one year unless the president of the Joint Commission, for good cause, waives all or a portion of this waiting period. (Accreditation Participation Requirement 10)

PDA04 The organization has been conditionally accredited on two consecutive full surveys in relation to an issue or issues in the same primary priority focus area(s).

Note: *Priority focus areas (PFAs) are processes, systems, or structures in a health care organization that significantly impact the safety and/or quality of care provided. The PFAs are as follows:*

- *Assessment and Care/Services*
- *Communication*
- *Credentialed Practitioners*
- *Equipment Use*
- *Infection Control*
- *Information Management*
- *Medication Management*
- *Organizational Structure*
- *Orientation and Training*
- *Patient Safety*
- *Physical Environment*
- *Quality Improvement Expertise/Activities*
- *Rights and Ethics*
- *Staffing*

PDA05 A number of not compliant standards at the time of survey of three or more standard deviations above the mean.

PDA06 The organization does not possess a license, certificate, and/or permit, as, or when, required by applicable law and regulation, to provide the health care services for which the organization is seeking accreditation. (Standard LD.1.30)

PDA07 The organization with a decision of Conditional Accreditation, as the result of a survey event, has failed to clear not compliant standards after two opportunities to do so as the result of:

- two failed Evidence of Standards Compliance (ESC) submissions
- two failed Measure of Success (MOS) submissions
- a combination of one failed ESC submission, one failed MOS submission and/or a failed Conditional Accreditation follow-up survey.

Note: *The opportunity is considered failed when the organization has not demonstrated resolution of all not compliant standards and continues to meet any of the decision rules requiring additional monitoring in the form of on-site follow-up, an Evidence of Standards Compliance submission, or a Measure of Success submission. In addition, a Conditional Accreditation follow-up survey is considered an opportunity to clear not compliant standards.*

PDA08 The result of a Conditional Accreditation follow-up survey is unacceptable.

Note: *The result of the Conditional Accreditation follow-up survey will be considered unacceptable if the organization continues to meet any of the rules or an exception to the rules that caused a recommendation of Conditional Accreditation or Preliminary Denial of Accreditation.*

PDA09 The organization has knowingly used Joint Commission full-time, part-time, or intermittent surveyors to provide any accreditation-related consulting services. (Accreditation Participation Requirement 12)

Conditional Accreditation

Conditional Accreditation will be recommended when one or more of the following conditions are met:

CON01 A number of not compliant standards at the time of survey of one and one-half standard deviations above the mean.

CON02 An individual who does not possess a license, registration, or certification is providing or has provided health care services in the organization that would, under applicable law or regulation, require such a license, registration, or certification. (Standard HR.4.10)

Note: *Except as provided under rule PDA02.*

CON03 The organization has failed to clear not compliant standards after two opportunities to do so (as the result of two failed Evidence of Standards Compliance [ESC] submissions, two failed Measure of Success [MOS] submissions, or a combination of one failed ESC submission and one failed MOS submission).

Note: *The opportunity is considered failed when the organization has not demonstrated resolution of all not compliant standards and continues to meet any of the decision rules requiring additional monitoring in the form of on-site follow-up, an Evidence of Standards Compliance submission, or a Measure of Success submission.*

CON04 The organization has failed to implement or make sufficient progress toward the corrective actions described in a Statement of Conditions™, Part 4, Plan for Improvement, which was previously accepted by the Joint Commission, or has failed to implement or enforce applicable interim life safety measures.

CON05 The organization, which was previously in Provisional Accreditation for failure to submit data and information to the Joint Commission within 31 days of the due date(s), did not meet all requirements for timely submission of data and information to the Joint Commission within 61 days of the due date(s). The submissions include, but are not limited to, the Accreditation Contract, annual updates to the organization's application for accreditation, annual PPR updates, and the electronic Statement of Conditions. (Accreditation Participation Requirement 19)

CON06 The organization, which was previously in Provisional Accreditation for failure to submit the Periodic Performance Review 31 days after the due date, has failed to submit a Periodic Performance Review, and corrective action plan as appropriate, 61 days after the due date. The organization may also be required to participate in a scheduled consultative phone call with Central Office staff as specified in the description of the full Periodic Performance Review and the Periodic Performance Review options. (Accreditation Participation Requirement 14)

Conditional Accreditation Follow-up

A Conditional Accreditation Follow-up survey will be recommended when one or more of the following conditions are met:

CONF01 A conditional follow-up survey will be scheduled for organizations with a Conditional Accreditation decision.

Note: *The date of the survey will be established at the time the final Conditional Accreditation decision is awarded (conditional follow-up surveys typically occur approximately six months from the date when the organization is notified of its official Conditional Accreditation decision).*

CONF02 A second Conditional Accreditation follow-up survey will be scheduled when, as the result of a conditional follow-up survey, one or more of the original Requirements for Improvement remain unresolved.

Note: *This accreditation decision results when the organization that was awarded Conditional Accreditation as the result of an on-site survey has passed its first ESC submission, but the Conditional Accreditation follow-up survey finds that one or more of the original Requirements for Improvement remain unmet, and none of the other rules for Preliminary Denial of Accreditation or Conditional Accreditation have been met.*

Provisional Accreditation

Provisional Accreditation will be recommended when one or more of the following conditions are met:

PROV01 The organization has failed to demonstrate resolution of all Requirements for Improvement at the time of its first ESC or first MOS submission. This accreditation decision results when at least one standard is scored not compliant and none of the rules for Preliminary Denial of Accreditation or Conditional Accreditation have been met.

Note 1: *Not compliant standards must be resolved within stipulated time frames (through an on-site MOS as provided in rule MOS03, submission of an ESC, or submission of an MOS by the organization) to maintain accreditation.*

Note 2: *When an organization is placed in Provisional Accreditation as the result of a failed first ESC or failed first MOS submission, it will remain in Provisional Accreditation until an MOS submission has been determined to be acceptable.*

PROV02 The organization did not meet all requirements for timely submission of data and information to the Joint Commission within 31 days of the due date(s). The submissions include, but are not limited to, the Accreditation Contract, annual updates to the organization's application for accreditation, and annual PPR updates. (Accreditation Participation Requirement 19)

PROV03 The organization has failed to submit a Periodic Performance Review, and corrective action plan as appropriate, 31 days after the due date. The organization may also be required to participate in a scheduled consultative phone call with Central Office staff as specified in the description of the full Periodic Performance Review and the Periodic Performance Review options. (Accreditation Participation Requirement 14)

One-Month Survey

A one-month survey will be scheduled when the following condition is met:

FOC01 A full laboratory survey will be conducted when an organization providing laboratory services cannot demonstrate to the Joint Commission their laboratory accreditation decision is in good standing with a Joint Commission–recognized accreditor, or the accreditation is more than 30 months old.

Evidence of Standards Compliance (ESC)

An Evidence of Standards Compliance (ESC) is a report submitted by a surveyed organization within 45 days of its survey, which details the action(s) that it took to bring itself into compliance with a standard or clarifies why the organization believes that it was in compliance with the standard for which it received a Requirement for Improvement. An ESC must address compliance at the EP level and include a Measure of Success (MOS) for all applicable EP corrections.

An ESC will be required when one or more of the following conditions are met:

ESC01 An organization has one or more standards scored not compliant at the time of a survey event.

ESC02 Failure to demonstrate continued compliance with all not compliant standards in the first ESC submission will result in Provisional Accreditation. The organization will be required to submit a second ESC within 30 days of the official notification that the first ESC was unacceptable.

On-Site ESC Survey

An on-site ESC survey, due in 45 days, will be scheduled when the following condition is met:

ESC03 If a determination is made that on-site evaluation is required to assess compliance with the relevant standards, the assigned follow-up activity may be in the form of an on-site ESC survey rather than an ESC submission.

Note: *A written ESC submission may still be required.*

Measure of Success (MOS)

A Measure of Success (MOS) is a numerical or quantifiable measure, usually related to an audit that determines if an action was effective and sustained, due four months after Evidence of Standards Compliance approval.

An MOS for all applicable EP corrections will be required when one or more of the following conditions are met:

MOS01 An organization has submitted a successful ESC.

MOS02 Failure to demonstrate continued compliance with all not compliant standards in the first MOS submission will require the submission of a second MOS four months after official notification of the failure of the first MOS.

Note: *If the organization determines that the corrective action documented in its first ESC submission was not effective, the organization may elect to submit a second ESC that identifies new corrective action, rather than submitting a second MOS. In this case, the first MOS submission will be considered failed. If this second ESC or the second MOS fails, the organization's decision will be changed to Conditional Accreditation or Preliminary Denial of Accreditation, as appropriate.*

On-Site MOS Survey

A four-month on-site MOS survey will be scheduled when the following condition is met:

MOS03 If a determination is made that on-site evaluation is required to assess compliance with the relevant standards, the assigned follow-up activity may be in the form of an on-site MOS survey rather than an MOS submission.

Note: *A written ESC submission may still be required.*

Preliminary Accreditation

Preliminary Accreditation will be recommended when one or more of the following conditions are met:

PA01 Preliminary Accreditation will be recommended when an organization has demonstrated compliance with the selected standards used in the first of two surveys conducted under the Early Survey Policy Option 1.

Note: *The first survey is conducted using a defined subset of applicable standards. The second survey is a full survey conducted approximately six months later. Preliminary Accreditation remains until the organization completes the second—that is, initial—survey.*

Accredited

Accreditation will be recommended when one or more of the following conditions are met:

A01 An organization's accreditation decision will be changed to Accredited when it is in compliance with all standards at the time of the on-site survey or has successfully addressed all requirements for improvement in its first ESC submission.

Note: *Organizations that are in Provisional Accreditation as a result of a failed ESC will have their accreditation decision changed to Accredited when their MOS submission has been determined to be acceptable.*

A02 An organization's accreditation decision will be changed to Accredited when, as a result of a Conditional Accreditation follow-up survey, all of the original requirements for improvement have been met.

Note: *The organization must provide Evidence of Standards Compliance for standards, that were not the subject of the Conditional Accreditation follow-up survey, that are identified as not compliant at the time of the follow-up survey. An organization that is in Conditional Accreditation as a result of two failed ESC submissions will have its accreditation status changed to Accredited when its MOS submission has been determined to be acceptable.*

Administrative Rules

Administrative rules will be used when one or more of the following conditions are met:

ADM01 The follow-up time frames and nature of follow-up activity for demonstrating compliance with all not compliant standards may be changed from that stated in these decision rules when the severity of the issue requires an earlier response.

ADM02 If the primary program meets a rule for Provisional Accreditation, Conditional Accreditation, or Preliminary Denial of Accreditation, the overall decision for the organization is Provisional Accreditation, Conditional Accreditation, or Preliminary Denial of Accreditation, respectively.

ADM03 If the primary or any secondary program meets a rule for Provisional Accreditation, the overall decision for the organization is Provisional Accreditation.

ADM04 If one of the secondary programs meets a rule for Preliminary Denial of Accreditation, the overall decision for the organization is Conditional Accreditation.

Note: *This rule is not applicable when the laboratory is the secondary program and the hospital is the primary program.*

ADM05 If one of the secondary programs meets a rule for Conditional Accreditation, the overall decision for the organization is Provisional Accreditation.

Note: *This rule is not applicable when the laboratory is the secondary program and the hospital is the primary program.*

ADM06 If two or more of the secondary programs meet rules for Preliminary Denial of Accreditation, the overall decision for the organization is Preliminary Denial of Accreditation.

ADM07 If two or more of the secondary programs meet rules for Conditional Accreditation, the overall decision for the organization is Conditional Accreditation.

Sentinel Event Policy Follow-up

SE01 An organization that has experienced a sentinel event subject to review under the Sentinel Event Policy is required to complete a thorough and credible root cause analysis and action plan and submit them to the Joint Commission, or otherwise provide evidence of an acceptable response to the sentinel event, in a manner and time frame acceptable to the Joint Commission as specified in the Sentinel Event Policy.

SE02 Follow-up will be scheduled, per the Sentinel Event policy, when a sentinel event, subject to review under the Sentinel Event Policy, has occurred and the Joint Commission has determined that the organization has completed a thorough and credible root cause analysis and action plan. The purpose of the follow-up activity is to assess the implementation and effectiveness of the organization's action plan.

The Quality Report

Quality Reports are publicly available and include relevant and useful information about the quality and safety of care provided in individual Joint Commission–accredited organization(s).

Quality Reports are created at the organization level, and contain information respecting an organization's accreditation status, its compliance with National Patient Safety Goals, and performance measurement results, as appropriate.

Joint Commission Quality Reports for each accredited organization include the following information:

- The date of the most recent full on-site survey.
- The accreditation decision based on the most recent full onsite survey.
- The organization's current accreditation decision. If an organization has been denied accreditation, this information will be posted on Quality Check® for one year.
- The date of the most recent on-site evaluation of the organization, if not a full survey.
- Standards areas with requirements for improvement, if the organization has a decision of Provisional Accreditation, Conditional Accreditation, or Preliminary Denial of Accreditation or has been denied accreditation.
- Subsequent satisfaction of requirements for improvement and the date(s) of resolution for specific standards areas.
- Subsequent new requirements for improvement and the date(s) assigned.
- Services included in the accreditation survey.
- Joint Commission policies or rules which lead to a Provisional Accreditation, Conditional Accreditation, Preliminary Denial of Accreditation, or Denial of Accreditation decision.
- Disease-specific care certification(s) and the effective date of each certification.
- The receipt of Special Quality Recognition awards, as recognized by the Board of Commissioners (for example, the Ernest A. Codman Awards, Magnet Status).
- Compliance with National Patient Safety Goal requirements.
- Performance against National Quality Improvement Goals.
- Performances in relation to Patient Experience of Care Measures, as data becomes available.

Each accredited organization is afforded the opportunity to prepare a commentary of up to two pages regarding its Quality Report. The commentary accompanies any Quality Reports distributed by the Joint Commission, whether via hard copy or the Joint Commission's Web site.

Each Quality Report released by the Joint Commission will also include appropriate background information.

When performance measurement data are included in Quality Reports, such data must be accompanied by information regarding their source of derivation; accuracy, reliability and validity; appropriate uses; and limitations and potential misuses.

An organization's Quality Report may be obtained via the Customer Service Department or through Quality Check.

Information That Is Publicly Disclosed on Request

In addition to information provided in a Quality Report, the following information may be obtained by writing or calling the Joint Commission:

- The organization's accreditation history.
- Survey fees paid by an accredited organization.
- The organization's scheduled survey date(s) once the organization has been surveyed.
- Applicable standards used for an accreditation survey.
- For a tailored survey, the organizational component(s) contributing to a Conditional Accreditation or Denial of Accreditation decision.
- Requirements for improvement for which the Joint Commission had no or insufficient evidence of resolution when an organization withdrew from accreditation.
- The standards areas for which the Joint Commission had no or insufficient evidence of resolution of requirements for improvement when an organization withdrew from accreditation.
- As applicable, confirmation of the occurrence of a sentinel event at an accredited organization and the Joint Commission's intent to apply its Sentinel Event Policy to this occurrence.

Release of Complaint-Related Information on Request

The Joint Commission addresses all complaints that pertain to patient safety or quality-of-care issues within the scope of Joint Commission standards. Complaints may be forwarded by the Centers for Medicare & Medicaid Services (CMS) or other federal or state agencies having oversight responsibilities for health care organizations, or may be received directly from consumers, payers, or health care professionals.

The Joint Commission has a toll-free hotline to provide patients, families, caregivers, and others with an opportunity to share concerns regarding quality-of-care issues at accredited health care organizations. The toll free number is 800/994-6610 and is available 24 hours a day, seven days a week; however, staff members are available to answer calls only on weekdays between 8:30 A.M. and 5:00 P.M. central standard time.

Upon request from any party, the Joint Commission releases the following aggregate information relating to complaints about an accredited organization for the three-year period prior to receipt of the request:

- The number of standards-related written complaints filed against an accredited organization that have met criteria for review.
- The applicable standards areas involved in a specific complaint review.
- The standards areas in which requirements for improvement were issued as a result of complaint evaluation activities.
- When an unannounced or unscheduled survey is based on information derived from a complaint or public sources, the standards areas related to the complaint.

The Joint Commission also provides the following information as appropriate to complainants regarding their complaints:

- Any determination that the complaint is not related to Joint Commission standards.
- If the complaint is related to standards, the course of action to be taken regarding the complaint.

- Whether the Joint Commission has decided to take action regarding an organization's accreditation decision following completion of the complaint investigation.
  - If the Joint Commission has decided to take no action, the complainant is to be so advised.
  - If the Joint Commission has taken action, the complainant is to be advised in conformance with the guidelines for release of complaint information as set forth above.
- Any change in an organization's accreditation decision following completion of the complaint investigation.

Release of Aggregate Performance Data

The Joint Commission reserves the right to publish or release aggregate performance data; however, no case-identifiable or protected health information is ever made publicly available. Performance data displayed on Quality Check are available to any interested party at no cost. Performance data on Quality Check may be downloaded electronically in a series of predefined report formats through a linked webpage called "Quality Data."

Data Release to Government Agencies and Organizations with Which the Joint Commission Performs Coordinated Survey Activities*

The Joint Commission makes available to federal, state, local, or other government certification or licensing agencies and organizations with which the Joint Commission performs survey activities specific to accreditation-related information under the following circumstances:

- When the Joint Commission identifies a serious situation in an organization that may jeopardize the health or safety of patients or the public and immediately takes action to deny accreditation
- Upon request, when the request involves otherwise publicly available information

Additional information is made available when an organization is certified for participation in a federal or state program or licensed to operate by a state agency on the basis of its accreditation. In addition, the Joint Commission may make available information to organizations with which the Joint Commission performs coordinated survey activities. The Joint Commission so advises the organization's chief executive officer and provides timely notice to local, state, and federal authorities having jurisdiction. The information available to government agencies and organizations with which the Joint Commission performs coordinated survey activities includes the following:

---

* Section 92, PL 96-499, the Omnibus Budget Reconciliation Act of 1980, requires that Medicare providers include, in all their contracts for services costing $10,000 or more in any 12-month period, a clause allowing the Secretary of the U.S. Department of Health and Human Services (DHHS), the U.S. Comptroller General, or their representatives to examine the contract and the contractor's books and records. The Joint Commission herein stipulates that if its charges to any such provider amount to $10,000 or more in any 12-month period, the contract or any agreement on which such charges are based and any of the Joint Commission's books, documents, and records that may be necessary to verify the extent and nature of Joint Commission costs will be available to the Secretary of DHHS, the Comptroller General, or any of their duly authorized representatives for four years after the survey. The same conditions will apply to any subcontracts the Joint Commission has with related organizations if the payments under such contracts amount to $10,000 or more in any 12-month period.

- The official accreditation decision, and any subsequent change in this decision
- Complaint information requested by CMS or state agencies in accordance with deemed status or other recognition requirements, including the following:
  - Actual complaint if the allegation(s) results in the classification of the complaint as high priority* and the governmental entity or organization with which the Joint Commission conducts a coordinate survey has entered into a written information-sharing agreement
  - Action taken on the complaint
  - The standards area(s) in which a requirement for improvement was issued as a result of the complaint evaluation
  - The status of the case
- Specific information when an organization is assigned a Conditional Accreditation, Preliminary Denial of Accreditation, or Denial of Accreditation decision. This includes the following:
  - All final requirements for improvement
  - A statement, if any, from the organization regarding its views on the validity of the Joint Commission survey findings
  - A copy of the approved Plan of Action and the results of the Plan of Action follow-up survey
- Notification of upcoming full surveys and retrospective dates of other surveys conducted, such as random unannounced, or for-cause, only if the governmental agency enters into an information-sharing agreement with the Joint Commission and agrees to maintain the confidentiality of the unannounced survey dates
- A copy of the Official Accreditation Decision Report
  - For CMS upon request respecting deemed status determinations
  - For state agencies that have entered into specific information sharing agreements that permit provider-authorized release of such reports to the state agency.

Data Release to Cooperative Accrediting Bodies

The Joint Commission makes available to accrediting bodies with which it has formal cooperative agreements relevant portions of the Official Accreditation Decision Report and complaint-related information which are pertinent to the accrediting activities of the cooperative partner. Judgments as to pertinence are made solely by the Joint Commission.

---

* High priority incidents are defined as harm that impairs mental, physical, and/or psychosocial status. This level of priority is assigned to an incident if the organization's alleged noncompliance with one or more standards may have caused harm that negatively impacts the patient's/resident's/client's mental, physical, and/or psychosocial status. Usually, specific rather than general information factors into the assignment of this priority level. Examples include the following:

- Allegation of a sentinel event (Complaints alleging the occurrence of a sentinel event will not be shared with CMS or state agencies if the alleged event has already been self-reported to the Joint Commission.)
- Allegation of an identification of a serious situation involving the potential jeopardy to the safety of patients
- Allegation of falsification of medical records or other information presented in the accreditation process
- Allegation of patient abuse/inappropriate use of restraints
- Allegation of unethical treatment of patients/families
- Allegation of patient-dumping
- Allegation of denial of care
- Allegation of failure to obtain surgical consent

Joint Commission Right to Clarify. The Joint Commission reserves the right to clarify information, even if the information involved would otherwise be considered confidential, when an organization disseminates inaccurate information regarding its accreditation.

Confidential Information. The Joint Commission keeps confidential the following information received or developed during the accreditation process:

- The Official Accreditation Decision Report unless its submission is required by a government agency (*see* "Data Release to Government Agencies", page 84), required by organizations with which the Joint Commission performs coordinating surveys, or is requested by an accrediting body with which the Joint Commission has a formal agreement (*see* "Data Release to Cooperative Accrediting Bodies", page 85)
- Information learned from the organization before, during, or following the accreditation survey, which is used to determine compliance with specific accreditation standards
- An organization's root cause analysis prepared in response to a sentinel event or in response to other circumstances specified by the Joint Commission
- All other materials that may contribute to the accreditation decision (for example, medical records, surveyor notes)
- Written staff analyses and Accreditation Committee minutes and agenda materials
- The algorithms used in the Priority Focus Process
- The Priority Focus Process information used in an organization's survey, other than that provided to the organization's staff prior to survey
- An organization's self-assessment and related corrective Plan of Action
- The identity of any individual who files a complaint about an accredited organization, except when the complaint is shared by the Joint Commission with a governmental entity, an organization with which the Joint Commission performs coordinated surveys, or accrediting organizations with which the Joint Commission has formal complaint-sharing agreements and the receiving organization has agreed to maintain the confidentiality of the complainant. In instances when the receiving organization cannot assure the confidentiality of the complainant, any complainant-identifying information shall be redacted by the Joint Commission prior to sharing.

This policy applies to all organizations with an accreditation history, subject to any requirements of any applicable laws.

Review and Appeal Procedures

After any Preliminary Denial of Accreditation decision, the organization has the right to make a detailed presentation before a Review Hearing Panel. The Accreditation Committee then reviews the findings of the Review Hearing Panel and either denies accreditation to the organization or selects an appropriate alternative accreditation decision. The organization may appeal any decision of the Accreditation Committee to deny accreditation before the decision becomes the final decision of the Joint Commission.

The following outline details the review and appeal procedures:

I. Evaluation by Joint Commission Staff

A. Review and Determination by Joint Commission Staff.

Following any survey activity, the Joint Commission staff shall review survey findings, survey documents, and any other relevant materials or information received from any source. Except as provided in paragraphs I.B, I.C, and I.D, Joint Commission staff shall, in accordance with decision rules approved by the Accreditation Committee of the Board of Commissioners, do the following:

1. Determine or recommend to the Accreditation Committee that the organization be accredited, as described in paragraph VII of these procedures
   or
2. Recommend to the Accreditation Committee that the organization be conditionally accredited
   or
3. Determine that the organization be conditionally accredited, if the organization does not submit Evidence of Standards Compliance (ESC) in accordance with paragraph I.B.I.a or I.B.I.b
   or
4. Recommend to the Accreditation Committee that the organization be preliminarily denied accreditation
   or
5. Defer consideration while additional information regarding the organization's compliance status is reviewed by the Joint Commission staff
   or
6. Determine or recommend to the Accreditation Committee that the organization be preliminarily accredited in accordance with the Early Survey Policy set forth on pages 24–28
   or
7. Recommend to the Accreditation Committee that the organization be initially denied Preliminary Accreditation in accordance with the Early Survey Policy set forth on pages 24–28

B. Determination to Recommend Conditional Accreditation Based on Full Surveys.

1. **Notification to Organization of Areas of Noncompliance with Standards.** In the case of a full survey, if Joint Commission staff, based on survey findings, survey documents and any other relevant materials or information received from any source, determine to recommend that the organization be conditionally accredited, it will outline its findings and determination. The organization may do the following:
   a. Accept the findings and determination of the staff through submission of the ESC
      or
   b. Submit to the Joint Commission, through ESC, any clarification of its compliance with Joint Commission standards at the time of the sur-

ACC

vey that is not reflected in the Accreditation Survey Findings Report, along with an explanation of why such documentation was not available for review at the time of the survey

2. **Consideration of the Organization's Response.** Joint Commission staff shall review the organization's submission of any additional information and shall, in accordance with decision rules approved by the Accreditation Committee, do the following:
   a. Recommend to the Accreditation Committee that the organization be conditionally accredited
   or
   b. Recommend to the Accreditation Committee that the organization be preliminarily denied accreditation
   or
   c. Recommend to the Accreditation Committee that the organization be accredited, as described in paragraph VII of these procedures

C. Determination to Recommend that Accreditation Be Preliminarily Denied Based on Full or Other Survey Activity.

1. **Notification to Organization of Areas of Noncompliance with Standards.** In the case of a full survey, if Joint Commission staff, based on survey findings, survey documents, and any other relevant materials or information received from any source, determine, in accordance with decision rules approved by the Accreditation Committee, to recommend to the Accreditation Committee that the organization be preliminarily denied accreditation, it will outline its findings and determination. The organization may do the following:
   a. Accept the findings and determination of the staff through submission of the ESC
   or
   b. Submit to the Joint Commission, through the ESC, any clarification of its compliance with Joint Commission standards at the time of the survey that is not reflected in the Accreditation Survey Findings Report, along with an explanation of why such information was not available for review at the time of the survey
2. **Consideration of the Organization's Response.** Joint Commission staff members shall review the organization's submission of any additional information and shall, in accordance with decision rules approved by the Accreditation Committee, do the following:
   a. Recommend to the Accreditation Committee that the organization be conditionally accredited
   or
   b. Recommend to the Accreditation Committee that the organization be preliminarily denied accreditation
   or
   c. Recommend to the Accreditation Committee that the organization be accredited, as described in paragraph VII of these procedures.

D. Decisions by the President of the Joint Commission. Notwithstanding anything outlined in paragraphs I.A–I.C.1 of these procedures to the contrary, if the findings of any survey identify any condition that poses a threat to public or patient safety, the president of the Joint Commission, or, if the president is not available, a vice president of the Joint Commission designated by the president to do so, may promptly decide that the organization be immediately placed in Preliminary Denial of Accreditation. This action and the findings that led to this action shall be reported by telephone and in writing to the organization's chief executive officer and in writing to the authorities having jurisdiction. The president's or his or her designee's decision shall be promptly reviewed by the Accreditation Committee in accordance with paragraph II of these procedures.

II. Review by the Accreditation Committee

A. Scope of Review. The Accreditation Committee shall consider the Joint Commission president's, or the president's designee's, decision and Joint Commission staff's report and recommendation and may review the survey findings, survey documents, and any other relevant materials or information received from any source, including any additional information supplied by the organization in response to this information or, in the case of a Preliminary Denial of Accreditation decision by the president or his or her designee, information supplied by the organization regarding corrective actions taken in response to the identification of a serious threat to patient or public health or safety.

B. Decision. Following such consideration, the Accreditation Committee shall do the following:

1. Accredit the organization, as described in paragraph VII of these procedures
   or
2. Conditionally accredit the organization
   or
3. Preliminarily deny accreditation to the organization or confirms a decision by the president or his or her designee to preliminarily deny accreditation
   or
4. Defer consideration while additional information regarding the organization's compliance status is gathered and reviewed by Joint Commission staff
   or
5. Order a resurvey or partial resurvey of the organization and an evaluation of the results, to the extent appropriate, by the Joint Commission staff. Thereafter, Joint Commission staff shall transmit its report and recommendation to the Accreditation Committee for action, as provided in paragraph II.C of these procedures.
   or
6. Preliminarily accredit the organization

or

7. Initially deny Preliminary Accreditation to those organizations that apply for Early Survey Policy Option 1

C. Deferred Consideration. When the Accreditation Committee defers consideration pursuant to paragraph II.B.4 or II.B.5 of these procedures, Joint Commission staff shall review and report to the Accreditation Committee concerning the organization's compliance decision. The Accreditation Committee may order any resurvey or partial resurvey necessary to determine such decision.

Following such consideration and review, the Accreditation Committee shall do the following:

1. Accredit the organization, as described in paragraph VII of these procedures

   or
2. Conditionally accredit the organization

   or
3. Preliminarily deny accreditation or confirm a decision of the president or his or her designee to preliminarily deny accreditation to the organization

   or
4. Defer consideration while additional information regarding the organization's compliance status is gathered and reviewed by the Joint Commission staff

   or
5. Order an additional resurvey or partial resurvey of the organization and an evaluation of the results, to the extent appropriate, by the Joint Commission staff. Thereafter, Joint Commission staff shall transmit its report and recommendations to the Accreditation Committee for action, as provided in paragraph II.C of these procedures.

   or
6. Preliminarily accredit the organization

   or
7. Preliminarily deny Preliminary Accreditation to those organizations applying under Early Survey Policy Option 1

III. Conditional Accreditation

A. Survey to Determine Implementation of the Evidence of Standards Compliance (ESC). Within approximately six months from the date the organization is notified of its Conditional Accreditation decision, the Joint Commission shall conduct a survey of the organization to determine the degree to which deficiencies have been corrected or improvements implemented, although the Joint Commission upon occasion may shorten that time period, as appropriate.

B. Review and Determination by Joint Commission Staff. Joint Commission staff shall review the survey findings, survey documents, and any other relevant materials or information received from any source. In accordance with decision rules approved by the Accreditation Committee, the Joint Commission staff shall do the following:

1. Determine or recommend to the Accreditation Committee that the organization be accredited, as described in paragraph VII of these procedures
   or
2. Recommend to the Accreditation Committee that the organization be preliminarily denied accreditation
   or
3. Defer consideration while additional information regarding the organization's compliance status is gathered and reviewed by the Joint Commission staff. At the conclusion of this review, one of the recommendations outlined in paragraph III.C of these procedures shall be made to the Accreditation Committee.

C. Action by the Accreditation Committee. Following review of the recommendations of the Joint Commission staff, the Accreditation Committee shall do the following:

1. Accredit the organization, as described in paragraph VII of these procedures
   or
2. Preliminarily deny accreditation to the organization
   or
3. Defer consideration while additional information regarding the organization's compliance status is gathered and reviewed by the Joint Commission staff
   or
4. Order a resurvey or partial resurvey of the organization and an evaluation of the results, to the extent appropriate, by the Joint Commission staff. Thereafter, Joint Commission staff shall transmit its report and recommendation to the Accreditation Committee for action, as provided in paragraph III.C of these procedures.

D. Charges to the Organization. The full costs of the Conditional Accreditation process shall be paid by the organization that receives Conditional Accreditation.

IV. Review Hearing Panels

A. Right to a Hearing Before a Review Hearing Panel. An organization that has been preliminarily denied accreditation* or initially denied Preliminary Accreditation pursuant to paragraph II.B.3, II.B.7, II.C.3, II.C.7, or III.C.2 of these procedures is entitled to a hearing in which to make a detailed presentation before a Review Hearing Panel if the Joint Commission receives the organization's written request for the hearing within five

* The Preliminary Denial of Accreditation decision, if subsequently changed to other than Denial of Accreditation, following review and action by the Accreditation Committee, is no longer disclosable as part of the organization's accreditation decision history.

business days after the organization receives the written notice of the Accreditation Committee's decision, including confirmation of a decision by the president, or his or her designee, to preliminarily deny accreditation, as provided in paragraph I.D of these procedures. A Review Hearing Panel shall be composed of two health care professionals not on the Accreditation Committee and one member of the Accreditation Committee who is familiar with the organization's decision.

B. Notice of the Time and Place of the Presentation Before a Review Hearing Panel. The presentation before the Review Hearing Panel shall be held at the Joint Commission's headquarters except when the president of the Joint Commission, or his or her designee, determines otherwise for good cause shown. At least 30 calendar days before the presentation, the Joint Commission shall send the organization written notice of the time and place of the hearing and copies of any supplemental materials or information received from any source that the organization does not already have and that may affect any accreditation decision. The notice shall advise the organization of the agenda to be followed and, if feasible, of the identity and professional qualifications of the panel members. At least 10 calendar days before the scheduled hearing date, the organization must submit to the Joint Commission any materials it wishes to be considered by the Review Hearing Panel.

C. Procedure for the Conduct of a Hearing. A Review Hearing Panel may proceed with only two of the three panel members present, provided one of them is the member of the Accreditation Committee. Representatives of the organization may make oral and written presentations and may be accompanied by legal counsel. The organization's representatives may present information relevant to the facts at the time of survey to the panel members. Presentations or information concerning actions taken by the organization subsequent to the survey upon which the Preliminary Denial of Accreditation decision was based are not considered relevant to the validity of the decision. A Joint Commission surveyor who participated in the survey will ordinarily appear at the hearing.

D. Report of Review Hearing Panel. After a hearing has been completed, the Review Hearing Panel shall review the facts regarding the original Preliminary Denial of Accreditation decision. The panel will submit a written report of its findings on factual matters for consideration by the Accreditation Committee. The Joint Commission shall send the organization a copy of the report of the Review Hearing Panel at least 15 calendar days before the meeting of the Accreditation Committee at which the report will be considered. The notice shall inform the organization of the meeting date and of the organization's right to submit written responses or comments for consideration by the Accreditation Committee. Any such written responses or comments must be received by the Joint Commission at least 10 calendar days before the meeting of the Accreditation Committee.

E. Charges to the Organization. The organization will be charged a nominal fee for the conduct of a Review Hearing Panel.

V. Second Consideration by the Accreditation Committee

A. Scope of Review. The report of the Review Hearing Panel shall be considered by the Accreditation Committee.

B. Decision. Following such consideration, the Accreditation Committee shall do the following:

1. Accredit or preliminarily accredit the organization, as described in paragraph VII of these procedures
   or
2. Conditionally accredit the organization
   or
3. Deny accreditation to the organization
   or
4. Defer consideration while additional information regarding the organization's compliance status is gathered and reviewed by Joint Commission staff
   or
5. Order a resurvey or partial resurvey of the organization and an evaluation of the results, to the extent appropriate, by the Joint Commission staff

VI. Review by the Board Appeal Review Committee

A. Review Request. An organization that has been denied accreditation or Preliminary Accreditation pursuant to paragraph V.B.3 of these procedures is entitled to request a review of the decision by the Board Appeal Review Committee if the Joint Commission receives the organization's request for review within five business days after the organization receives the written notice of the Accreditation Committee's decision. The Board Appeal Review Committee is composed of four members of the Board of Commissioners who are not members of the Accreditation Committee.

B. Notice of Time and Procedure for Review. The Joint Commission shall send the organization a copy of the report of the Review Hearing Panel at least 20 business days before the meeting of the Board Appeal Review Committee at which the organization's request for review will be considered. Two members of the Board Appeal Review Committee will constitute a quorum. This meeting will generally be held by telephone conference, except when it is held in conjunction with meetings of the Board of Commissioners or other committee(s) of the Board of Commissioners. The organization must submit any materials that it wishes the Board Appeal Review Committee to consider at least 10 calendar days before the scheduled meeting date. The Board Appeal Review Committee shall review the decision of the Accreditation Committee, which considered the report of the Review Hearing Panel, and any written materials submitted by the organization, and shall do one of the following:

1. Deny accreditation or Preliminary Accreditation to the organization, after finding that there is substantial evidence to support the Accreditation Committee's decision

   or

2. Make an independent evaluation of the Accreditation Committee's decision and then decide to conditionally accredit, preliminarily accredit, or accredit the organization, as described in paragraph VII of these procedures

The action taken by the Board Appeal Review Committee shall constitute the final accreditation decision of the Joint Commission.

C. Participation. No member of the Accreditation Committee or of the Review Hearing Panel who participated in an accreditation decision or review of findings on factual matters concerning an organization shall participate in any deliberations or vote of the Board Appeal Review Committee in its review of that accreditation decision or report of findings on factual matters. This provision shall not preclude any commissioner who participated in a review hearing as a member of the Review Hearing Panel from presenting and responding to questions about the report of that Review Hearing Panel to the Board Appeal Review Committee.

VII. Procedure Relating to Not Compliant Standards and Determination of Corrected Not Compliant Standards

A. A decision of the Joint Commission staff pursuant to paragraph I.A.1, I.B.2.c, or I.C.2.c of these procedures, of the Accreditation Committee pursuant to paragraph II.B.1, II.C.1, or III.C.1 of these procedures, or of a Board Appeal Review Committee, as provided in paragraph VI.B of these procedures, to accredit an organization may be made contingent upon satisfactory correction of not compliant standards or, when appropriate, upon compliance with interim life safety measures. The organization may be conditionally accredited or its accreditation may be withdrawn if it does not correct or document the correction of the specified not compliant standards within the time specified in the notice of the decision to the organization, or, when applicable, fails to demonstrate compliance with the interim life safety measures. Joint Commission staff, through the use of surveys or partial surveys or through other means, such as ESC and MOS, shall determine whether the organization has corrected the not compliant standards within the time provided or, when applicable, has demonstrated compliance with interim life safety measures, and shall report its findings to the organization. If the Joint Commission staff determines that the organization has not corrected the not compliant standards within the time provided or, when applicable, has not demonstrated compliance with interim life safety measures, the organization's status will change to Provisional Accreditation. The Joint Commission shall report its findings to the organization, and, after reviewing any comments of the organization, as appropriate and in accordance with decision rules approved by the Accreditation Committee, do the following:

1. Provide another opportunity to the organization to correct or document the correction of not compliant standards, as provided in any applicable decision rules approved by the Accreditation Committee
   or
2. Determine or recommend that the organization be placed in Conditional Accreditation status with a conditional follow-up survey in approximately four months or other time as appropriate
   or
3. Recommend to the Accreditation Committee that the organization be preliminarily denied accreditation, if certain not compliant standards, specified in decision rules approved by the Accreditation Committee, have not been corrected or the correction of which has not been documented after the specified number of opportunities given to the organization to do so, and, when applicable and as specified in decision rules approved by the Accreditation Committee, the organization has failed to demonstrate compliance with interim life safety measures

B. If the Joint Commission staff determines to recommend to the Accreditation Committee that the organization be preliminarily denied accreditation in accordance with paragraph VII.A.3, or be conditionally accredited in accordance with VII.A.2, the staff shall submit its recommendation and any comments of the organization to the Accreditation Committee for action, as provided in paragraph II.B.1 through II.B.7.

VIII. Final Accreditation Decision

A. The action taken by the Joint Commission staff shall constitute the final decision of the Joint Commission to do the following:

1. Accredit the organization, when taken pursuant to paragraph I.A.1, I.B.2.c, or I.C.2.c of these procedures
   or
2. Conditionally accredit the organization, when taken pursuant to paragraph I.A.3 or VII.A.2 of these procedures
   or
3. Preliminarily accredit the organization, when taken pursuant to paragraph I.A.6 of these procedures

B. The action taken by the Accreditation Committee shall constitute the final decision of the Joint Commission to do the following:

1. Accredit the organization, when taken pursuant to paragraph II.B.1, II.C.1, or III.C.1 of these procedures
   or
2. Conditionally accredit the organization, when taken pursuant to paragraph II.B.2 or II.C.2 of these procedures
   or
3. Deny accreditation to the organization, when taken pursuant to paragraph II.B.3, II.C.3, III.C.2, or VII.B of these procedures, and the organiza-

tion does not request the opportunity to make a presentation before a Review Hearing Panel pursuant to paragraph IV.A of these procedures
or
4. Preliminarily accredit the organization, when taken pursuant to paragraph II.B.6 of these procedures
or
5. Deny Preliminary Accreditation to the organization, when taken pursuant to paragraph II.B.7 of these procedures, and the organization applying for Early Survey Policy Option 1 or 2 does not request the opportunity to make a presentation before a Review Hearing Panel pursuant to paragraph IV.A of these procedures

C. The action taken by the Board Appeal Review Committee shall constitute the final decision of the Joint Commission to do the following:
1. Accredit the organization, conditionally accredit the organization, or deny accreditation, when taken pursuant to paragraph VI.B of these procedures

IX. Status of the Organization Pending a Final Decision and Effective Date of a Final Decision

A. The accreditation status of an accredited organization shall continue in effect pending any final accreditation decision.

B. A final decision to accredit, preliminarily accredit, or conditionally accredit an organization that follows an initial Accreditation Committee decision of Preliminary Denial of Accreditation pursuant to paragraph II.B shall be considered effective as of the first day after completion of the organization's survey from which the decision results.

C. A final decision to deny accreditation or Provisional Accreditation to an organization shall become effective as follows:
1. As of the date of the decision made by the Board Appeal Review Committee pursuant to paragraph VI.B of these procedures
or
2. At the expiration of the time during which an organization may, but does not, request a review by the Board Appeal Review Committee, pursuant to paragraph VI.A of these procedures
or
3. At the expiration of the time during which an organization may, but does not, request the opportunity to make a presentation before a Review Hearing Panel pursuant to paragraph IV.A of these procedures
or
4. On receipt by the Joint Commission, before a final decision, of notification from the organization that it withdraws its request for review of a Preliminary Denial of Accreditation decision before a Review Hearing Panel or its request for appeal of a Denial of Accreditation decision before the Board Appeal Review Committee

X. Notice

Any notice required by these accreditation procedures to be given to an organization shall be addressed to the organization at its post office address as shown in Joint Commission records and shall be sent to the organization by certified letter as forwarded by a recognized package delivery service. Any notice required to be given to the Joint Commission by the organization shall be sent by the organization in the same manner and shall be addressed to the Office of the Executive Vice President for Accreditation Operations, Joint Commission on Accreditation of Healthcare Organizations, One Renaissance Boulevard, Oakbrook Terrace, IL 60181.

Sentinel Events

I. Sentinel Events

In support of its mission to continuously improve the safety and quality of health care provided to the public, the Joint Commission reviews organizations' activities in response to sentinel events in its accreditation process, including all full accreditation surveys and random unannounced surveys and, as appropriate, for-cause surveys.

SE

- A sentinel event is an unexpected occurrence involving death or serious physical or psychological injury, or the risk thereof. Serious injury specifically includes loss of limb or function. The phrase "or the risk thereof" includes any process variation for which a recurrence would carry a significant chance of a serious adverse outcome.
- Such events are called "sentinel" because they signal the need for immediate investigation and response
- The terms "sentinel event" and "medical error" are not synonymous; not all sentinel events occur because of an error and not all errors result in sentinel events

II. Goals of the Sentinel Event Policy

The policy has four goals:

1. To have a positive impact in improving patient care, treatment, and services and preventing sentinel events
2. To focus the attention of an organization that has experienced a sentinel event on understanding the causes that underlie the event, and on changing the organization's systems and processes to reduce the probability of such an event in the future
3. To increase the general knowledge about sentinel events, their causes, and strategies for prevention
4. To maintain the confidence of the public and accredited organizations in the accreditation process

III. Standards Relating to Sentinel Events

Standards

Each Joint Commission accreditation manual contains standards in the "Improving Organization Performance" (PI) chapter that relate specifically to the management of sentinel events. These standards are PI.1.10, PI.2.20, PI.2.30, and PI.3.10.

Organization-Specific Definition of Sentinel Event

The Improving Organization Performance standard PI.2.30 requires each accredited organization to define "sentinel event" for its own purposes in establishing mechanisms to identify, report, and manage these events. While this definition must be consistent with the general definition of sentinel event as published by the Joint Commission, accredited organizations have some latitude in setting more specific parameters to define "unexpected," "serious," and "the risk thereof." At a minimum, an organization's definition must include those events that are subject to review under the Sentinel Event Policy as defined in Section IV of this chapter.

Expectations Under the Standards for an Organization's Response to a Sentinel Event

Accredited organizations are expected to identify and respond appropriately to all sentinel events (as defined by the organization in accordance with the preceding paragraph) occurring in the organization or associated with services that the organization provides, or provides for. Appropriate response includes conducting a timely, thorough, and credible root cause analysis; developing an action plan designed to implement improvements to reduce risk; implementing the improvements; and monitoring the effectiveness of those improvements.

Root Cause Analysis

Root cause analysis is a process for identifying the basic or causal factors that underlie variation in performance, including the occurrence or possible occurrence of a sentinel event. A root cause analysis focuses primarily on systems and processes, not on individual performance. It progresses from special causes in clinical processes to common causes in organizational processes and systems and identifies potential improvements in processes or systems that would tend to decrease the likelihood of such events in the future or determines, after analysis, that no such improvement opportunities exist.

Action Plan

The product of the root cause analysis is an action plan that identifies the strategies that the organization intends to implement in order to reduce the risk of similar events occurring in the future. The plan should address responsibility for implementation, oversight, pilot testing as appropriate, time lines, and strategies for measuring the effectiveness of the actions.

Survey Process

When conducting an accreditation survey, the Joint Commission seeks to evaluate the organization's compliance with the applicable standards and to score those standards based on performance throughout the organization over time (for example, the preceding 12 months for a full accreditation survey or the preceding 4 months for an initial survey). Surveyors are instructed not to seek out specific sentinel events beyond those already known to the Joint Commission.

If, in the course of conducting the usual survey activities, a sentinel event is identified, the surveyor will take the following steps:

- Inform the CEO that the event has been identified
- Inform the CEO the event will be reported to the Joint Commission for further review and follow-up under the provisions of the Sentinel Event Policy

During the onsite survey, the surveyor(s) will assess the organization's compliance with sentinel event-related standards in the following ways:

- Review the organization's process for responding to a sentinel event
- Interview the organization's leaders and staff about their expectations and responsibilities for identifying, reporting, and responding to sentinel events
- Ask for an example of a root cause analysis that has been conducted in the past year to assess the adequacy of the organization's process for responding to a sentinel event. Additional examples may be reviewed if needed to more fully assess the organization's understanding of, and ability to conduct, root cause analyses. In selecting an example, the organization may choose a "closed case" or a "near miss" to demonstrate its process for responding to a sentinel event.

IV. Reviewable Sentinel Events

Definition of Occurrences That Are Subject to Review by the Joint Commission Under the Sentinel Event Policy

The definition of a reviewable sentinel event takes into account a wide array of occurrences applicable to a wide variety of health care organizations. Any or all occurrences may apply to a particular type of health care organization. Thus, not all of the following occurrences may apply to your particular organization. The subset of sentinel events that is subject to review by the Joint Commission includes any occurrence that meets any of the following criteria:

- The event has resulted in an unanticipated death or major permanent loss of function, not related to the natural course of the patient's illness or underlying condition*†

  or
- The event is one of the following (even if the outcome was not death or major permanent loss of function unrelated to the natural course of the patient's illness or underlying condition):
  - Suicide of any patient receiving care, treatment, or services in a staffed around-the-clock care setting or within 72 hours of discharge
  - Unanticipated death of a full-term infant
  - Abduction of any patient receiving care, treatment, or services
  - Discharge of an infant to the wrong family

---

* A distinction is made between an adverse outcome that is primarily related to the natural course of the patient's illness or underlying condition (not reviewable under the Sentinel Event Policy) and a death or major permanent loss of function that is associated with the treatment (including "recognized complications") or lack of treatment of that condition, or otherwise not clearly and primarily related to the natural course of the patient's illness or underlying condition (reviewable). In indeterminate cases, the event will be presumed reviewable and the organization's response will be reviewed under the Sentinel Event Policy according to the prescribed procedures and time frames without delay for additional information such as autopsy results.

† *Major permanent loss of function* means sensory, motor, physiologic, or intellectual impairment not present on admission requiring continued treatment or lifestyle change. When major permanent loss of function cannot be immediately determined, applicability of the policy is not established until either the resident is discharged with continued major loss of function, or two weeks have elapsed with persistent major loss of function, whichever occurs first.

- Rape*
- Hemolytic transfusion reaction involving administration of blood or blood products having major blood group incompatibilities
- Surgery on the wrong patient or wrong body part†
- Unintended retention of a foreign object in a patient after surgery or other procedure
- Severe neonatal hyperbilirubinemia (bilirubin > 30 milligrams/deciliter)
- Prolonged fluoroscopy with cumulative dose > 1,500 rads to a single field or any delivery of radiotherapy to the wrong body region or > 25% above the planned radiotherapy dose

Examples of reviewable sentinel events and nonreviewable events are provided in Table 1 (page103–104).

How the Joint Commission Becomes Aware of a Sentinel Event

Each organization is encouraged, but not required, to report to the Joint Commission any sentinel event meeting the above criteria for reviewable sentinel events. Alternatively, the Joint Commission may become aware of a sentinel event by some other means such as communication from a patient, a family member, an employee of the organization, a surveyor, or through the media.

Reasons for Reporting a Sentinel Event to the Joint Commission

Although self-reporting a sentinel event is not required and there is no difference in the expected response, time frames, or review procedures, whether the organization voluntarily reports the event or the Joint Commission becomes aware of the event by some other means, there are several advantages to the organization that self-reports a sentinel event:

- Reporting the event enables the addition of the "lessons learned" from the event to be added to the Joint Commission's Sentinel Event Database, thereby contributing to the general knowledge about sentinel events and to the reduction of risk for such events in many other organizations
- Early reporting provides an opportunity for consultation with Joint Commission staff during the development of the root cause analysis and action plan
- The organization's message to the public that it is doing everything possible to ensure that such an event will not happen again is strengthened by its acknowl-

* *Rape*, as a reviewable sentinel event, is defined as unconsented sexual contact involving a patient and another patient, staff member, or other perpetrator while being treated or on the premises of the health care organization, including oral, vaginal, or anal penetration or fondling of the patient's sex organ(s) by another individual's hand, sex organ, or object. One or more of the following must be present to determine reviewability:

- Any staff-witnessed sexual contact as described above
- Sufficient clinical evidence obtained by the organization to support allegations of unconsented sexual contact
- Admission by the perpetrator that sexual contact, as described above, occurred on the premises

† All events of surgery on the wrong patient or wrong body part are reviewable under the policy, regardless of the magnitude of the procedure or the outcome.

SE

Table 1. Examples of Sentinel Events That Are Reviewable and Events That Are Not Reviewable Under The Joint Commission's Sentinel Event Policy*

Examples of Sentinel Events That Are Reviewable Under the Joint Commission's Sentinel Event Policy

Any patient death, paralysis, coma, or other major permanent loss of function associated with a medication error.

A patient commits suicide within 72 hours of being discharged from an ambulatory care setting that provides staffed around-the-clock care.

Any elopement, that is unauthorized departure, of a patient from an around-the-clock care setting resulting in a temporally related death (suicide, accidental death, or homicide) or major permanent loss of function.

An ambulatory care organization operates on the wrong side of the patient's body.

Any intrapartum (related to the birth process) maternal death.

Any perinatal death unrelated to a congenital condition in an infant having a birth weight greater than 2,500 grams.

A patient is abducted from the organization where he or she receives care, treatment, or services.

Assault, homicide, or other crime resulting in patient death or major permanent loss of function.

A patient fall that results in death or major permanent loss of function as a direct result of the injuries sustained in the fall.

Hemolytic transfusion reaction involving major blood group incompatibilities.

A foreign body, such as a sponge or forceps, is left in a patient after surgery.

> **Note:** An adverse outcome that is *directly related* to the natural course of the patient's illness or underlying condition (for example, terminal illness present at the time of presentation) is **not** reportable **except** for suicide in, or following elopement from, a 24-hour care setting (see above).

Examples of Events That Are Not Reviewable Under the Joint Commission's Sentinel Event Policy

Any "near miss."

Full or expected return of limb or bodily function to the same level as prior to the adverse event by discharge or within two weeks of the initial loss of said function.

continued on next page

* **Note:** *This list may not apply to all settings.*

SE

Table 1. Examples of Sentinel Events That Are Reviewable and Events That Are Not Reviewable Under The Joint Commission's Sentinel Event Policy *(continued)*

Any sentinel event that has not affected a recipient of care (patient, client, resident).

Medication errors that do not result in death or major permanent loss of function.

Suicide other than in an around-the-clock care setting or following elopement from such a setting.

A death or loss of function following a discharge "against medical advice (AMA)."

Unsuccessful suicide attempts unless resulting in major permanent loss of function.

Minor degrees of hemolysis not caused by a major blood group incompatibility and with no clinical sequelae.

> **Note:** In the context of its performance improvement activities, an organization may choose to conduct intensive assessment (for example, root cause analysis) for some nonreviewable events. Please refer to the "Improving Organization Performance" chapter of this Joint Commission accreditation book.

edged collaboration with the Joint Commission to understand how the event happened and what can be done to reduce the risk of such an event in the future

Required Response to a Reviewable Sentinel Event

If the Joint Commission becomes aware (either through voluntary self-reporting or otherwise) of a sentinel event that meets the previous criteria (*see* pages 101–102) and the event has occurred in an accredited organization, the organization is expected to do the following:

- Prepare a thorough and credible root cause analysis and action plan within 45 calendar days of the event or of becoming aware of the event
- Submit to the Joint Commission its root cause analysis and action plan, or otherwise provide for Joint Commission evaluation of its response to the sentinel event under an approved protocol (*see* Section VI), within 45 calendar days of the known occurrence of the event

The Joint Commission will then determine whether the root cause analysis and action plan are acceptable. If the determination that an event is reviewable under the Sentinel Event Policy occurs more than 45 calendar days following the known occurrence of the event, the organization will be allowed 15 calendar days for its response. If the organization fails to submit an acceptable root cause analysis within the 45 calendar days (or within 15 calendar days, if the 45 calendar days have already elapsed), the following consequences will result (depending on the length of time the organization fails to submit a root cause analysis):

- If the organization has failed to submit a root cause analysis within an additional 30 days following its due date, its accreditation decision will automatically be changed to Provisional Accreditation, and both the organization and the Accreditation Committee will be notified.
- If the organization has failed to submit a root cause analysis within 60 days following its due date, its accreditation decision will automatically be changed to Conditional Accreditation, and both the organization and the Accreditation Committee will be notified.
- If the organization then continues to fail to submit a root cause analysis for 90 days following its due date, a recommendation for Denial of Accreditation will be presented to the Accreditation Committee. The organization would then be given the opportunity to submit a response to the Accreditation Committee. However, if the Committee were to reach a Denial of Accreditation Decision because the organization has failed to submit any root cause analysis, the organization would not have access to the appeals process.

Please note that an organization that experiences a sentinel event as defined by the organization, but that does not meet the criteria for review under the Sentinel Event Policy, is still expected to complete a root cause analysis (as required by standard PI.2.30) but does not need to submit it to the Joint Commission.

Review of Root Cause Analyses and Action Plans

A root cause analysis will be considered *acceptable* if it has the following characteristics:

- The analysis focuses primarily on systems and processes, not on individual performance
- The analysis progresses from special causes in clinical processes to common causes in organizational processes
- The analysis repeatedly digs deeper by asking "Why?"; then, when answered, "Why?" again, and so on
- The analysis identifies changes that could be made in systems and processes (either through redesign or development of new systems or processes) which would reduce the risk of such events occurring in the future
- The analysis is thorough and credible

To be *thorough*, the root cause analysis must include the following:

- A determination of the human and other factors most directly associated with the sentinel event and the process(es) and systems related to its occurrence
- An analysis of the underlying systems and processes through a series of "Why?" questions to determine where redesign might reduce risk
- An inquiry into all areas appropriate to the specific type of event as described in Table 2 (*see* page 106)
- An identification of risk points and their potential contributions to this type of event

SE

Table 2. Minimum Scope of Root Cause Analysis for Specific Types of Sentinel Events

Detailed inquiry into these areas is expected when conducting a root cause analysis for the specified type of sentinel event. Inquiry into areas not checked (or listed) should be conducted as appropriate to the specific event under review.

	Suicide (24-Hour Care)	Medication Error	Procedural Complication	Wrong-Site Surgery	Treatment Delay	Restraint Death	Elopement Death	Assault/Rape/Homicide	Transfusion Death	Patient Abduction	Unanticipated Death of Full-Term Infant	Unintended Retention of Foreign Body	Fall Related
Behavioral assessment process*	X					X	X	X					
Physical assessment process†	X	X	X	X	X	X	X				X		X
Patient identification process		X		X					X				
Patient observation procedures	X				X	X	X	X	X		X		X
Care planning process	X		X			X	X				X		X
Continuum of care	X	X			X	X							X
Staffing levels	X	X	X	X	X	X	X	X	X	X		X	X
Orientation and training of staff	X	X	X	X	X	X	X	X	X	X	X	X	X
Competency assessment/ credentialing	X	X	X	X	X	X	X	X	X	X	X	X	X
Supervision of staff‡	X	X	X		X	X			X			X	
Communication with patient/family	X	X		X	X	X	X			X			X
Communication among staff members	X	X	X	X	X	X	X	X	X	X	X	X	X
Availability of information	X	X	X	X	X	X			X		X		X
Adequacy of technological support		X	X										
Equipment maintenance/ management		X	X		X	X					X		X
Physical environment§	X	X	X	X		X	X	X	X	X			X
Security systems and processes	X						X	X		X			
Medication management‖		X	X		X				X		X		X

* Includes the process for assessing patient's risk to self (and to others, in cases of assault, rape, or homicide where a patient is the assailant).

† Includes search for contraband.

‡ Includes supervision of physicians-in-training.

§ Includes furnishings, hardware (for example, bars, hooks, rods), lighting, distractions.

‖ Includes selection and procurement; storage, ordering, and transcribing; preparing and dispensing; administration; and monitoring.

- A determination of potential improvement in processes or systems that would tend to decrease the likelihood of such events in the future, or a determination, after analysis, that no such improvement opportunities exist

To be *credible*, the root cause analysis must do the following:

- Include participation by the leadership of the organization and by individuals most closely involved in the processes and systems under review
- Be internally consistent (that is, not contradict itself or leave obvious questions unanswered)

- Provide an explanation for all findings of "not applicable" or "no problem"
- Include consideration of any relevant literature

An action plan will be considered *acceptable* if it does the following:
- Identifies changes that can be implemented to reduce risk, or formulates a rationale for not undertaking such changes
- Identifies, in situations where improvement actions are planned, who is responsible for implementation, when the action will be implemented (including any pilot testing), and how the effectiveness of the actions will be evaluated

All root cause analyses and action plans will be considered and treated as confidential by the Joint Commission. A detailed listing of the minimum scope of root cause analysis for specific types of sentinel events is included in Table 2.

Follow-up Activities

After the Joint Commission has determined that an organization has conducted an acceptable root cause analysis and developed an acceptable action plan, the Joint Commission will notify it that the root cause analysis and action plan are acceptable and will assign an appropriate follow-up activity, typically one or more sentinel event measures of success (SE MOS) due in four months (*see* page 111 for more details).

V. The Sentinel Event Database

To achieve the third goal of the Sentinel Event Policy, "to increase the general knowledge about sentinel events, their causes, and strategies for prevention," the Joint Commission collects and analyzes data from the review of sentinel events, root cause analyses, action plans, and follow-up activities. These data and information form the content of the Joint Commission's Sentinel Event Database.

The Joint Commission is committed to developing and maintaining this Sentinel Event Database in a fashion that will protect the confidentiality of the organization, the caregiver, and the patient. Included in this database are three major categories of data elements:
1. Sentinel event data
2. Root cause data
3. Risk reduction data

De-identified aggregate data relating to root causes and risk-reduction strategies for sentinel events that occur with significant frequency will form the basis for future error-prevention advice to organizations through *Sentinel Event Alert* and other media. The Sentinel Event Database is also a major component of the evidence base for the National Patient Safety Goals.

VI. Procedures for Implementing the Sentinel Event Policy

SE

Voluntary Self Reporting of Reviewable Sentinel Events to the Joint Commission

If an organization wishes to report an occurrence in the subset of sentinel events that are subject to review by the Joint Commission, the organization will be asked to complete a form accessible through its extranet home page. From the home page, select "Self Report Sentinel Event" from the "Continuous Compliance Tools" section.

Reviewable Sentinel Events That Are Not Reported by the Organization

If the Joint Commission becomes aware of a sentinel event subject to review under the Sentinel Event Policy that was not reported to the Joint Commission by the organization, the CEO of the organization is contacted, and a preliminary assessment of the sentinel event is made. An event that occurred more than one year before the date the Joint Commission became aware of the event will not, in most cases, be reviewed under the Sentinel Event Policy. In such a case, a written response will be requested from the organization, including a summary of processes in place to prevent similar occurrences.

Determination That a Sentinel Event Is Reviewable Under the Sentinel Event Policy

Based on available factual information received about the event, Joint Commission staff will apply the previous definition (pages 101–102) to determine whether the event is reviewable under the Sentinel Event Policy. Challenges to a determination that an event is reviewable will be resolved through consultation with senior staff in the Division of Accreditation and Certification Operations.

Initial On-Site Review of a Sentinel Event

An initial on-site review of a sentinel event will usually not be conducted unless it is determined that there is a potential ongoing immediate threat to patient health or safety or potentially significant noncompliance with Joint Commission standards. Immediate Threat to Life incidents include situations in which the organization's noncompliance with one or more standards has caused, or is likely to cause, serious injury, harm, impairment, or death to a patient and is likely to continue. Complaints are assigned this priority if the information indicates immediate corrective action is necessary. All are immediately referred to Joint Commission Executive Leadership for authorization to conduct an unannounced for-cause survey. If an on-site ("for-cause") review is conducted, the organization will be billed an appropriate amount based on the established fee schedule to cover the costs of conducting such a survey.

Disclosable Information

If the Joint Commission receives an inquiry about the accreditation status of an organization that has experienced a reviewable sentinel event, the organization's accreditation status will be reported in the usual manner without making reference to the sentinel event. If the inquirer specifically references the specific sentinel event, the Joint Commission will acknowledge that it is aware of the event and currently is working or has worked with the organization through the sentinel event review process.

SE

Submission of Root Cause Analysis and Action Plan

The organization that experiences a sentinel event subject to the Sentinel Event Policy is asked to submit two documents (in addition to the sentinel event reporting form discussed on page 108): (1) the complete root cause analysis, including its findings; and (2) the resulting action plan that describes the organization's risk reduction strategies and a strategy for evaluating their effectiveness. This information will be submitted to the Joint Commission Central Office using an online root cause analysis collection tool, also accessible from the "Continuous Compliance Tools" section of the extranet home page, under the "Sentinel Event Activities" link.

The root cause analysis and action plan are not to include the name(s) of caregivers and patients involved in the sentinel event.

Alternatively, if the organization has concerns about waivers of confidentiality protections as a result of sending the root cause analysis documents to the Joint Commission, the following alternative approaches to a review of the organization's response to the sentinel event are acceptable:

1. A review of the root cause analysis and action plan documents brought to Joint Commission headquarters by organization staff and then taken back to the organization on the same day
2. An on-site visit by a specially trained surveyor to review the root cause analysis and action plan
3. An on-site visit by a specially trained surveyor to review the root cause analysis and findings without directly viewing the root cause analysis documents through a series of interviews and a review of relevant documentation. For purposes of this review activity, *relevant documentation* includes, at a minimum, any documentation relevant to the organization's process for responding to sentinel events, the patient's medical record, and the action plan resulting from the analysis of the subject sentinel event. The latter serves as the basis for appropriate follow-up activity.
4. When the organization affirms that it meets specified criteria respecting the risk of waiving confidentiality protections for root cause analysis information shared with the Joint Commission, an on-site visit by a specially trained surveyor to conduct the following:
   a. Interviews and reviews of relevant documentation, including the patient's medical record, to obtain information about the following:

- The *process* the organization uses in responding to sentinel events
- The relevant policies and procedures preceding and following the organization's review of the specific event, and the implementation thereof, sufficient to permit inferences about the adequacy of the organization's response to the sentinel event

b. A standards-based survey that traces a patient's care, treatment, and services and the organization management functions relevant to the sentinel event under review.

SE

Any one of the four alternatives will result in a charge to the organization sufficient to cover the average direct costs of the visit. Inquiries about the fee should be directed to the Joint Commission's pricing unit at 630/792-5115.

The Joint Commission must receive a request for review of an organization's response to a sentinel event using any of these alternative approaches within at least five business days of the self-report of a reviewable event or of the initial communication by the Joint Commission to the organization that it has become aware of a reviewable sentinel event.

The Joint Commission's Response

Staff assesses the acceptability of the organization's response to the reviewable sentinel event, including the thoroughness and credibility of any root cause analysis information reviewed and the organization's action plan. If the root cause analysis and action plan are found to be thorough and credible, the response will be accepted and one or more sentinel event Measures of Success (SE MOS) will be assigned (*see* page 111 for more details).

If the response is unacceptable, staff will provide consultation to the organization on the criteria that have not yet been met and will allow an additional 15 calendar days beyond the original submission period for the organization to resubmit its response.

If the response does not meet established criteria, the organization's accreditation decision automatically will be changed to Provisional Accreditation, and both the organization and the Accreditation Committee will be notified. The Joint Commission staff will provide additional consultative support to the organization and allow an additional 10 business days to submit an acceptable root cause analysis and action plan. The organization's accreditation decision reverts to Accredited when the root cause analysis and action plan are determined to be acceptable.

If the third submission continues to not meet established criteria, the Joint Commission staff will recommend that the organization's accreditation decision be changed to Conditional Accreditation, and both the organization and the Accreditation Committee will be notified. The organization will have one final 45-day period in which to submit an acceptable root cause analysis and action plan. If the submitted root cause analysis and action plan still do not meet established criteria, the Accreditation Commmittee of the Joint Commission will be requested to change the organization's accreditation decision to Preliminary Denial of Accreditation.

When the organization's response (initial or revised) is found to be acceptable, the Joint Commission issues a letter that does the following:

- Reflects the Joint Commission's determination to continue or modify the organization's current accreditation decision
- Assigns an appropriate follow-up activity, typically one or more sentinel event Measures of Success due in four months

Sentinel Event Measure of Success

The organization's follow-up activity will be conducted through the Measure of Success (MOS) process. An MOS is a numerical or quantifiable measure, usually related to an audit, that determines if a planned action was effective and sustained. The sentinel event Measures of Success (SE MOS) are due four months after the root cause analysis and action plan are determined acceptable. If the planned action can be associated with a standard or National Patient Safety Goal requirement, it will have a level of compliance expectation based on the type of element of performance (EP) for the associated standard or National Patient Safety Goal requirement. That is, if the action is equivalent to an EP that is identified as an "A" EP, the minimum required level of compliance for the SE MOS for that action will be 100%. If the action is equivalent to an EP that is identified as a "C" EP, the minimum required level of compliance expectation for the SE MOS for that action will be 90%.* If the action cannot be associated with an existing standard or National Patient Safety Goal requirement, the organization will identify the level of compliance expectation, which must be at least 85%, subject to approval by the Joint Commission. The following information further outlines the SE MOS requirement:

- If an SE MOS is 30 or more days late, the organization's accreditation status will automatically be changed to Provisional Accreditation and both the organization and the Accreditation Committee will be notified.
- If an SE MOS is 60 or more days late, the Joint Commission staff will recommend that the organization's accreditation decision be changed to Conditional Accreditation, and both the organization and the Accreditation Committee will be notified.
- If an SE MOS is 90 or more days late, the Joint Commission staff will recommend to the Accreditation Committee that the organization decision be changed to Denial of Accreditation. In accordance with the Accreditation Committee policy, such an organization will not be afforded any appeal.
- If an SE MOS of success is submitted on time but does not meet established levels of compliance, the Joint Commission staff will request an additional four months of data. The organization's accreditation decision will be changed to Provisional Accreditation, and both the organization and the Accreditation Committee will be notified.
- If the second set of data meet established levels of compliance, the organization will be restored to Accredited.
- If the second set of data does not meet established levels of compliance, the Joint Commission staff will recommend that the organization's accreditation decision will be changed to Conditional Accreditation, and both the organization and the

Accreditation Committee will be notified. Any further actions will be based on the standards-based measures of success decision rules.

A decision to maintain or change the organization's accreditation decision as a result of the follow-up activity or to assign additional follow-up requirements will be based on existing decision rules unless otherwise determined by the Accreditation Committee.

Handling Sentinel Event–Related Documents

Handling of any submitted root cause analysis and action plan is restricted to specially trained staff in accordance with procedures designed to protect the confidentiality of the documents.

Upon completion of the Joint Commission review of any submitted root cause analysis and action plan and the abstraction of the required data elements for the Joint Commission's Sentinel Event Database, the original root cause analysis documents and any copies will be destroyed. Upon request, the original documents will be returned to the organization. With the new electronic process, the information contained in the electronically submitted RCA tool will be de-identified once the review is completed.

The action plan resulting from the analysis of the sentinel event will initially be retained to serve as the basis for the SE MOS. Once the action plan has been implemented and meets the established levels of compliance as determined through the SE MOS, the Joint Commission will destroy the action plan. If the SE MOS was submitted electronically, the information will likewise be de-identified upon completion of the review.

Oversight of the Sentinel Event Policy

The Accreditation Committee of the Joint Commission's Board of Commissioners is responsible for overseeing the implementation of this policy and procedure. In addition to reviewing and deciding individual cases involving changes in an organization's accreditation decision, the senior staff in Accreditation and Certification Operations will periodically audit the root cause analyses and sentinel event measures of success and report these findings to the Accreditation Committee. For the purposes of these audits, the Joint Commission temporarily retains random samples of these documents. Upon completion of the audit, these documents are also destroyed.

For more information about the Joint Commission's Sentinel Event Policy and Procedures, visit the Joint Commission's Web site at http://www.jointcommission.org or call the Sentinel Event Hotline at 630/792-3700.

National Patient Safety Goals

NP SG

This chapter addresses the 2008 National Patient Safety Goals, requirements, rationales, and implementation expectations. The purpose of The Joint Commission's National Patient Safety Goals is to promote specific improvements in patient safety. The goals highlight problematic areas in health care and describe evidence and expert-based consensus to solutions to these problems. Recognizing that sound system design is intrinsic to the delivery of safe, high-quality health care, the goals generally focus on systemwide solutions, wherever possible.

A broadly representative Sentinel Event Advisory Group works with Joint Commission staff on a continuing basis to prioritize and develop goals, requirements, and implementation expectations. As part of this development process, candidate goals, requirements, and implementation expectations are sent to the field for review and comment. The Advisory Group annually recommends selected existing and new goals, requirements, and implementation expectations to the Joint Commission's Board of Commissioners for review and approval.

If an organization thinks that an alternative approach meets the intent of the requirement and wishes to implement such an alternative, the organization must obtain Joint Commission approval of the alternative. The Sentinel Event Advisory Group also assists the Joint Commission in evaluating potential alternatives to goal requirements that have been suggested by individual organizations.

Ambulatory care organizations providing care, treatment, and services relevant to these goals are responsible for implementing the applicable requirements or effective alternatives. Compliance with these requirements is assessed throughout the accreditation cycle, through on-site surveys, and the Periodic Performance Review (PPR).* When an organization does not fully comply with a requirement, the organization will be assigned a Requirement for Improvement in the same way that noncompliance with an element of performance (EP) generates a Requirement for Improvement at a standard. All Requirements for Improvement must be addressed in an Evidence of Standards Compliance (ESC) report. Failure to resolve a Requirement for Improvement affects an organization's accreditation decision, which could ultimately lead to a loss of accreditation.

For a grid listing National Patient Safety Goals and requirements applicability for ambulatory care services and/or settings, please *see* pages 130–131.

* For those programs required to complete a PPR.

The Joint Commission provides guidance on how to effectively comply with each goal's requirements. This guidance includes detailed answers to Frequently Asked Questions (FAQs), which are posted on the Joint Commission Web site (http://www.jointcommission.org).

Goal 1
Improve the accuracy of patient identification.

Requirement 1A

Use at least two patient identifiers when providing care, treatment, or services.

Rationale for Requirement 1A

Wrong-patient errors occur in virtually all aspects of diagnosis and treatment. The intent for this goal is two-fold; first, to reliably identify the individual as the person for whom the service or treatment is intended; second, to match the service or treatment to that individual.

Implementation Expectations for Requirement 1A

C Ⓜ 1. Two patient identifiers are used when administering medications or blood products.

A Ⓜ 2. Two patient identifiers are used when collecting blood samples and other specimens for clinical testing.

C Ⓜ 3. Two patient identifiers are used when providing other treatments or procedures.

A 4. The patient's room number or physical location is not used as an identifier.

A Ⓜ 5. Containers used for blood and other specimens are labeled in the presence of the patient.

Requirement 1B

Not applicable

Goal 2
Improve the effectiveness of communication among caregivers.

Requirement 2A

For verbal or telephone orders or for telephonic reporting of critical test results, verify the complete order or test result by having the person receiving the information record and "read-back" the complete order or test result.

Rationale for Requirement 2A

Ineffective communication is the most frequently cited category of root causes of sentinel events. Effective communication, which is timely, accurate, complete, unambiguous, and understood by the recipient, reduces error and results in improved patient safety.

Implementation Expectations for Requirement 2A

C Ⓜ 1. The receiver of the information **writes** down the complete order or test result or enters it into a computer.

C Ⓜ 2. The receiver of the information **reads** back the order or test result.

C Ⓜ 3. The receiver of the information **receives** confirmation from the individual who gave the order or test result.

Requirement 2B

Standardize a list of abbreviations, acronyms, symbols, and dose designations that are not to be used throughout the organization.

Implementation Expectations for Requirement 2B

A 1. The organization develops a standardized a list of abbreviations, acronyms, symbols, and dose designations that are not to be used throughout the organization.

A 2. The list of abbreviations not to be used includes the following:

- U, u
- IU
- Q.D., QD, q.d., qd
- Q.O.D., QOD, q.o.d, qod
- Trailing zero (X.0 mg)*
- Lack of leading zero (.X mg)
- MS
- MSO_4
- $MgSO_4$

C Ⓜ 3. The organization implements the "do not use" list and applies this list to all orders and all medication-related documentation when handwritten or entered as free text into a computer.

* **Exception:** A "trailing zero" may be used only where required to demonstrate the level of precision of the value being reported, such as for laboratory results, studies that report sizes of lesions, or catheter/tube sizes. It may not be used in medication orders or other medication-related documentation.

A 4. Preprinted forms do not include any abbreviations identified as not to be used.

Requirement 2C

Measure and assess and, if appropriate, take action to improve the timeliness of reporting, and the timeliness of receipt by the responsible licensed caregiver, of critical tests and critical results and values.

Implementation Expectations for Requirement 2C

A 1. The organization defines critical tests and critical results and values.

A 2. The organization defines the acceptable length of time between the ordering of critical tests and reporting the critical tests and critical results and values.

A 3. The organization defines the acceptable length of time between the availability of critical tests and critical results and values and receipt by the responsible licensed caregiver.

A 4. The organization collects data on the timeliness of reporting critical tests and critical results and values.

A 5. The organization assesses the data and determines whether there is a need for improvement.

A 6. The organization takes appropriate action to improve and measure the effectiveness of those actions.

Requirement 2D

Not applicable

Requirement 2E

Implement a standardized approach to "hand-off" communications, including an opportunity to ask and respond to questions.

Rationale for Requirement 2E

The primary objective of a "hand off" is to provide accurate information about a patient's care, treatment, and services, current condition, and any recent or anticipated changes. The information communicated during a hand off must be accurate in order to meet patient safety goals.

In health care there are numerous types of patient "hand offs," including but not limited to nursing shift changes, physicians transferring complete responsibility for a patient, physicians transferring on-call responsibility, temporary responsibility for staff leaving the unit for a short time, anesthesiologist report to post-anesthesia recovery room nurse, nursing and physician "hand off" from the emergency department to inpatient units, different hospitals, nursing homes and home health care, and critical laboratory and radiology results sent to physician offices.

Implementation Expectations for Requirement 2E

C Ⓜ 1. The organization's process for effective "hand off" communication includes: Interactive communications allowing for the opportunity for questioning between the giver and receiver of patient information.

C Ⓜ 2. The organization's process for effective "hand off" communication includes: Up-to-date information regarding the patient's care, treatment, and services; condition; and any recent or anticipated changes.

C Ⓜ 3. The organization's process for effective "hand off" communication includes: A process for verification of the received information, including repeat-back or read-back, as appropriate.

A 4. The organization's process for effective "hand off" communication includes: An opportunity for the receiver of the hand off information to review relevant patient historical data, which may include previous care, treatment, and services.

C Ⓜ 5. Interruptions during hand offs are limited to minimize the possibility that information would fail to be conveyed or would be forgotten.

Goal 3
Improve the safety of using medications.

Requirement 3A

Not applicable

Requirement 3B

Not applicable

Requirement 3C

Identify and, at a minimum, annually review a list of look-alike/sound-alike drugs used by the organization, and take action to prevent errors involving the interchange of these drugs.

Implementation Expectations for Requirement 3C

A 1. Identify a list of look-alike/sound-alike (LASA) drugs used by the organization. (The list must include a minimum of 10 look-alike/sound-alike drug combinations selected from the tables of LASA drugs posted on the Joint Commission Web site.)

A 2. Review the list of look-alike/sound-alike drugs used by the organization at least annually.

A 3. The organization takes action to prevent errors involving the interchange of these drugs.

Requirement 3D

Label all medications, medication containers (for example, syringes, medicine cups, basins), or other solutions on and off the sterile field.

NP SG

Rationale for Requirement 3D

This risk reduction activity is consistent with safe medication practices and addresses a recognized risk point in the safe administration of medications in perioperative and other procedural settings.

Errors, sometimes tragic, have resulted from medications and other solutions removed from their original containers and placed into unlabeled containers. Medications or other solutions in unlabeled containers are unidentifiable. This unsafe practice neglects basic principles of medication management safety, yet has been routine in many organizations with respect to medications transferred to the sterile field.

Implementation Expectations for Requirement 3D

A 1. Medications and solutions both on and off the sterile field are labeled even if there is only one medication being used.

A 2. Labeling occurs when any medication or solution is transferred from the original packaging to another container.

A 3. Labels include the drug name, strength, amount (if not apparent from the container), expiration date when not used within 24 hours, and expiration time when expiration occurs in less than 24 hours.

C Ⓜ 4. All labels are verified both verbally and visually by two qualified individuals when the person preparing the medication is not the person administering the medication.

A 5. No more than one medication or solution is labeled at one time.

A 6. Any medications or solutions found unlabeled are immediately discarded.

C Ⓜ 7. All original containers from medications or solutions remain available for reference in the perioperative/procedural area until the conclusion of the procedure.

A 8. All labeled containers on the sterile field are discarded at the conclusion of the procedure.

C Ⓜ 9. At shift change or break relief, all medications and solutions both on and off the sterile field and their labels are reviewed by entering and exiting personnel.

Anticoagulation Therapy

Requirement 3E

Reduce the likelihood of patient harm associated with the use of anticoagulation therapy.

Note: *This requirement applies only to organizations that provide anticoagulation therapy.*

Rationale for Requirement 3E

Anticoagulation is a high-risk treatment, which commonly leads to adverse drug events due to the complexity of dosing these medications, monitoring their effects, and ensuring patient compliance with outpatient therapy. The use of standardized practices that include patient involvement can reduce the risk of adverse drug events associated with the use of heparin (unfractionated), low molecular weight heparin (LMWH), warfarin, and other anticoagulants.

Note: *This requirement has a one-year phase-in period that includes defined expectations for planning, development, and testing ("milestones") at three, six, and nine months in 2008, with the expectation of full implementation by January 1, 2009.*

A 1. As of April 1, 2008, the organization's leadership has assigned responsibility for oversight and coordination of the development, testing, and implementation of Requirement 3E.

A 2. As of July 1, 2008, an implementation work plan is in place that identifies adequate resources, assigned accountabilities, and a time line for full implementation of Requirement 3E by January 1, 2009.

A 3. As of October 1, 2008, pilot testing in at least one clinical unit is under way.

A 4. As of January 1, 2009, the process is fully implemented across the organization.

The Implementation Expectations that will apply beginning January 1, 2009, are provided below.

Implementation Expectations for Requirement 3E

A 1. The organization implements a defined anticoagulant management program to individualize the care provided to each patient receiving anticoagulant therapy.

A 2. To reduce compounding and labeling errors, the organization uses ONLY oral unit dose products and pre-mixed infusions, when these products are available.

C Ⓜ 3. When pharmacy services are provided by the organization, warfarin is dispensed for each patient in accordance with established monitoring procedures.

C Ⓜ 4. The organization uses approved protocols for the initiation and maintenance of anticoagulation therapy appropriate to the medication used, to the condition being treated, and to the potential for drug interactions.

A Ⓜ 5. For patients being started on warfarin, a baseline International Normalized Ratio (INR) is available, and for all patients receiving warfarin therapy, a current INR is available and is used to monitor and adjust therapy.

C Ⓜ 6. When dietary services are provided by the organization, the service is notified of all patients receiving warfarin and responds according to its established food/drug interaction program.

A 7. When heparin is administered intravenously and continuously, the organization uses programmable infusion pumps.

C Ⓜ 8. The organization has a policy that addresses baseline and ongoing laboratories tests that are required for heparin and low molecular weight heparin therapies.

C Ⓜ 9. The organization provides education regarding anticoagulation therapy to staff, patients, and families.

C Ⓜ 10. Patient/family education includes the importance of follow-up monitoring, compliance issues, dietary restrictions, and potential for adverse drug reactions and interactions.

A 11. The organization evaluates anticoagulation safety practices (*see* MM.8.10).

Goal 4
Not applicable

Goal 5
Not applicable

Goal 6
Not applicable

Goal 7
Reduce the risk of health care–associated infections.

Requirement 7A
Comply with current World Health Organization (WHO) Hand Hygiene Guidelines or Centers for Disease Control and Prevention (CDC) hand hygiene guidelines.

Rationale for Requirement 7A
Compliance with the WHO Hand Hygiene Guidelines or CDC hand hygiene guidelines will reduce the transmission of infectious agents by staff to patients, thereby decreasing the incidence of health care–associated infections.

Implementation Expectation for Requirement 7A
C Ⓜ 1. Comply with current WHO Hand Hygiene Guidelines or Centers for Disease Control and Prevention (CDC) hand hygiene guidelines.*

Requirement 7B
Manage as sentinel events all identified cases of unanticipated death or major permanent loss of function associated with a health care–associated infection.

Rationale for Requirement 7B
A significant percentage of patients who unexpectedly die or suffer major permanent loss of function have health care–associated infections. These unanticipated deaths and injuries meet the definition of a sentinel event and, therefore, are required to undergo a root cause analysis. The root cause analysis should attempt to answer the questions (1) Why did the patient acquire an infection and, (2) Given the fact of the infection, why did the patient die or suffer permanent loss of function?

Implementation Expectations for Requirement 7B
C Ⓜ 1. The organization manages all identified cases of unanticipated death or major permanent loss of function associated with a health care–associated infection as sentinel events (that is, conducts a root cause analysis).

A 2. The root cause analysis addresses the management of the patient before and after the identification of infection.

Goal 8
Accurately and completely reconcile medications across the continuum of care.

* Organizations are required to comply with all 1A, 1B, 1C CDC recommendations or WHO guidelines.

Requirement 8A

There is a process for comparing the patient's current medications with those ordered for the patient while under the care of the organization.

Rationale for Requirement 8A

Patients are most at risk during transitions in care (hand offs) across settings, services, providers, or levels of care. The development, reconciliation, and communication of an accurate medication list throughout the continuum of care is essential in the reduction of transition-related adverse drug events.

Implementation Expectations for Requirement 8A

C Ⓜ 1. The organization, with the patient's involvement, creates a complete list of the patient's current medications at admission/entry.

C Ⓜ 2. The medications ordered for, administered to, or dispensed to the patient while under the care of the organization are compared to those on the list and any discrepancies (for example, omissions, duplications, potential interactions) are resolved.

Requirement 8B

A complete list of the patient's medications is communicated to the next provider of service when a patient is referred or transferred to another setting, service, practitioner, or level of care within or outside the organization. The complete list of medications is also provided to the patient on discharge from the organization.

Implementation Expectations for Requirement 8B

C Ⓜ 1. The patient's accurate medication reconciliation list (complete with medications prescribed by the first provider of service) is communicated to the next provider of service, whether it be within or outside the organization.

C Ⓜ 2. The next provider of service checks the medication reconciliation list again to make sure it is accurate and in concert with any new medications to be ordered/prescribed.

C Ⓜ 3. The complete list of medications is also provided to the patient on discharge from the organization.

Goal 9
Not applicable

Goal 10
Not applicable

Goal 11
Reduce the risk of surgical fires.

Requirement 11A

Educate staff, including operating licensed independent practitioners and anesthesia providers, on how to control heat sources and manage fuels with enough time for patient preparation, and establish guidelines to minimize oxygen concentration under drapes.

Rationale for Requirement 11A

When surgical fires occur, they often result in serious injury and sometimes death. The unique circumstances in the surgical environment (oxygen-rich atmosphere, flammable materials, and ignition sources) require response and prevention strategies to be specific to the setting. Educating surgical staff to these distinctions is crucial in reducing/eliminating surgical fires.

Implementation Expectations for Requirement 11A

A 1. Organizations assess the risk for surgical fires based on equipment and procedures used.

A 2. The organization establishes guidelines to minimize oxygen concentrations under drapes.

C Ⓜ 3. Organizations that identify themselves at risk provide staff training on methods to minimize oxygen concentration under drapes.

C Ⓜ 4. Organizations that identify themselves at risk provide staff training on methods to avoid the use of flammable solutions and materials.

C Ⓜ 5. Organizations that identify themselves at risk provide staff training on actions to take in the event of a surgical fire.

Goal 12
Not applicable

Goal 13
Encourage patients' active involvement in their own care as a patient safety strategy.

Requirement 13A

Define and communicate the means for patients and their families to report concerns about safety and encourage them to do so.

Rationale for Requirement 13A

Communication with patients and families about all aspects of their care, treatment, or services is an important characteristic of a culture of safety. When patients know what to expect, they are more aware of possible errors and choices. Patients can be an important source of information about potential adverse events and hazardous conditions.

Implementation Expectation for Requirement 13A

C Ⓜ 1. Patients and families are educated on methods available to report concerns related to care, treatment, services and patient safety issues.

C Ⓜ 2. The organization encourages patients and their families to report concerns about safety.

Goal 14
Not applicable

Goal 15
Not applicable

Universal Protocol

Wrong site, wrong procedure, wrong person surgery can be prevented. This Universal Protocol for Preventing Wrong Site, Wrong Procedure, Wrong Person Surgery™ is intended to achieve that goal. It is based on the consensus of experts from the relevant clinical specialties and professional disciplines and is endorsed by more than 40 professional medical associations and organizations.

In developing this universal protocol, consensus was reached on the following principles:

- Wrong site, wrong procedure, wrong person surgery can and must be prevented.
- A robust approach—using multiple, complementary strategies—is necessary to achieve the goal of eliminating wrong site, wrong procedure, wrong person surgery.
- Active involvement and effective communication among all members of the surgical team is important for success.
- To the extent possible, the patient (or legally designated representative) should be involved in the process.

- Consistent implementation of a standardized approach using a universal, consensus-based protocol will be most effective.
- The protocol should be flexible enough to allow for implementation with appropriate adaptation when required to meet specific patient needs.
- A requirement for site marking should focus on cases involving right/left distinction, multiple structures (fingers, toes), or levels (spine).
- The universal protocol should be applicable or adaptable to all operative and other invasive procedures that expose patients to harm, including procedures done in settings other than the operating room.

In concert with these principles, the following steps, taken together, comprise the Universal Protocol for eliminating wrong site, wrong procedure, wrong person surgery:

- Pre-operative verification process
  - Purpose: To ensure that all of the relevant documents and studies are available prior to the start of the procedure and that they have been reviewed and are consistent with each other and with the patient's expectations and with the team's understanding of the intended patient, procedure, site, and, as applicable, any implants. Missing information or discrepancies must be addressed before starting the procedure.
  - Process: An ongoing process of information gathering and verification, beginning with the determination to do the procedure, continuing through all settings and interventions involved in the preoperative preparation of the patient, up to and including the "time out" just before the start of the procedure.
- Marking the operative site
  - Purpose: To identify unambiguously the intended site of incision or insertion.
  - Process: For procedures involving right/left distinction, multiple structures (such as fingers and toes), or multiple levels (as in spinal procedures), the intended site must be marked such that the mark will be visible after the patient has been prepped and draped.
- "Time out" immediately before starting the procedure
  - Purpose: To conduct a final verification of the correct patient, procedure, site, and, as applicable, implants.
  - Process: Active communication among all members of the surgical/procedure team, consistently initiated by a designated member of the team, conducted in a "fail-safe" mode, i.e., the procedure is not started until any questions or concerns are resolved.

Universal Protocol 1

The organization fulfills the expectations set forth in the Universal Protocol.

Requirement 1A

Conduct a pre-operative verification process as described in the Universal Protocol.

Implementation Expectations for Requirement 1A

A Ⓜ 1. Verification of the correct person, procedure, and site should occur during the following (as applicable):
- At the time the surgery/procedure is scheduled
- At the time of admission or entry into the facility
- Anytime the responsibility for care of the patient is transferred to another caregiver
- With the patient involved, awake and aware, if possible
- Before the patient leaves the preoperative area or enters the procedure/surgical room

NP SG

A Ⓜ 2. The following is reviewed prior to the start of the procedure:
- Relevant documentation (for example, history and physical, consent)
- Relevant images, properly labeled and displayed
- Any required implants and special equipment

Requirement 1B

Mark the operative site as described in the Universal Protocol.

Implementation Expectations for Requirement 1B

C Ⓜ 1. Make the mark at or near the incision site; do not mark any non-operative site(s) unless necessary for some other aspect of care.

A 2. The mark must be unambiguous. (**Note:** *For example, use initials or "YES" or a line representing the proposed incision; consider that "X" may be ambiguous.*)

C Ⓜ 3. The mark must be positioned to be visible after the patient is prepped and draped.

A 4. The method of marking and type of mark should be consistent throughout the organization.

C Ⓜ 5. At a minimum, mark all cases involving laterality, multiple structures (fingers, toes, lesions), or multiple levels (spine). (**Note:** *In addition to pre-operative skin marking of the general spinal region, special intraoperative radiographic techniques are used for marking the exact vertebral level.*)

C Ⓜ 6. The person performing the procedure should do the site marking.

C Ⓜ 7. Marking must take place with the patient involved, awake and aware, if possible.

Requirement 1C

Conduct a "time out" immediately before starting the procedure as described in the Universal Protocol.

Implementation Expectations for Requirement 1C

C Ⓜ 1. The final verification process must be conducted in the location where the procedure will be done, just before starting the procedure.

A Ⓜ 2. The process must involve the entire operative team, use active communication, and must, at least, include:
- Correct patient identity
- Correct side and site
- Agreement on the procedure to be done
- Correct patient position
- Availability of correct implants and any special equipment or special requirements

C Ⓜ 3. The process is briefly documented, such as in a checklist. (**Note:** *The organization should determine the type and amount of documentation.*)

A 4. The organization should have processes and systems in place for reconciling differences in staff responses during the final verification process.

NP SG

Guidelines for the Universal Protocol for Preventing Wrong Site, Wrong Procedure, Wrong Person Surgery™

These guidelines provide detailed implementation requirements, exemptions, and adaptations for special situations.

1. **Pre-operative verification process**

   Verification of the correct person, procedure, and site should occur (as applicable):
   - At the time the surgery/procedure is scheduled
   - At the time of admission or entry into the facility
   - Anytime the responsibility for care of the patient is transferred to another caregiver
   - With the patient involved, awake and aware, if possible
   - Before the patient leaves the preoperative area or enters the procedure/surgical room

   A pre-operative verification checklist may be helpful to ensure availability and review of the following, prior to the start of the procedure:
   - Relevant documentation (for example, history and physical, consent)
   - Relevant images, properly labeled and displayed
   - Any required implants and special equipment
2. **Marking the operative site**
   - Make the mark at or near the incision site. Do NOT mark any non-operative site(s) unless necessary for some other aspect of care.

- The mark must be unambiguous (for example, use initials or "YES" or a line representing the proposed incision; consider that "X" may be ambiguous).
- The mark must be positioned to be visible after the patient is prepped and draped.
- The mark must be made using a marker that is sufficiently permanent to remain visible after completion of the skin prep. Adhesive site markers should not be used as the sole means of marking the site.
- The method of marking and type of mark should be consistent throughout the organization.
- At a minimum, mark all cases involving laterality, multiple structures (fingers, toes, lesions), or multiple levels (spine). **Note:** *In addition to pre-operative skin marking of the general spinal region, special intraoperative radiographic techniques are used for marking the exact vertebral level.*
- The person performing the procedure should do the site marking.
- Marking must take place with the patient involved, awake and aware, if possible.
- Final verification of the site mark must take place during the "time out."
- A defined procedure must be in place for patients who refuse site marking.
- **Exemptions:**
  - Single organ cases (for example, Cesarean section, cardiac surgery)
  - Interventional cases for which the catheter/instrument insertion site is not predetermined (for example, cardiac catheterization)
  - Teeth—BUT, indicate operative tooth name(s) on documentation *OR* mark the operative tooth (teeth) on the dental radiographs or dental diagram
  - Premature infants, for whom the mark may cause a permanent tattoo

3. **"Time out" immediately before starting the procedure**

   Must be conducted in the location where the procedure will be done, just before starting the procedure. It must involve the entire operative team, use active communication, be briefly documented, such as in a checklist (the organization should determine the type and amount of documentation) and must, at the least, include:
   - Correct patient identity
   - Correct side and site
   - Agreement on the procedure to be done
   - Correct patient position
   - Availability of correct implants and any special equipment or special requirements

   The organization should have processes and systems in place for reconciling differences in staff responses during the "time out."

4. **Procedures for non-OR settings, including bedside procedures.**
   - Site marking must be done for any procedure that involves laterality, multiple structures, or levels (even if the procedure takes place outside of an OR).
   - Verification, site marking, and "time out" procedures should be as consistent as possible throughout the organization, including the OR and other locations where invasive procedures are done.

- Exception: Cases in which the individual doing the procedure is in continuous attendance with the patient from the time of decision to do the procedure and consent from the patient through to the conduct of the procedure may be exempted from the site marking requirement. The requirement for a "time out" final verification still applies.

NP SG

Ambulatory Care Applicability Grid

2008 National Patient Safety Goals

National Patient Safety Goal requirements applicable to ambulatory settings are marked by an "X." This grid is intended to provide general applicability information only. Applicability in each setting is determined by whether or not the setting provides a specific type of care/service/treatment.

Goals and Requirements	ASCs/ OBS	Cath. Lab	Endoscopy	Diagnostic Imaging	Diagnostic Sleep	Therapeutic OT/PT	Correctional Care	Primary Care	Group Practices
1. Patient Identification									
1a (two patient identifiers)	X	X	X	X		X	X	X	X
2. Communication									
2a ("read-back")	X	X	X	X	X	X	X	X	X
2b (abbreviations)	X	X	X	X	X	X	X	X	X
2c (timeliness of reporting critical test results)	X	X	X	X	X	X	X	X	X
2e ("hand-off" communications)	X	X	X	X	X	X	X	X	X
3. Safety of Medications									
3c (list of look-alike/ sound-alike drugs)	X	X	X	X		X	X	X	X
3d (label all medications, medication containers, or other solutions in perioperative and other procedural settings)	X	X	X	X					
7. Health Care–Associated Infections									
7a (CDC guidelines)	X	X	X	X	X	X	X	X	X
7b (sentinel event for deaths associated with infections)	X	X	X	X	X	X	X	X	X
8. Reconcile Medications									
8a (compare current medications with those ordered)	X	X	X	X	X	X	X	X	X
8b (communicate complete list of medications to next provider and patient at discharge)	X		X	X	X	X	X	X	X

Goals and Requirements	ASCs/ OBS	Cath. Lab	Endoscopy	Diagnostic Imaging	Diagnostic Sleep	Therapeutic OT/PT	Correctional Care	Primary Care	Group Practices
11. Reduce Risk of Surgical Fires									
11a (educate staff on managing heat sources and fuels)	X		X		X				
13. Patient Involvement									
13a (communication with patients and families)	X	X	X	X	X	X	X	X	X
Universal Protocol (UP)									
UP 1 Preventing Wrong Site, Wrong Procedure, Wrong Person Surgery	X	X	X	X					
1a (preoperative verification process)	X	X	X	X				X	
1b (mark the operative site)	X	X	X	X				X	
1c (conduct a "time out")	X	X	X	X				X	

NP SG

The following services and settings are listed in the grid:

ASCs/OBS—Ambulatory Surgical Center/Office-Based Surgery Practices (Includes oral/maxillofacial surgery, podiatric surgery, ophthalmology surgery, plastic surgery, and orthopedics.)

Cath. Lab—Catheterization Lab

Endoscopy—Endoscopic/Gastrointestinal Services

Diagnostic Imaging—Diagnostic Imaging Centers

Diagnostic Sleep—Diagnostic Sleep Centers and Labs [**Note:** 11a applies to sleep centers because of oxygen use.]

Therapeutic OT/PT—Occupational Therapy/Physical Therapy Services (includes therapeutic services such as occupational health, rehabilitation, and infusion therapy.) [**Note:** Goal 3 applies to infusion therapy.]

Correctional Care—Includes federal and other prisons, and immigration services.

Primary Care—Includes Community Health Centers, Department of Defense (DOD), Veterans Administration (VA) Clinics, and Medical/Dental Services.

Group Practices

NP
SG

Accreditation Participation Requirements

This chapter includes specific requirements for participation in the accreditation process and for maintaining an accreditation award. These differ from survey eligibility criteria in that the accreditation process may be initiated even when all accreditation participation requirements (APRs) have not yet been met.

For an organization seeking accreditation for the first time, compliance with the APRs is assessed during the initial survey, including the Early Survey Policy Option. For the accredited organization, compliance with these requirements is assessed throughout the accreditation cycle through on-site surveys, the Periodic Performance Review (PPR), Evidence of Standards Compliance (ESCs), and periodic updates of organization-specific data and information. Organizations are either compliant or not compliant with APRs. When an organization does not comply with an APR, the organization will be assigned a requirement for improvement (RFI) in the same context that noncompliance with a standard or element of performance generates an RFI. However, refusal to permit performance of a survey (APR 3) or falsification of information (APR 10), will immediately lead to Preliminary Denial of Accreditation. All RFIs can affect the accreditation decision and follow-up requirements, as determined by established accreditation decision rules. Failure to resolve an RFI can ultimately lead to loss of accreditation.

Application for Accreditation

APR 1

When requested, the organization provides the Joint Commission with all official records and reports of public or publicly recognized licensing (for example, a state license), examining, reviewing, or planning bodies.*

Element of Performance for APR 1

A 1. The organization provides the Joint Commission with all official records and reports of licensing, examining, reviewing, or planning bodies.

APR 2

The organization immediately reports any changes in the information provided in the application for accreditation and any changes made between surveys.†

Rationale for APR 2

An organization that experiences a significant change in ownership or control, location, capacity, or the categories of services offered must notify the Joint Commission in writing not more than 30 days after such changes. The Joint Commission may decide that the organization must be resurveyed when a significant merger or consolidation has taken place. The Joint Commission continues the organization's accreditation until it determines whether a resurvey is necessary. Failure to provide timely notification to the Joint Commission of ownership, merger or consolidation, and service changes may result in interruption or loss of accreditation.

Element of Performance for APR 2

A 1. The organization notifies the Joint Commission not more than 30 days after a significant change in ownership or control, location, capacity, or the categories of services offered.

Acceptance of Survey

APR 3

An organization permits the performance of a survey at the discretion of the Joint Commission.

---

* *See also* page 84 in "The Accreditation Process" chapter.

† *See also* page 64.

Element of Performance for APR 3

A 1. The organization permits the performance of a survey.

Performance Measurement

APRs 4 Through 7

Not applicable

Public Information Interviews

APR 8

The organization provides notices to its publics that when an individual has any concerns about patient care and safety in the organization, that the organization has not addressed, he or she is encouraged to contact the organization's management.

Rationale for APR 8

Methods of notice may include, but are not limited to, distribution of information about The Joint Commission, including contact information in published materials such as admission brochures and/or posting of this information on the organization's Web site.

Element of Performance for APR 8

A 1. The organization provides notices to its publics that when an individual has any concerns about patient care and safety in the organization, that the organization has not addressed, he or she is encouraged to contact the organization's management. If the concerns cannot be resolved through the organization, the individual is to be encouraged by the organization to contact the Joint Commission.*

APR 9

Not applicable

* The public may contact The Joint Commission's Office of Quality Monitoring to report any concerns or register complaints about a Joint Commission–accredited health care organization by either calling 1/800-994-6610 or e-mailing complaint@jointcommission.org.

Misrepresentation of Information

APR 10

The organization does not misrepresent information in the accreditation process.*

Rationale for APR 10

Information provided by the organization and used by the Joint Commission for the accreditation process must be accurate and truthful. Such information may be the following:

- Provided orally
- Obtained through direct observation by Joint Commission surveyors
- Derived from documents supplied by the organization to the Joint Commission

The Joint Commission requires each organization seeking accreditation to engage in the accreditation process in good faith. Any organization that fails to participate in good faith by falsifying information presented in the accreditation process or by failing to exercise due care and diligence to ensure the accuracy of such information may have its accreditation denied or removed by the Joint Commission.

For the purpose of this requirement, falsification is defined as the fabrication, in whole or in part, and through commission or omission, of any information provided by an applicant or accredited organization to the Joint Commission. This includes any redrafting, reformatting, or content deletion of documents. However, the organization may submit additional material that summarizes or otherwise explains the original information submitted to the Joint Commission. These additional materials must be properly identified, dated, and accompanied by the original documents.

Element of Performance for APR 10

A 1. The organization provides accurate and truthful information throughout the accreditation process.

APR 11

The organization does not publicly misrepresent its accreditation status or the scope of facilities and services to which the accreditation applies.*

Rationale for APR 11

Organizations accredited by the Joint Commission must be accurate when describing to the public the nature and meaning of their accreditation. On request, the Joint Commission's Department of Communications will provide accredited organizations with appropriate guidelines for characterizing the accreditation award. An organization may not engage in any false or misleading advertising with respect to

* *See also* pages 22–23

the accreditation award. Any such advertising may be grounds for denying or revoking accreditation.

Elements of Performance for APR 11

A 1. The organization accurately represents its accreditation status as to the scope of facilities and services to which the accreditation applies.

A 2. The organization does not engage in any false or misleading advertising with respect to the accreditation award.

APR 12

Accredited organizations or organizations seeking accreditation are not permitted to use Joint Commission full-time, part-time, or intermittent surveyors to provide any accreditation-related consulting services.

Rationale for APR 12

Consulting services include, but are not limited to, the following:

- Helping an organization to meet Joint Commission standards
- Helping an organization to complete its PPR
- Assisting an organization to remedy areas identified in its PPR as needing improvements
- Conducting mock surveys for an organization
- Providing consultation to an organization to address Priority Focus Process information

Element of Performance for APR 12

A 1. The organization does not use Joint Commission full-time, part-time, or intermittent surveyors to provide any accreditation-related consulting services.

Survey Observers

APR 13

An organization that applies for survey is obligated to accept the Joint Commission's surveyor management staff and/or a member of the Board of Commissioners to observe a survey under the following two specific circumstances:

- Observation and mentoring of surveyors as part of surveyor management and development
- Preceptorship of new surveyors

The observer will not participate in the on-site survey process in any fashion, including the scoring of standards compliance. The presence of an observer will not result in any additional charge to the organization nor will it be accepted as de facto grounds for score revisions or decision appeal.

Element of Performance for APR 13

A 1. The organization accepts the Joint Commission's surveyor management staff and/or a member of the Board of Commissioners to observe a survey under either of the two specific circumstances.

Periodic Performance Review

APR 14

The organization fulfills the Periodic Performance Review requirement annually.

Rationale for APR 14

Full Periodic Performance Review

If the organization does not select one of the options set forth below, it must annually update and transmit to the Joint Commission its Periodic Performance Review (PPR) and, if appropriate, its Plan of Action and identify relevant Measures of Success (MOS). The Plan of Action must address all standards areas identified during the PPR as being not in compliance. Following this submission, the organization may elect to participate in a conference call with Joint Commission staff to reach agreement on the elements of the Plan of Action and MOS and discuss other standards-related issues of their choosing. When an organization's approach to standards compliance is approved by the Joint Commission staff, its design cannot be challenged by surveyors. However, surveyors will evaluate its execution. At the time of the organization's full survey, the surveyors will validate whether the MOS data indicate that performance has been achieved and sustained.

The results of the PPR do not affect an organization's accreditation decision. In the unlikely event that the Joint Commission or the organization identifies a continuing situation that represents a potential immediate threat to health or safety through the PPR, a special announced survey will be initiated to facilitate resolution of the situation.

Option 1

If the organization selects option 1 as an alternative to the full PPR, the organization must annually attest that, after careful consideration with legal counsel, the organization has decided not to participate in the full PPR and instead will complete a PPR and Plan of Action and identify appropriate MOS. The plan of action must address all standards areas identified as being not in compliance. Following completion of these tasks, the organization may elect to participate in a conference call related to standards issues with Joint Commission staff. At the time of the organization's full survey, the surveyors will validate whether the MOS data indicate that performance has been achieved and sustained.

Option 2
If the organization selects option 2 as an alternative to the full PPR, it must annually attest that, after careful consideration with legal counsel, the organization has decided not to participate in the full PPR and instead intends to undergo a limited or full survey. Following the survey, the organization must submit a Plan of Action with appropriate MOS for any recommendation cited as a result of the survey. The organization may elect to participate in a conference call with Joint Commission staff to reach final agreement on the elements of the Plan of Action and MOS. At the time of the organization's full survey, the surveyors will validate whether the MOS data indicate that performance has been achieved and sustained.

Option 3
If the organization selects option 3 as an alternative to the full PPR, it must annually attest that, after careful consideration with legal counsel, it has decided not to participate in the full PPR and instead intends to undergo a limited or full survey with no written report left with the organization. Following the survey, the organization may elect to participate in a conference call to discuss standards-related issues with Joint Commission staff. At the time of the organization's full survey, the surveyors will receive no information relating to the organization's option 3 survey findings.

Element of Performance for APR 14

A 1. The organization annually updates and transmits to the Joint Commission the full PPR and, if appropriate, its Plan of Action.

OR

The organization annually attests that after careful consideration with legal counsel, it has decided not to participate in the full PPR and completes option 1.

OR

The organization annually attests that, after careful consideration with legal counsel, it has decided not to participate in the full PPR and completes option 2.

OR

The organization annually attests that, after careful consideration with legal counsel, it has decided not to participate in the full PPR and completes option 3.

APR 15
Not applicable

APR 16

Not applicable

APR 17

The organization educates its staff that any employee who has concerns about the safety or quality of care provided in the organization may report these concerns to the Joint Commission.

Elements of Performance for APR 17

A 1. The organization educates its staff that any employee who has concerns about the safety or quality of care provided in the organization may report these concerns to the Joint Commission.

A 2. The organization further informs its staff that it will take no disciplinary action because an employee reports safety or quality-of-care concerns to the Joint Commission.

A 3. The organization demonstrates this commitment by taking no retaliatory disciplinary action against employees when they do report safety or quality-of-care concerns to the Joint Commission.

APR 18

The organization adheres to the Joint Commission's published guidelines for describing information in its Quality Report.

Rationale for APR 18

Each organization accredited by the Joint Commission must be truthful and accurate when describing to the public information in its Quality Report. Whether intentionally or otherwise, an organization is not to provide a misleading interpretation or suggest a conclusion other than what the information in its Quality Report conveys.

Element of Performance for APR 18

A 1. The organization adheres to the Joint Commission's published guidelines for describing information in its Quality Report.

APR 19

The organization meets all requirements for timely submissions of data and information to the Joint Commission.

Rationale for APR 19

The cornerstone of the Joint Commission's new accreditation process is the shift from the previous episodic process to a continuous process. As such, in order to realize the full benefit of a more continuous accreditation process, accredited organizations will be required to have regular interactions with the Joint Commission.

Element of Performance for APR 19

A 1. The organization meets all requirements for timely submissions of data and information to the Joint Commission.

Note: *The Joint Commission will impose the following consequences for failure to comply with this APR:*

- *If the organization continues not to comply with the requirement after 31 days, the organization will be placed in Provisional Accreditation*
- *If the organization continues not to comply with the requirement after 61 days, the organization's accreditation decision will be changed from Provisional Accreditation to Conditional Accreditation*
- *If the organization continues not to comply with the requirement after 91 days, the organization's accreditation decision will be changed from Conditional Accreditation to Denial of Accreditation. In accordance with the Accreditation Committee policy, such organizations will not be afforded any appeal.*

The proposed consequences address only compliance with the requirement itself. It does not address the content of the organization's submissions to the Joint Commission. For example, if information in an organization's electronic application leads to inaccuracies in the appropriate length of the survey and a longer survey is required, the organization will incur the additional costs of the longer survey. In addition, if there is evidence that the organization has intentionally falsified the information submitted to the Joint Commission, the *Information Accuracy and Truthfulness Policy* and its consequences will be applicable.

Standards Applicability Grid

Standards Applicability Grid for Ambulatory Care: Ambulatory Care Organizations and Specialized Services and/or Circumstances

Introduction

Not all of the standards in the SAC *apply to all ambulatory care organizations.* Based on the particular services provided by your organization, you should use this grid to identify which standards apply to your organization.

Services/settings are listed horizontally along the top of this grid, while the **functional standards chapters** in this manual are listed vertically along the left margin. Applicability is indicated with "All" and also with "Exceptions," which are not applicable requirements for that particular setting/service.

SA

The following services and settings are listed in the grid:

ASCs—Ambulatory Surgical Centers/Office-Based Surgery Practices (includes oral/maxillofacialsurgery, podiatric surgery, opthalmology surgery, plastic surgery, and orthopedics)
Cath. Labs—Catheterization Labs
Endoscopy—Endoscopic/Gastrointestinal Services
Diagnostic Imaging—Diagnostic Imaging Centers
Diagnostic Sleep—Diagnostic Sleep Centers and Labs
Therapeutic OT/PT—Occupational Therapy/ Physical Therapy Services (includes therapeutic services such as occupational health, rehabilitation, and infusion)
Community Health—Community Health Services
Correctional Care—Includes federal and other prisons, and immigration services
Primary Care—Includes Community Health Centers, Department of Defense, and VA Clinics
Group Practices

Note: *For additional segment-specific applicability information, please consult the Joint Commission's Web site at http://www.jointcommission.org/AccreditationPrograms/AmbulatoryCare/.*

The applicability tables posted online contain element of performance (EP)-specific applicability for each standard, listed by service/setting. The direct link to these tables is as follows: http://www.jointcommission.org/AccreditationPrograms/AmbulatoryCare/Standards/amb_stds_app_grid.htm. This information is updated in January and July.

Standards Applicability Grid for Ambulatory Care: Ambulatory Care Organizations and Specialized Services and/or Circumstances

This applicability grid is provided for general guidance. It indicates the applicability of all the standards and elements of performance (EPs) to each ambulatory care service/setting. However, each organization should review the services and activities it provides against the standards in the *SAC*. Applicability questions may be directed to the Joint Commission's Standards Interpretation Group at 630/792-5900.

Standards Functional Chapters	Standards and EP Applicability by Service/Setting							
	ASCs	Cath Labs/ Endoscopy	Diagnostic Imaging	Diagnostic Sleep	Therapeutic OT/PT	Community Health	Correctional Care	Primary Care/ Group Practices
Ethics, Rights, and Responsibilities (RI)	All	All RI.2.180*	All Except: RI.1.40; RI.2.180* RI.2.160	All RI.2.180*	All RI.2.180*	All RI.2.180*	All RI.2.180*	All RI.2.180*
Provision of Care, Treatment, and Services (PC)	All	All Except: PC.3.230 EP 4; PC.9.10, EP 13; PC.13.20, EPs 15, 16, 17, 18; PC.15.10, EPs 16, 17, 18, 19; PC.15.20; EPs 2, 3, 8 PC.16.10–PC.17.30 PC.13.40 EP 6	All Except: PC.3.230 EP 4; PC.4.10 EPs 12, 13; PC.5.10 EP 4; PC.6.10; PC.7.10; PC.9.10; PC.13.10 EP 1 (last bullet); PC.13.20 EPs 15, 16, 17, 18; PC.13.40 EP 6; PC.15.10 EP 1 (first 3 bullets) & EPs 16, 17, 18, 19; PC.15.20 EPs 2, 3, 8; PC.17.10–PC.17.30	All Except: PC.11.70; PC.11.100; PC.13.10; PC.13.20; PC.13.30; PC.13.40; PC.15.10; PC.15.20; PC.16.10–PC.17.30 PC.3.230 EP 4 PC.9.10 EP 13	All Except: PC.11.70; PC.11.100; PC.13.10; PC.13.20; PC.13.30; PC.13.40; PC.15.10; PC.15.20; PC.16.10–PC.17.30 PC.3.230 EP 4 PC.9.10 EP 13	All Except: PC.13.20, EPs 15, 16, 17, 18; PC.15.10, EPs 16, 17, 18, 19 PC.13.40 EP 6 PC.3.230 EP 4 PC.9.10 EP 13	All Except: PC.13.10; PC.13.20; PC.15.10 EPs 16, 17, 18, 19 PC.13.30 PC.13.40 PC.3.230 EP 4 PC.9.10 EP 13	All Except: PC.11.70; PC.11.100; PC.13.10; PC.13.20; PC.15.10 EPs 16, 17, 18, 19
Medication Management (MM)	All Except: MM.4.50; MM.4.60 EP 2	All Except: MM.3.20 EP 12 MM.6.20 EP 5 MM.7.40 EPs 2, 3	All Except: MM.3.20 EP 12 MM.6.20 EP 5 MM.7.40 EPs 2, 3	All Except: MM.2.10; MM.2.20; MM.3.20; MM.4.10; MM.4.20; MM.4.30; MM.4.40; MM.4.50; MM.4.60; MM.4.70; MM.4.80; MM.5.10; MM.6.10;	All Except: MM.2.10; MM.2.20; MM.3.20; MM.4.10; MM.4.20; MM.4.30; MM.4.40; MM.4.50; MM.4.60; MM.4.70; MM.4.80; MM.5.10; MM.6.10;	All Except: MM.6.20 EP 5 MM.3.20 EP 12	All Except: MM.6.20 EP 5 MM.3.20 EP 12	All Except: MM.6.20 EP 5 MM.3.20 EP 12

* May apply to some settings.

Standards Functional Chapters	Standards and EP Applicability by Service/Setting							
	ASCs	Cath Labs/ Endoscopy	Diagnostic Imaging	Diagnostic Sleep	Therapeutic OT/PT	Community Health	Correctional Care	Primary Care/ Group Practices
MM *(continued)*				MM.6.20; MM.7.10; MM.7.40; MM.8.10	MM.6.20; MM.7.10; MM.7.40; MM.8.10			
Surveillance, Prevention, and Control of Infection (IC)	All	All Except: IC.4.10 EP 8	All	All	All	All	All	All
Improving Organization Performance (PI)	All	All Except: PI.1.10 EPs 23, 24	All Except: PI.1.10 EPs 5, 23, 24; PI.2.20 EPs 4, 7	All Except: PI.1.10 EPs 23, 24	All Except: PI.1.10 EPs 23, 24	All Except: PI.1.10 EPs 23, 24	All Except: PI.1.10 EPs 23, 24	All Except: PI.1.10 EPs 23, 24
Leadership (LD)	All	All	All	All	All	All	All	All
Management of the Environment of Care (EC)	All	All Except: EC.5.10 EP 5; EC.7.20 EPs 5, 9, 10, 14, 15; EC.8.10 EPs 12, 14	All Except: EC.5.10 EP 5; EC.7.20 EPs 5, 9, 10, 14, 15; EC.8.10 EPs 12, 14	All Except: EC.5.10 EP 5; EC.7.20 EPs 5, 9, 10, 14, 15; EC.8.10 EPs 12, 14	All Except: EC.5.10 EP 5; EC.7.20 EPs 5, 9, 10, 14, 15; EC.8.10 EPs 12, 14	All Except: EC.5.10 EP 5; EC.7.20 EPs 5, 14, 15; EC.8.10 EPs 12, 14	All Except: EC.5.10 EP 5; EC.7.20 EPs 5; EC.8.10 EPs 12, 14	All Except: EC.5.10 EP 5; EC.7.20 EPs 5, 14,† 15;† EC.8.10 EPs 12, 14
Management of Human Resources (HR)	All	All Except: HR.1.10 EPs 5, 12, 13, 14, 15; HR.4.10 EPs 9, 10; HR.4.20 EPs 15, 16; HR.4.20 EPs 17–22;* HR.4.32;* HR.4.33; HR.4.34; HR.4.35	All Except: HR.1.10 EPs 5, 12, 13, 14, 15; HR.4.10 EPs 9, 10; HR.4.20 EPs 15, 16; HR.4.20 EPs 17–22;* HR.4.32;* HR.4.33; HR.4.34; HR.4.35	All Except: HR.1.10 EPs 5, 12, 13, 14, 15; HR.4.10 EPs 9, 10; HR.4.20 EPs 15, 16; HR.4.20 EPs 17–22;* HR.4.32;* HR.4.33; HR.4.34; HR.4.35	All Except: HR.1.10 EPs 5, 12, 13, 14, 15; HR.4.10 EPs 9, 10; HR.4.20 EPs 15, 16; HR.4.20 EPs 17–22;* HR.4.32;* HR.4.33; HR.4.34; HR.4.35	All Except: HR.1.10 EPs 5, 12, 13, 14, 15; HR.4.10 EPs 9, 10; HR.4.20 EPs 15, 16; HR.4.20 EPs 17–22;* HR.4.32;* HR.4.33; HR.4.34	All Except: HR.1.10 EPs 5, 12, 13, 14, 15; HR.4.10 EPs 9, 10; HR.4.20 EPs 15, 16; HR.4.20 EPs 17–22;* HR.4.32;* HR.4.33; HR.4.34; HR.4.35	All Except: HR.1.10 EPs 5, 15, 16, 17, 18; HR.4.10 EPs 9, 10; HR.4.20 EPs 15, 16; HR.4.20 EPs 17–22;* HR.4.32;* HR.4.33; HR.4.34; HR.4.35
Management of Information (IM)	All	All Except: IM.6.20 EP 5; IM.6.30 EP 9	All Except: IM.6.20 EP 5; IM.6.30	All Except: IM.6.20 EP 5; IM.6.30	All Except: IM.6.20 EP 5; IM.6.30	All Except: IM.6.20 EP 5; IM.6.30	All Except: IM.6.20 EP 5; IM.6.30	All Except: IM.6.20 EP 5; IM.6.30

* May apply to some settings.

† May be applicable to some group practices.

Ethics, Rights, and Responsibilities

Overview

The **goal** of the ethics, rights, and responsibilities function is to improve care, treatment, services, and outcomes by recognizing and respecting the rights of each patient and by conducting business in an ethical manner. Care, treatment, and services are provided in a way that respects and fosters dignity, autonomy, positive self-regard, civil rights, and involvement of patients. Care, treatment, and services consider the patient's abilities and resources, the relevant demands of his or her environment, and the requirements and expectations of the providers and those they serve. The family is involved in care, treatment, and service decisions with the patient's approval.

An organization's adherence to ethical care and business practices significantly affects the patient's experience of and response to care, treatment, and services. The standards in this chapter address the following processes and activities related to ethical care and business practices:

- Managing the organization's relationships with patients and the public in an ethical manner
- Considering the values and preferences of patients, including the decision to discontinue care, treatment, and services
- Helping patients understand and exercise their rights
- Informing patients of their responsibilities in care, treatment, and services
- Recognizing the organization's responsibilities under law

Patients deserve care, treatment, and services that safeguard their personal dignity and respect their cultural, psychosocial, and spiritual values. These values often influence the patient's perceptions and needs. By understanding and respecting these values, providers can meet care, treatment, and service needs and preferences.

Standards

The following is a list of all standards for this function. They are presented here for your convenience without footnotes or other explanatory text. If you have a question about a term used here, please check the Glossary.

Note: *A revised standard numbering system is being used with the reformatted standards. This revised numbering system will allow for more flexibility to add standards while maintaining the current label for each standard.*

Organization Ethics

RI.1.10 The organization follows ethical behavior in its care, treatment, and services and business practices.

RI.1.20 The organization addresses conflicts of interest.

RI.1.30 The integrity of decisions is based on identified care, treatment, and service needs of the patients.

RI.1.40 When internal or external review results in the denial of care, treatment, services, or payment, the organization makes decisions regarding the ongoing provision of care, treatment, and services, discharge or transfer based on the assessed needs of the patients.

Individual Rights

RI.2.10 The organization respects the rights of patients.

RI.2.20 Patients receive information about their rights.

RI.2.30 Patients are involved in decisions about care, treatment, and services provided.

RI.2.40 Informed consent is obtained.

RI.2.50 Consent is obtained for recording or filming made for purposes other than the identification, diagnosis, or treatment of the patients.

RI.2.60 Patients receive adequate information about the person(s) responsible for the delivery of their care, treatment, and services.

RI.2.70 Patients have the right to refuse care, treatment, and services in accordance with law and regulation.

RI.2.80 The organization addresses the wishes of the patient relating to end-of-life decisions.

RI.2.90 Patients and, when appropriate, their families are informed about the outcomes of care, treatment, and services that have been provided, including unanticipated outcomes.

RI.2.100 The organization respects the patient's right to and need for effective communication.

RI.2.110 Not applicable

RI.2.120 The organization addresses the resolution of complaints from patients and their families.

RI.2.130 The organization respects the needs of patients for confidentiality, privacy, and security.

RI.2.140 Not applicable

RI.2.150 Patients have the right to be free from mental, physical, sexual, and verbal abuse, neglect, and exploitation.

RI.2.160 Patients have the right to pain management.

RI.2.170 Not applicable

Applicable to Ambulatory Care Organizations Participating in Research

RI.2.180 The organization protects research subjects and respects their rights during research, investigation, and clinical trials involving human subjects.

RI.2.190 Through RI.2.320 Not applicable

Individual Responsibilities

RI.3.10 Patients are given information about their responsibilities while receiving care, treatment, and services.

Standards, Rationales, Elements of Performance, and Scoring

Organization Ethics

Introduction

An organization has an ethical responsibility to the patients and community it serves. To fulfill this responsibility, ethical care, treatment, and service practices and ethical business practices must go hand in hand. Furthermore, the organization provides care, treatment, and services within its scope, stated mission and philosophy, and applicable law and regulation.

The organization's system of ethics supports honest and appropriate interactions with patients. The system of ethics also includes patients whenever possible in decisions about their care, treatment, and services, including ethical issues.

Standard RI.1.10

The organization follows ethical behavior in its care, treatment, and services and business practices.

Elements of Performance for RI.1.10

B 1. The organization identifies ethical issues and issues prone to conflict.

B 2. The organization develops a process to handle these ethical issues that are prone to conflict and implements a process when these issues arise.

B 3. The organization's policies and procedures reflect ethical practices for marketing, admission, transfer, discharge, and billing.

B 4. Marketing materials accurately represent the organization and address the care, treatment, and services that the organization can provide, directly or by contractual arrangement.

C Ⓜ 5. Patients receive information about charges for which they will be responsible.

B 6. The effectiveness and safety of care, treatment, and services does not depend on the patient's ability to pay.

C Ⓜ 7. The leaders ensure that care, treatment, and services are not negatively affected when the organization grants a staff member's request to be excused from participating in an aspect of the care, treatment, and services.

Standard RI.1.20

The organization addresses conflicts of interest.

Rationale for RI.1.20

Potential conflicts of interest can arise in subtle and obvious circumstances. The organization needs to be aware of potential conflicts of interest and review relationships with other entities carefully to ensure that its mission and responsibility to the patients and community it serves are not harmed by any professional, ownership, contractual, or other relationships.

Elements of Performance for RI.1.20

A 1. The organization defines what constitutes a *conflict of interest*.

C Ⓜ 2. The organization discloses existing or potential conflicts of interest for those who provide care, treatment, and services as well as governance.

B 3. The organization reviews its relationship and its staff's relationships with other care providers, educational institutions, and payers to ensure that those relationships are within law and regulation and determine if conflicts of interest exist.

B 4. The organization addresses conflicts of interest when they arise.

RI

Standard RI.1.30

The integrity of decisions is based on identified care, treatment, and service needs of the patients.

Rationale for RI.1.30

Decisions are based on the patients' care, treatment, and service needs, regardless of how the organization compensates or shares financial risk with its leaders, managers, staff, and licensed independent practitioners.

Elements of Performance for RI.1.30

B 1. The organization has policies and procedures that address the integrity of clinical decision making.

C Ⓜ 2. To avoid compromising the quality of care, decisions are based on the patient's identified care, treatment, and service needs and in accordance with organization policy.

B 3. Policies, procedures, information about the relationship between the use of care, treatment, and services, and financial incentives, as they relate to either referring to or using services, are available to all patients, staff, licensed independent practitioners, and contracted providers, when requested.

Standard RI.1.40

When internal or external review results in the denial of care, treatment, services, or payment, the organization makes decisions regarding the ongoing provision of care, treatment, and services, discharge or transfer based on the assessed needs of the patients.

Rationale for RI.1.40

When an individual requests or presents for care, treatment, and services, the organization is professionally and ethically responsible for providing care, treatment, and services within its capability, mission, and applicable law and regulation. At times, indications for such care, treatment, and services can contradict the recommendations of an external entity performing a utilization review (for example, insurance companies, managed care reviewers, and federal or state payers). If such a conflict arises, care, treatment, service, and discharge decisions are made based on the patients' identified needs, regardless of the recommendations of the external agency.

Elements of Performance for RI.1.40

C Ⓜ 1. The organization makes decisions regarding the provision of ongoing care, treatment, services, or discharge based on the care, treatment, and services required by the patient.

C Ⓜ 2. The patient and/or the family is involved in these decisions.

Individual Rights

Introduction

A mere list of rights cannot guarantee those rights. Rather, an organization shows its support of rights by how its staff interacts with patients and involves them in decisions about their care, treatment, and services. These standards focus on how the organization respects the culture and rights of patients during those interactions. This begins with respecting their right to treatment, care, and service.

Standard RI.2.10

The organization respects the rights of patients.

Elements of Performance for RI.2.10

B 1. The organization's policies and practices address the rights of patients to care, treatment, and services within its capability and mission and in compliance with law and regulation.

C Ⓜ 2. Each patient has a right to have his or her cultural, psychosocial, spiritual, and personal values, beliefs, and preferences respected.

C Ⓜ 3. The organization supports the right of each patient to personal dignity.

Standard RI.2.20

Patients receive information about their rights.

Elements of Performance for RI.2.20

1. Not applicable

B 2. Information about patient rights is readily accessible.

3. Not applicable

4. Not applicable

5. Not applicable

C Ⓜ 6. The patient has the right to access, request amendment to, and receive an accounting of disclosures regarding his or her own health information as permitted under applicable law.

Standard RI.2.30

Patients are involved in decisions about care, treatment, and services provided.

Rationale for RI.2.30

Making decisions about care, treatment, and services sometimes presents questions, conflicts, or other dilemmas for the organization and the patients, family, or other decision makers. These dilemmas may involve issues about admission; care, treatment, and services; or discharge. The organization works with patients, and when appropriate, their families, to resolve such dilemmas.

Elements of Performance for RI.2.30

C Ⓜ 1. Patients are involved in decisions about their care, treatment, and services.

C Ⓜ 2. Patients are involved in resolving dilemmas about care, treatment, and services.

C Ⓜ 3. A surrogate decision maker, as allowed by law, is identified when a patient cannot make decisions about his or her care, treatment, and service.

C Ⓜ 4. The legally responsible representative approves care, treatment, and service decisions.*

* In some states, law dictates that urgent care, family planning, and/or behavioral health services can be provided to a minor without the approval or consent of a parent or guardian.

C Ⓜ 5. The family, as appropriate and as allowed by law, with permission of the patient or surrogate decision maker, is involved in care, treatment, and service decisions.

C Ⓜ 6. Information about diagnosis and prognosis is provided to the patient and family.

Standard RI.2.40

Informed consent is obtained.

Rationale for RI.2.40

The goal of the informed consent process is to establish a mutual understanding between the patient and the physician or other licensed independent practitioner who provides the care, treatment, and services about the care, treatment, and services that the patient receives. This process allows each patient to fully participate in decisions about his or her care, treatment, and services.

Elements of Performance for RI.2.40

B 1. The organization's policies describe the following:
- Which, if any, procedures or care, treatment, and services provided require informed consent
- The process used to obtain informed consent
- How informed consent is to be documented in the record
- When a surrogate decision maker, rather than the patient, may give informed consent
- When procedures or care, treatment, and services normally requiring informed consent may be given without informed consent

C Ⓜ 2. Informed consent is obtained and documented in accordance with the organization's policy.

B 3. A complete informed consent process includes a discussion of the following elements:*
- The nature of the proposed care, treatment, services, medications, interventions, or procedures
- Potential benefits, risks, or side effects, including potential problems that might occur during recuperation
- The likelihood of achieving goals
- Reasonable alternatives
- The relevant risks, benefits, and side effects related to alternatives, including the possible results of not receiving care, treatment, and services
- When indicated, any limitations on the confidentiality of information learned from or about the patient

* Documentation of the items listed in EP 3 may be in a form, progress notes, or elsewhere in the record.

Standard RI.2.50

Consent is obtained for recording or filming* made for purposes other than the identification, diagnosis, or treatment of the patients.

Rationale for RI.2.50

Recording or filming of care, treatment, and services provided to patients can be useful for many purposes, but such recording or filming is likely to compromise the patient's privacy and confidentiality. Therefore, the organization should obtain consent from the patient for recording or filming.

Elements of Performance for RI.2.50

C Ⓜ 1. When recording or filming are to be used only for internal organizational purposes (for example, performance improvement and education), there is documentation of consent, which may be obtained as part of general consent to treatment or another form, if a statement is included in the form regarding the use of recording or filming for such internal purposes.

C Ⓜ 2. When recordings or films are made for external purposes that will be heard or seen by the public (for example, commercial filming, television programs, marketing), there is documentation of a specific, separate consent that includes the circumstances of the use of the recording or film.

C Ⓜ 3. Except for the circumstances set forth in EP 4 (below), there is documentation of consent before recording or filming.

C Ⓜ 4. The following occurs in situations in which the patient is unable to give informed consent before recording or filming:

- The recording or filming may occur before consent, provided it is within the established policy of the organization and the policy is established through an appropriate ethical mechanism (for example, an ethics committee) that includes community input
- The recording or film remains in the organization's possession and is not used for any purpose until and unless consent is obtained
- If consent for use cannot subsequently be obtained, the recording or film is either destroyed or the nonconsenting patient must be removed from the recording or film

A 5. Patients have the right to request cessation of recording or filming.

A 6. Patients have the right to rescind consent for use up until a reasonable time before the recording or film is used.

C Ⓜ 7. Anyone who engages in recording or filming (who is not already bound by the organization's confidentiality policy) signs a confidentiality statement to protect the patient's identity and confidential information.

---

* Recording or filming refers to photographic, video, electronic, or audio media.

Standard RI.2.60

Patients receive adequate information about the person(s) responsible for the delivery of their care, treatment, and services.

Elements of Performance for RI.2.60

C Ⓜ 1. The information provided includes the following:
- The name of the physician or other practitioner primarily responsible for their care, treatment, and services
- The name of the physician or other practitioner who will provide the care, treatment, and services

C Ⓜ 2. The information is given to the patient on a timely basis as defined by the organization.

Standard RI.2.70

Patients have the right to refuse care, treatment, and services in accordance with law and regulation.

Elements of Performance for RI.2.70

A 1. Patients have the right to refuse care, treatment, and services in accordance with law and regulation.

A 2. When the patient is not legally responsible, the surrogate decision maker, as allowed by law, has the right to refuse care, treatment, and services on the patient's behalf.

Standard RI.2.80

The organization addresses the wishes of the patient relating to end-of-life decisions.

Elements of Performance for RI.2.80

1. Through 9. Not applicable

B 10. The organization's policies address advance directives and specify whether the organization will honor the directives.

C Ⓜ 11. The policies are communicated to patients and families when asked about or as appropriate to the care, treatment, and services provided.

C Ⓜ 12. Upon request, the organization helps patients formulate medical advance directives or refers them for assistance.

13. Through 20. Not applicable

C Ⓜ 21. The policies are consistently implemented.

Standard RI.2.90

Patients and, when appropriate, their families are informed about the outcomes of care, treatment, and services that have been provided, including unanticipated outcomes.

Elements of Performance for RI.2.90

At a minimum, the patient and, when appropriate, his or her family, is informed about the following (EPs 1–2):

C Ⓜ 1. Outcomes of care, treatment, and services that have been provided that the patient (or family) must be knowledgeable about to participate in current and future decisions affecting the patient's care, treatment, and services

C Ⓜ 2. Unanticipated outcomes of care, treatment, and services that relate to sentinel events considered reviewable* by the Joint Commission

C Ⓜ 3. The responsible licensed independent practitioner or his or her designee informs the patient (and, when appropriate, his or her family) about those unanticipated outcomes of care, treatment, and services related to sentinel events, when the patient is not already aware of the occurrence, or further discussion is needed (*see* EP 2 above).†

Standard RI.2.100

The organization respects the patient's right to and need for effective communication.

Rationale for RI.2.100

The patient has the right to receive information in a manner that he or she understands. This includes communication between the organization and the patient, as well as communication between the patient and others outside the organization.

Elements of Performance for RI.2.100

B 1. The organization respects the right and need of patients for effective communication.

B 2. Written information provided is appropriate to the age, understanding, and, as appropriate to the population served, the language of the patient.

C Ⓜ 3. The organization provides interpretation (including translation) services as necessary.

C Ⓜ 4. The organization addresses the needs of those with vision, speech, hearing, language, and cognitive impairments.

---

* *See* the "Sentinel Events" (SE) chapter of this book for a definition of reviewable sentinel events.

† In settings where there is no licensed independent practitioner, the staff member responsible for the care of the patient is responsible for sharing information about such outcomes.

Standard RI.2.110

Not applicable

Standard RI.2.120

The organization addresses the resolution of complaints from patients and their families.

Elements of Performance for RI.2.120

C Ⓜ 1. The organization informs patients, families, and staff about the complaint resolution process.

C Ⓜ 2. The organization receives, reviews, and, when possible, resolves complaints from patients and their families.

Standard RI.2.130

The organization respects the needs of patients for confidentiality, privacy, and security.

Rationale for RI.2.130

This standard and its EPs allow flexibility in how an organization can accomplish this requirement. Privacy, safety, and security can be demonstrated in various ways, for example, via policies and procedures, practices, or the design of the environment.

Elements of Performance for RI.2.130

C Ⓜ 1. The organization protects confidentiality of information about patients.

C Ⓜ 2. The organization respects the privacy of patients.

3. Not applicable

C Ⓜ 4. The organization provides for the safety and security of patients and their property.

Standard RI.2.140

Not applicable

Standard RI.2.150

Patients have the right to be free from mental, physical, sexual, and verbal abuse, neglect, and exploitation.*

Note: See *standard PC.3.10, which addresses assessing and reporting of abuse, neglect, and exploitation.*

* Taking advantage of another for one's own advantage or benefit.

Elements of Performance for RI.2.150

B 1. The organization addresses how it will, to the best of its ability, protect patients from real or perceived abuse, neglect, or exploitation from anyone, including staff, students, volunteers, other patients, visitors, or family members.

C Ⓜ 2. All allegations, observations, or suspected cases of abuse, neglect, or exploitation that occur in the organization are explored by the organization and, based on the type of event, are referred to the appropriate authorities for investigation.

Standard RI.2.160

Patients have the right to pain management.

Rationale for RI.2.160

Patients may experience pain. Unrelieved pain has adverse physical and psychological effects. The organization respects and supports the right of patients to pain management. In accordance with the organization's mission, this may occur through referral.

Element of Performance for RI.2.160

B 1. The organization plans, supports, and coordinates activities and resources to ensure that pain is recognized and addressed appropriately and in accordance with the care, treatment, and services provided including the following:
- Assessing for pain
- Educating all relevant providers about assessing and managing pain
- Educating patients and families, when appropriate, about their roles in managing pain and the potential limitations and side effects of pain treatments

Standard RI.2.170

Not applicable

Applicable to Ambulatory Care Organizations Participating in Research

Standard RI.2.180

The organization protects research subjects and respects their rights during research, investigation, and clinical trials involving human subjects.

Rationale for RI.2.180

An organization that conducts research, investigations, or clinical trials involving human subjects knows that its first responsibility is to the health and well being of the research subjects. To protect and respect the research subjects' rights, the organization reviews all research protocols. If another institution's Institutional Review Board (IRB) reviews the research protocols, the organization does not need to perform this activity.

Elements of Performance for RI.2.180

C Ⓜ 1. The organization reviews all research protocols in relation to its mission, values, and other guidelines and weighs the relative risks and benefits to the research subjects.

C Ⓜ 2. The organization provides patients who are potential subjects in research, investigation, and clinical trials with adequate information* to participate or refuse to participate in research.

C Ⓜ 3. Patients are informed that refusing to participate or discontinuing participation at any time will not compromise their access to care, treatment, and services not related to the research.

C Ⓜ 4. Consent forms address the above elements of performance; indicate the name of the person who provided the information and the date the form was signed; and address the participant's right to privacy, confidentiality, and safety.

C Ⓜ 5. Subjects are told the extent to which their personally identifiable private information will be held in confidence.

C Ⓜ 6. All information given to subjects is in the medical record or research file along with the consent forms.

C Ⓜ 7. If a research-related injury (that is, physical, psychological, social, financial, or otherwise) occurs, the principal investigator attempts to address any harmful consequences the subject may have experienced as a result of research procedures.

Individual Responsibilities

Introduction

The safety of health care delivery is enhanced when patients, as appropriate to their condition, are partners in the health care process. Additionally, organizations are entitled to reasonable and responsible behavior on the part of the patients, within their capabilities, and their families. The organization identifies the responsibilities of the patients and their families and educates them about these responsibilities, particularly in regard to facilitating the safe delivery of care, treatment, and services.

---

* **Adequate information** includes an explanation of the purpose of the research and expected duration of the subject's participation; a description of expected benefits, potential discomforts, and risks; alternative services that might prove advantageous to the individual; and a full explanation of the procedures to be followed.

The statement of responsibilities includes at least the following:

- **Providing information.** Patients and families, as appropriate, must provide, to the best of their knowledge, accurate and complete information about present complaints, past illnesses, hospitalization, medications, and other matters relating to their health. Patients and their families must report perceived risks in their care and unexpected changes in their condition. They can help the organization understand their environment by providing feedback about service needs and expectations.
- **Asking questions.** Patients and families, as appropriate, must ask questions when they do not understand their care, treatment, and service or what they are expected to do.
- **Following instructions.** Patients and their families must follow the care, treatment, and service plan developed. They should express any concerns about their ability to follow the proposed care plan or course of care, treatment, and services. The organization makes every effort to adapt the plan to the specific needs and limitations of the patients. When such adaptations to the care, treatment, and service plan are not recommended, patients and their families are informed of the consequences of the care, treatment, and service alternatives and not following the proposed course.
- **Accepting consequences.** Patients and their families are responsible for the outcomes if they do not follow the care, treatment, and service plan.
- **Following rules and regulations.** Patients and their families must follow the organization's rules and regulations.
- **Showing respect and consideration.** Patients and their families must be considerate of the organization's staff and property, as well as other patients and their property.
- **Meeting financial commitments.** Patients and their families should promptly meet any financial obligation agreed to with the organization.

Standards RI.2.190 Through RI.2.320

Not applicable

Standard RI.3.10

Patients are given information about their responsibilities while receiving care, treatment, and services.

Elements of Performance for RI.3.10

B 1. The organization has a policy that defines the mechanism for communicating responsibilities of patients.

B 2. The policy includes the responsibilities for providing information, asking questions, following instructions, accepting consequences, following rules and regulations, showing respect and consideration, and meeting financial commitments.

C Ⓜ 3. Patients are informed about their responsibilities verbally, in writing, or both, based on organization policy.

C Ⓜ 4. Patients are informed about their responsibilities initially and as needed thereafter.

Provision of Care, Treatment, and Services*

Overview

Care, treatment, and services are provided through the successful coordination and completion of a series of processes that include appropriate initial assessment of needs; development of a plan for care, treatment, and services; the provision of care, treatment, and services; ongoing assessment of whether the care, treatment, and services provided are meeting the patient's needs; and either the successful discharge of the patient or referral or transfer of the patient for continuing care, treatment, and services.

The provision of care, treatment, and services to patients is composed of four core processes or elements:

1. Assessing patient needs
2. Planning care, treatment, and services
3. Providing the care, treatment, and services the patient needs
4. Coordinating care, treatment, and services

These core elements may also include the following activities:

- Providing access to the appropriate levels of care and/or disciplines for patients
- Providing interventions based on the plan for care, treatment, and services
- Teaching patients what they need to know about their care, treatment, and services
- Coordinating care, treatment, and services, if needed, when the patient is referred, transferred, or discharged

The elements that make up the provision of care, treatment, and services are related to each other through an integrated and cyclical process that may occur over minutes, hours, days, weeks, months, or years, depending on the setting and the needs of the patient. This cyclical process may occur among multiple organizations or within a single organization. The standards in this chapter address the processes in this cycle, including those provided for patient populations with unique needs or patients who are receiving interventions or services that are problem prone.

The core processes or elements of the provision of care, treatment, and services should not be seen as separate steps, but rather as interrelated activities in an integrated and ongoing care process. The activities related to the provision of care, treatment, and services should be capable of moving easily between elements as required to meet patients' needs and maintain the continuity of care, treatment, and services.

---

* This chapter is a compilation of the former "Assessment," "Care," "Education," and "Continuum of Care" chapters.

Standards

The following is a list of all standards for this function. They are presented here for your convenience without footnotes or other explanatory text. If you have a question about a term used here, please check the Glossary.

Note: *A revised standard numbering system is being used with the reformatted standards. The revised numbering system will allow for more flexibility to add standards while maintaining the current number for each standard.*

Entry to Care, Treatment, and Services

PC.1.10 The organization accepts for care, treatment, and services only those patients whose identified care, treatment, and service needs it can meet.

Assessment

PC.2.10 Not applicable

PC.2.20 The organization defines in writing the data and information gathered during assessment and reassessment.

PC.2.30 Through PC.2.110 Not applicable

PC.2.120 The organization defines in writing the time frame(s) for conducting the initial assessment(s).

PC.2.130 Initial assessments are performed as defined by the organization.

PC.2.140 Not applicable

PC.2.150 Patients are reassessed as needed.

Additional Standards for Victims of Abuse

PC.3.10 Patients who may be victims of abuse or neglect are assessed. (*See* standard RI.2.150.)

PC.3.20 Through PC.3.220 Not applicable

Diagnostic Services

PC.3.230 Diagnostic testing necessary for determining the patient's health care needs is performed.

Planning Care, Treatment, and Services

PC.4.10 Development of a plan for care, treatment, and services is individualized and appropriate to the patient's needs, strengths, limitations and goals.

PC.4.20 Through PC.4.120 Not applicable

Providing Care, Treatment, and Services

PC.5.10 The organization provides care, treatment, and services for each patient according to the plan for care, treatment, and services.

PC.5.20 Not applicable

PC.5.30 Not applicable

PC.5.40 Not applicable

PC.5.50 Care, treatment, and services are provided in an interdisciplinary, collaborative manner.

PC.5.60 The organization coordinates the care, treatment, and services provided to a patient as part of the plan for care, treatment, and services and consistent with the organization's scope of care, treatment, and services.

PC

PC.5.70 Not applicable

Education

PC.6.10 The patient receives education and training specific to the patient's needs and as appropriate to the care, treatment, and services provided.

PC.6.20 Not applicable

PC.6.30 The patient receives education and training specific to the patient's abilities as appropriate to the care, treatment, and services provided by the organization.

PC.6.40 Through PC.6.180 Not applicable

Nutritional Care

PC.7.10 The organization has a process for preparing and/or distributing food and nutrition products as appropriate to the care, treatment, and services provided.

Pain

PC.8.10 Pain is assessed in all patients.

PC.8.20 Through PC.8.70 Not applicable

Specific Procedures

Administering Blood and Blood Components

PC.9.10 Blood and blood components are administered safely, as appropriate to the setting.

Responding to Life-Threatening Emergencies

PC.9.20 The organization responds to life-threatening emergencies according to organization policy and procedure.

PC.9.30 Through PC.10.130 Not applicable

Restraint and Seclusion

PC.11.10 Through PC.11.60 Not applicable

PC

PC.11.70 Patients in restraint are monitored.

PC.11.80 Not applicable

PC.11.90 Not applicable

PC.11.100 Each episode of restraint use is documented in the patient's medical record, consistent with organization policies and procedures.

PC.12.10 Through PC.12.190 Not applicable

Operative or Other High-Risk Procedures and/or the Administration of Moderate or Deep Sedation or Anesthesia

PC.13.10 Licensed independent practitioners define the scope of assessment for operative or other procedures and/or the administration of moderate or deep sedation or anesthesia.

PC.13.20 Operative or other procedures and/or the administration of moderate or deep sedation or anesthesia are planned.

PC.13.30 Patients are monitored during the procedure and/or administration of moderate or deep sedation or anesthesia.

PC.13.40 Patients are monitored immediately after the procedure and/or administration of moderate or deep sedation or anesthesia.

PC.13.50 Through PC.14.30 Not applicable

Discharge or Transfer from the Organization

PC.15.10 A process addresses the needs for continuing care, treatment, and services after discharge or transfer.

PC.15.20 The transfer or discharge of a patient to another level of care, treatment, and services, different professionals, or different settings is based on the patient's assessed needs and the organization's capabilities.

PC.15.30 When patients are transferred or discharged, appropriate information related to the care, treatment, and services provided is exchanged with other service providers.

PC.15.40 Not applicable

PC.15.50 Not applicable

Waived Testing

PC.16.10 The director named on the CLIA certificate establishes policies and procedures that define the context in which waived test results are used in patient care, treatment, and services.

PC.16.20 The director named on the CLIA certificate identifies the staff responsible for performing and supervising waived testing.

PC.16.30 Staff receive specific training and orientation for the tests they perform, and demonstrate satisfactory levels of competence.

PC.16.40 Policies and procedures governing specific testing-related processes are current, approved, and readily available.

PC.16.50 Quality control checks are conducted on each procedure.

PC.16.60 Quality control and test result records are maintained.

Tissue Storage and Issuance

PC.17.10 The organization uses standardized procedures to acquire, receive, store, and issue tissues.

PC.17.20 The organization's record keeping permits bi-directional traceability of all tissues.

PC.17.30 The organization has a defined process to investigate adverse events to tissue or donor infections.

Standards, Rationales, Elements of Performance, and Scoring

Entry To Care, Treatment, And Services

Introduction

Agreeing to provide care, treatment, and services for a patient should be based both on the patient's needs and the scope of the services provided by the organization. To do this, the organization does the following:

- Establishes criteria to determine entry eligibility
- Defines the minimum information necessary to determine the patient's eligibility for entry to a program or service
- Defines the appropriate professionals and settings needed to provide the services offered consistent with the organization's mission
- Makes entry decisions for appropriate care, treatment, and services offered by the organization based on these criteria

Standard PC.1.10

The organization accepts for care, treatment, and services only those patients whose identified care, treatment, and service needs it can meet.

Elements of Performance for PC.1.10

B 1. The organization has a defined written process that includes the following:
- The information to be gathered to determine eligibility for entrance into the organization
- The populations of patients accepted or not accepted by the organization (for example, programs designed to treat adults that do not treat young children)
- The criteria to determine eligibility for entry into the system
- The procedures for accepting referrals

2. Through 8. Not applicable

C Ⓜ 9. The organization accepts patients for care, treatment, and services according to established processes.

Assessment

Introduction

The goal of assessment is to determine the appropriate care, treatment, and services to meet a patient's initial needs as well as his or her changing needs while in the setting.

Identifying and delivering appropriate care, treatment, and services depends on three processes:

1. *Collecting data* about each patient's health history; physical, functional, and psychosocial status; and needs as appropriate to the setting and circumstances
2. *Analyzing data* to produce information about patients' needs for care, treatment, and services and to identify the need for additional data
3. *Making care, treatment, and service decisions* based on information developed about each patient's needs and his or her response to care, treatment, and services

Qualified staff assesses each patient's care needs throughout the patient's contact with the organization through assessments or screenings. These activities may also identify the need for additional assessments or planning. These assessments are as follows:

- Defined by the organization
- Individualized to meet each patient's needs
- Address the needs of special populations

The process defined by the organization identifies the patient's physical, cognitive, behavioral, emotional, and psychosocial status. This assessment identifies facilitating factors and possible barriers to the patient reaching his or her goals, including the presenting problems and needs, such as the following:

- Symptoms that might be associated with a disease, condition, or treatment (such as pain, nausea, or dyspnea)
- Social barriers, including cultural and language barriers
- Social and environmental factors
- Physical disabilities
- Vision and hearing impairments and disabilities
- Developmental disabilities
- Communicative disorders
- Cognitive disorders
- Emotional, behavioral, and mental disorders
- Substance abuse, dependence, and other addictive behaviors

The depth and frequency of the assessment or screening depend on a number of factors, including the patient's needs, program goals, and the care, treatment, and services provided. Assessment or screening activities may vary between settings, as defined by the clinical and other leaders of the organization. Patient screenings, assessments, and reassessments need to be done and documented within a reasonable time frame to identify the patient's needs and determine if these needs are being met.

Information is gathered through screening or assessment processes when the patient first contacts the program or service to identify the reasons for coming to the organization. The information to be collected is defined by the organization's policies and procedures and depends on the patient's emergent needs and the setting in which care, treatment, and services are sought. As appropriate, information gathered from the patient's family is included.

Information gathered at the first contact can indicate the need for more data or a more intensive assessment of the patient's physical, psychological, cognitive, and communicative skills or development or social functioning. At a minimum, the need for further assessment is determined by the care, treatment, and services sought; the patient's presenting condition(s); and whether the patient agrees to care, treatment, and services.

Information gathered at the first contact can indicate the need for more data or a more intensive assessment of the patient's vocational, educational, legal, and nutritional functioning. At a minimum, the need for further assessment is determined by the care, treatment, and services sought; the patient's presenting condition(s); and whether the patient agrees to care, treatment, and services.

Standard PC.2.10

Not applicable

Standard PC.2.20

The organization defines in writing the data and information gathered during assessment and reassessment.

Rationale for PC.2.20

A full assessment involves obtaining relevant information from multiple sources. This may include obtaining information from the patient, a family member, or other sources, including other providers. Sources might also include mediums that the patient has sought out to convey information to those who may provide care, treatment, or services. These include databases, medical jewelry, and paper or electronic documents. Whatever the source, information to complete a comprehensive assessment should be sought out from all available sources.

Elements of Performance for PC.2.20

B 1. The organization's written definition of the data and information gathered during assessment and reassessment includes the following:
- The scope of assessment and reassessment activities
- The content of the assessment and reassessment
- The criteria for when an additional or more in-depth assessment is done*

* For example, nutritional or functional risk assessments may be defined for at-risk patients. In such cases, nutritional risk criteria should be developed by dieticians or other qualified individuals, and functional risk criteria should be developed by rehabilitation specialists or other qualified individuals.

B 2. The screening, assessment, and reassessment activities described are within the scope of practice, state licensure laws, applicable regulations, or certification of the discipline doing the assessment.

A 3. If applicable, separate specialized assessment and reassessment information is identified for the various populations served.

B 4. The information defined by the organization to be gathered during the initial assessment includes the following, as relevant to the care, treatment, and services:
- Physical assessment, as appropriate
- Psychological assessment, as appropriate
- Social assessment, as appropriate
- Each patient's nutrition and hydration status, as appropriate
- Each patient's functional status, as appropriate
- For patients receiving end-of-life care, the social, spiritual, and cultural variables that influence the perceptions and expressions of grief by the patient, family members, or significant others

Standards PC.2.30 Through PC.2.110

Not applicable

Standard PC.2.120

The organization defines in writing the time frame(s) for conducting the initial assessment(s).

Elements of Performance for PC.2.120

A 1. The organization defines the time frame(s) for conducting the initial assessment(s).

2. Through 13. Not applicable

Some of these elements may have been completed ahead of time, but must meet the following criteria (EPs 14 and 15):

A 14. Updates to the patient's condition since the assessment(s) are recorded at the time of the visit

A 15. Findings from assessments conducted outside the organization are available in sufficient time to facilitate care, treatment, and services

Standard PC.2.130

Initial assessments are performed as defined by the organization.

Elements of Performance for PC.2.130

C Ⓜ 1. Each patient is assessed per organization policy.

C Ⓜ 2. Each patient's initial assessment is conducted within the time frame specified by the needs of the patient, organization policy, and law and regulation.

Standard PC.2.140

Not applicable

Standard PC.2.150

Patients are reassessed* as needed.

Rationale for PC.2.150

Each patient may be reassessed for many reasons including the following:

- To evaluate his or her response to care, treatment, and services
- To respond to a significant change in status and/or diagnosis or condition
- To satisfy legal or regulatory requirements
- To meet time intervals specified by the organization
  and/or
- To meet time intervals determined by the course of the care, treatment, and services for the patient

Element of Performance for PC.2.150

C Ⓜ 1. Each patient is reassessed as needed.

Additional Standards for Victims of Abuse

Standard PC.3.10

Patients who may be victims of abuse or neglect are assessed. (*See* standard RI.2.150.)

Rationale for PC.3.10

Victims of abuse or neglect may come to an organization in a variety of ways. The patient may be unable or may be reluctant to speak of the abuse, and it may not be obvious to the casual observer. Staff needs to be able to identify abuse or neglect, as well as the extent and circumstances of the abuse or neglect to give the patient appropriate care.

Criteria for identifying and assessing victims of abuse or neglect should be used throughout the organization. The assessment of the patient must be conducted

* The scope and intensity of any further assessments are based on the patient's diagnosis; the setting; the patient's desire for care, treatment, and services; and the patient's response to any previous care, treatment, and services.

within the context of the requirements of the law to preserve evidentiary materials and support future legal actions.

Elements of Performance for PC.3.10

A 1. The organization develops or adopts criteria* for identifying victims in each of the following situations:
- Physical assault
- Rape
- Sexual molestation
- Domestic abuse
- Elder neglect or abuse
- Child neglect or abuse

B 2. Appropriate staff† is educated about abuse or neglect and how to refer as appropriate.

A 3. A list of private and public community agencies that provide or arrange for assessment and care of abuse victims is maintained to facilitate appropriate referrals.

B 4. Victims of abuse or neglect are identified using the criteria developed or adopted by the organization at entry into the system and on an ongoing basis.

B 5. The organization's staff refers appropriately or conducts the assessment of victims of abuse or neglect.

A 6. All cases of possible abuse or neglect are reported to appropriate agencies according to organization policy and law and regulation.

A 7. All cases of possible abuse or neglect are immediately reported in the organization.

Standards PC.3.20 Through PC.3.220

Not applicable

PC

* The Family Violence Prevention Fund is one resource that can be contacted for further information at http://www.fvpf.org.

† Staff should be able to screen for abuse and neglect as indicated by the patient's needs or conditions. The organization may define who conducts the full assessment for alleged or suspected abuse or neglect or refer to another organization.

Diagnostic Services

Standard PC.3.230

Diagnostic testing* necessary for determining the patient's health care needs is performed.

Elements of Performance for PC.3.230

C Ⓜ 1. Diagnostic testing and procedures are performed as ordered.

C Ⓜ 2. Diagnostic testing and procedures are performed in a timely manner as defined by the organization.

C Ⓜ 3. When a test report requires clinical interpretation, relevant information is provided with the request.

For Medicare-Certified Ambulatory Surgical Centers

A 4. The Medicare-certified ambulatory surgical center has procedures for obtaining radiological services from a Medicare-approved facility to meet patients' needs.

Planning Care, Treatment, and Services

Introduction

Planning includes creating an initial plan for care, treatment, and services appropriate to the patient's specific assessed needs, and then revising or maintaining the plan based on the patient's response. Planning for care, treatment, and services is individualized to meet the patient's unique needs and circumstances. Performed by qualified individuals, planning for care, treatment, and services involves using an interdisciplinary approach when warranted and involving the patient to the extent possible.

The plan may be modified or terminated based on reassessment; the patient's need for further care, treatment, and services; or the achievement of plan of care goals. This modification may result in planning for the patient's transfer to another setting or service or discharge from the organization.

Standard PC.4.10

Development of a plan for care, treatment, and services is individualized and appropriate to the patient's needs, strengths, limitations, and goals.

Rationale for PC.4.10

Planning care, treatment, and services is not limited to developing a written plan. Rather, planning is a dynamic process that addresses the execution of care, treat-

* Diagnostic testing includes laboratory, radiologic, electrodiagnostic, and other functional tests and imaging technologies.

ment, and services. The plan for care, treatment, and services must be consistently reevaluated to ensure that the patient's needs are met. Planning for care, treatment, and services includes the following:

- Integrating assessment findings in the care-planning process
- Developing a plan for care, treatment, and services that includes patient care goals that are reasonable and measurable
- Regularly reviewing and revising the plan for care, treatment, and services
- Determining how the planned care, treatment, and services will be provided
- Documenting the plan for care, treatment, and services
- Monitoring the effectiveness of care planning and the provision of care, treatment, and services
- Involving patients and/or families in care planning

Elements of Performance for PC.4.10

B 1. Care, treatment, and services are planned to ensure that they are individualized to the patient's needs.

B 2. Development of a plan for care, treatment, and services is based on the data from assessments.

3. Through 11. Not applicable

C Ⓜ 12. Evaluation of the patient is based on the patient care goals and the patient's plan for care, treatment, and services.

C Ⓜ 13. The goals of care, treatment, and services are revised when necessary.

B 14. Plans for care, treatment, and services are revised when necessary.

PC

Standards PC.4.20 Through PC.4.120

Not applicable

Providing Care, Treatment, and Services

Introduction

Caring for patients involves providing individualized, planned, and appropriate interventions in settings responsive to specific individual needs. "Care" includes care, treatment, services, rehabilitation, habilitation, or another intervention provided to the patient by the organization.

The goal of providing effective care, treatment, and services is met when the following are performed well:

- Intervening in a collaborative manner (in light of assessed patient needs)
- Educating the patient
- Promoting health and providing appropriate preventive care

- Providing supportive care, treating a disease or condition, and/or treating symptoms (such as pain, nausea, or dyspnea) using accepted professional standards of practice
- Meeting the patient's nourishment needs, if appropriate to the setting
- Helping patients with appropriate restorative services, including assistance with activities of daily living, such as eating, dressing, grooming, bathing, oral hygiene, ambulation, and toilet activities
- Rehabilitating physical, communicative, or psychosocial impairment or maintaining the patient's level of functioning
- Coordinating the care, treatment, and services provided to a patient
- Optimizing comfort and dignity during end-of-life care
- Involving families as indicated and acceptable to the patient

All interventions should respect and encourage the patient's ability to make choices, to develop and maintain a sense of achievement about attaining their personal health goals, and to choose to continue or modify participation in the care process.

The activities comprising care, treatment, and services may be performed by a variety of staff whose roles and responsibilities are determined by the component of care, treatment, and service being provided; relevant licensure; law and regulation; registration; certification; scope of practice; job description; or privileges.

Standard PC.5.10

The organization provides care, treatment, and services for each patient according to the plan for care, treatment, and services.

Elements of Performance for PC.5.10

C Ⓜ 1. The organization provides care, treatment, and services for each patient according to the plan for care, treatment, and services.

2. Not applicable

3. Not applicable

4. Use at least two patient identifiers (neither to be the patient's physical location) whenever administering medications or blood products; taking blood samples and other specimens for clinical testing; or providing any other treatments or procedures.

   Note: *The preceding requirement is not scored here. It is scored at goal 1, requirement 1A.*

Standard PC.5.20

Not applicable

Standard PC.5.30

Not applicable

Standard PC.5.40

Not applicable

Standard PC.5.50

Care, treatment, and services are provided in an interdisciplinary, collaborative manner.

Rationale for PC.5.50

A collaborative, interdisciplinary approach to meeting the patient's needs and goals helps to coordinate care, treatment, and services and achieve optimal outcomes. The mix of disciplines involved and the intensity of the collaboration will vary as appropriate to each patient and the scope of services provided by the organization. An interdisciplinary approach should not be interpreted as a requirement for an interdisciplinary care plan or the signing of other individuals' notes. While an interdisciplinary care plan may be one method of accomplishing this goal, it is not required.

PC

Element of Performance for PC.5.50

B 1. Care, treatment, and services are provided in an interdisciplinary, collaborative manner as appropriate to the needs of the patient and the organization's scope of services.

Standard PC.5.60

The organization coordinates the care, treatment, and services provided to a patient as part of the plan for care, treatment, and services and consistent with the organization's scope of care, treatment, and services.

Rationale for PC.5.60

Throughout the provision of care, treatment, and services, patients should be matched with appropriate internal and external resources to meet their ongoing needs in a timely manner. Care, treatment, and services should be coordinated between providers and between settings, independent of whether they are provided directly or through written agreement.

Elements of Performance for PC.5.60

B 1. The organization coordinates the care, treatment, and services provided through internal resources to a patient.

B 2. When external resources are needed, the organization participates in coordinating care, treatment, and services with these resources.

B 3. The organization has a process to receive or share relevant patient information to facilitate appropriate coordination and continuity when patients are referred to other care, treatment, and service providers.

B 4. There is a process to resolve duplication or conflict with either internal or external resources.

B 5. The activities detailed in the plan of care, treatment, and services are designed to occur in a time frame that meets the patient's health needs.

Standard PC.5.70

Not applicable

Education

Standard PC.6.10

The patient receives education and training specific to the patient's needs and as appropriate to the care, treatment, and services provided.

Rationale for PC.6.10

Patients must be given sufficient information to make decisions and to take responsibility for self-management activities related to their needs. Patients and, as appropriate, their families are educated to improve individual outcomes by promoting healthy behavior and appropriately involving patients in their care, treatment, and service decisions.

Elements of Performance for PC.6.10

B 1. Education provided is appropriate to the patient's needs.

C Ⓜ 2. The assessment of learning needs addresses cultural and religious beliefs, emotional barriers, desire and motivation to learn, physical or cognitive limitations, and barriers to communication as appropriate.

B 3. As appropriate to the patient's condition and assessed needs and the organization's scope of services, the patient is educated about the following:
- The plan for care, treatment, and services
- Basic health practices and safety
- The safe and effective use of medications
- Nutrition interventions, modified diets, or oral health
- Safe and effective use of medical equipment or supplies when provided by the organization
- Understanding pain, the risk for pain, the importance of effective pain management, the pain assessment process, and methods for pain management

- Habilitation or rehabilitation techniques to help them reach the maximum independence possible

Standard PC.6.20
Not applicable

Standard PC.6.30
The patient receives education and training specific to the patient's abilities as appropriate to the care, treatment, and services provided by the organization.

Rationale for PC.6.30
Learning styles vary, and the ability to learn can be affected by many factors, including individual learning preferences and readiness to learn. Educational activities must be tailored to meet the patient's needs and abilities.

Elements of Performance for PC.6.30
B 1. Education provided is appropriate to the patient's abilities.

B 2. Education is coordinated among the disciplines providing care, treatment, and services.

B 3. The content is presented in an understandable manner.

B 4. Teaching methods accommodate various learning styles.

C Ⓜ 5. Comprehension is evaluated.

Standards PC.6.40 Through PC.6.180
Not applicable

Nutritional Care

Introduction
This standard focuses on providing appropriate nutritional care, including food and nutrition therapy, in a timely and efficient manner using appropriate resources. Elements of nutritional care, such as screening or assessment and education, are addressed in other standards in this book.

Standard PC.7.10
The organization has a process for preparing and/or distributing food and nutrition products as appropriate to the care, treatment, and services provided.

Elements of Performance for PC.7.10

B 1. Food and nutrition products are provided for the patient as appropriate to care, treatment, and services.

C Ⓜ 2. Food and nutrition products are stored under proper conditions of sanitation, temperature, light, moisture, ventilation, and security.

C Ⓜ 3. Patients' cultural, religious, and ethnic food preferences are honored, when possible, unless contraindicated.

4. Through 16. Not applicable

C Ⓜ 17. Food and nutrition products are prepared under proper conditions of sanitation, temperature, light, moisture, ventilation, and security.

Pain

Standard PC.8.10

Pain is assessed in all patients.

Rationale for PC.8.10

The identification and treatment of pain is an important component of the plan of care. Individuals are assessed based upon their clinical presentation, services sought, and in accordance with the care, treatment, and services provided.

Elements of Performance for PC.8.10

1. Not applicable

C Ⓜ 2. A referral for a comprehensive pain assessment is made or a comprehensive pain assessment is conducted when warranted by the patient's condition.

3. Not applicable

C Ⓜ 4. Reassessment and follow-up occur according to the criteria developed by the organization or as required by the organization assessing or treating the pain.

C Ⓜ 5. If conducted by the organization, the assessment and a measure of pain intensity and quality (for example, pain character, frequency, location, duration, exacerbating and relieving factors) appropriate to the patient's age are recorded.

6. Not applicable

C Ⓜ 7. When pain is identified, the patient is treated by the organization or referred for treatment.

Standards PC.8.20 Through PC.8.70

Not applicable

Specific Procedures

Administering Blood and Blood Components

Standard PC.9.10

Blood and blood components are administered safely, as appropriate to the setting.

Elements of Performance for PC.9.10

1. Through 10. Not applicable

B 11. The organization has detailed written procedures for how to obtain blood components or blood products.

A 12. The procedures describe at least the following:
- The source of the materials
- The time frames for obtaining them
- Accountability for procurement
- On-site storage

For Medicare-Certified Ambulatory Surgical Centers

A Ⓜ 13. Only physicians or registered nurses administer blood and blood products.

Responding to Life-Threatening Emergencies

Standard PC.9.20

The organization responds to life-threatening emergencies according to organization policy and procedure.

Elements of Performance for PC.9.20

B 1. The organization develops policy and procedures for responding to life-threatening emergencies such as respiratory arrest and cardiac arrest.

2. Not applicable

A 3. The organization responds to life-threatening emergencies according to organization policy and procedure.

PC

Standards PC.9.30 Through PC.10.130

Not applicable

Restraint and Seclusion

Standards PC.11.10 Through PC.11.60

Not applicable

Standard PC.11.70

Patients in restraint are monitored.

Rationale for PC.11.70

Monitoring determines the following:

- The patient's physical and emotional well-being
- That the patient's rights, dignity, and safety are maintained
- Whether less restrictive methods are possible
- Changes in the patient's behavior or clinical condition needed to initiate the removal of restraints
- Whether the restraint has been appropriately applied, removed, or reapplied

Elements of Performance for PC.11.70

B 1. Organization policies and procedures, applicable state law, protocols, individual orders, the setting, and individual patient needs are used to establish the frequency, nature, and extent of monitoring of a patient in restraints.

A 2. A patient in restraints is monitored at least every two hours or sooner according to patient need and organization policy.

C Ⓜ 3. Monitoring is accomplished by observation, interaction with the patient, or related direct examination of the patient by qualified staff.*

Standard PC.11.80

Not applicable

Standard PC.11.90

Not applicable

* Documentation of monitoring is in accordance with organization policies and procedures. Documentation is scored at standard PC.11.100.

Standard PC.11.100

Each episode of restraint use is documented in the patient's medical record, consistent with organization policies and procedures.

Elements of Performance for PC.11.100

B 1. Organization policies and procedures establish the frequency, format (if appropriate), and content of entries in the patient's record relative to each episode of restraint use.

C Ⓜ 2. Documentation includes the following:
- Relevant orders for use
- Results of patient monitoring
- Reassessment
- Significant changes in the patient's condition

Standards PC.12.10 Through PC.12.190

Not applicable

PC

Standards for Operative or Other High-Risk Procedures and/or the Administration of Moderate or Deep Sedation or Anesthesia

Introduction

Operative or other procedures and the administration of sedation or anesthesia often occur simultaneously. However, procedures do occur without sedation, and sedation or anesthesia is administered for noninvasive procedures (hyperbaric treatment, CT scan, MRI). Therefore, the following standards address both operative or other procedures and/or the administration of moderate or deep sedation or anesthesia.

Whenever an operative or other procedure is conducted, whether or not sedation or anesthesia is administered, appropriate staff must be involved in planning for and providing care to the patient. All procedures carry risk, but that risk is increased when sedation or anesthesia is administered.

The standards for sedation and anesthesia care apply when patients in any setting receive, for any purpose, by any route, the following:
- General, spinal, or other major regional anesthesia
  or
- Moderate or deep sedation (with or without analgesia) that, in the manner used, may be reasonably expected to result in the loss of protective reflexes

Because sedation is a continuum, it is not always possible to predict how an individual patient receiving sedation will respond. Therefore, each organization develops specific, appropriate protocols for the care of patients receiving sedation.

These protocols are consistent with professional standards and address at least the following:

- Sufficient qualified individuals present to perform the procedure and to monitor the patient throughout administration and recovery. The individuals providing moderate or deep sedation and anesthesia have at a minimum had competency-based education, training, and experience in the following:
    1. Evaluating patients before performing moderate or deep sedation and anesthesia
    2. Performing the moderate or deep sedation and anesthesia, including rescuing patients who slip into a deeper-than-desired level of sedation or analgesia. These include the following:
        a. Moderate sedation—are qualified to rescue patients from deep sedation and are competent to manage a compromised airway and to provide adequate oxygenation and ventilation
        b. Deep sedation—are qualified to rescue patients from general anesthesia and are competent to manage an unstable cardiovascular system as well as a compromised airway and inadequate oxygenation and ventilation
- Appropriate equipment for care and resuscitation
- Appropriate monitoring of vital signs, including, but not limited to, heart rates and oxygenation using pulse oximetry equipment, respiratory frequency and adequacy of pulmonary ventilation, the monitoring of blood pressure at regular intervals, and cardiac monitoring (by EKG or use of continuous cardiac monitoring device) in patients with significant cardiovascular disease or when dysrhythmias are anticipated or detected
- Documentation of care
- Monitoring of outcomes

PC

Definitions of four levels of sedation and anesthesia include the following:

- **Minimal sedation (anxiolysis)**
  A drug-induced state during which patients respond normally to verbal commands. Although cognitive function and coordination may be impaired, ventilatory and cardiovascular functions are unaffected.
- **Moderate sedation/analgesia ("conscious sedation")**
  A drug-induced depression of consciousness during which patients respond purposefully to verbal commands (note: reflex withdrawal from a painful stimulus is not considered a purposeful response)—either alone or accompanied by light tactile stimulation. No interventions are required to maintain a patent airway, and spontaneous ventilation is adequate. Cardiovascular function is usually maintained.
- **Deep sedation/analgesia**
  A drug-induced depression of consciousness during which patients cannot be easily aroused but respond purposefully after repeated or painful stimulation. The ability to independently maintain ventilatory function may be impaired. Patients may require assistance in maintaining a patent airway and spontaneous ventilation may be inadequate. Cardiovascular function is usually maintained.
- **Anesthesia**
  Consists of general anesthesia and spinal or major regional anesthesia. It does *not* include local anesthesia. General anesthesia is a drug-induced loss of con-

sciousness during which patients are not arousable, even by painful stimulation. The ability to independently maintain ventilatory function is often impaired. Patients often require assistance in maintaining a patent airway, and positive pressure ventilation may be required because of depressed spontaneous ventilation or drug-induced depression of neuromuscular function. Cardiovascular function may be impaired.

Standard PC.13.10

Licensed independent practitioners define the scope of assessment for operative or other procedures and/or the administration of moderate or deep sedation or anesthesia.

Rationale for PC.13.10

The scope of assessment is defined to enhance the safety of the procedures' performance.

Element of Performance for PC.13.10

B 1. The assessment includes the following:
- The patient's history
- The patient's physical status
- Diagnostic data
- The risks and benefits of procedures
- The possible need to administer blood or blood components

Standard PC.13.20

Operative or other procedures and/or the administration of moderate or deep sedation or anesthesia are planned.

Rationale for PC.13.20

Because the response to procedures is not always predictable and sedation-to-anesthesia is a continuum, it is not always possible to predict how an individual patient will respond. Therefore, qualified individuals are trained in professional standards and techniques to manage patients in the case of a potentially harmful event.

Elements of Performance for PC.13.20

B 1. Sufficient numbers of qualified staff (in addition to the individual performing the procedure) are present to evaluate the patient, help with the procedure, provide the sedation and/or anesthesia, monitor, and recover the patient.

A 2. Individuals administering moderate or deep sedation and anesthesia are qualified and have the appropriate credentials to manage patients at whatever level of sedation or anesthesia is achieved, either intentionally or unintentionally.

3. Not applicable

B 4. Appropriate equipment to monitor the patient's physiologic status is available.

B 5. Appropriate equipment to administer intravenous fluids and drugs, including blood and blood components, is available as needed.

B 6. Resuscitation capabilities are available.

The following must occur before the operative and other procedures or the administration of moderate or deep sedation or anesthesia (EPs 7–10):

C Ⓜ 7. The anticipated needs of the patient are assessed to plan for the appropriate level of postprocedure care.

C Ⓜ 8. Preprocedural education, treatments, and services are provided according to the plan for care, treatment, and services.

9. Conduct a "time out" immediately before starting the procedure as described in the Universal Protocol for eliminating wrong site, wrong procedure, wrong person surgery.

Note: *The preceding requirement is not scored here. It is scored at the Universal Protocol, requirement 1C, in the "National Patient Safety Goals" chapter.*

A 10. A presedation or preanesthesia assessment is conducted.

A 11. Before sedating or anesthetizing a patient, a licensed independent practitioner with appropriate clinical privileges plans or concurs with the planned anesthesia.

A 12. The patient is reevaluated immediately before moderate or deep sedation and before anesthesia induction.

A 13. Operative and other procedures are done only after completion and documentation of appropriate history and physical examination, any indicated diagnostic tests, and the preoperative diagnosis.

C Ⓜ 14. A history and physical examination are completed within 30 days before an operative or other procedure.

For Medicare-Certified Ambulatory Surgical Centers

A 15. A physician must examine patients immediately before surgery to evaluate the risk of moderate or deep sedation or anesthesia.

A 16. Results of any preoperative diagnostic studies performed are entered into the medical record before surgery to evaluate the risk of anesthesia.

A 17. Emergency provisions available to operating rooms include the following:
- An emergency call system
- Oxygen

- Mechanical ventilatory assistance equipment including airways, manual breathing bags, and ventilators
- Cardiac defibrillator
- Cardiac monitoring equipment
- A tracheotomy set
- Laryngoscopes and endotracheal tubes
- Suction equipment
- Emergency medical equipment and supplies specified by the ambulatory surgical center's physicians

A 18. Anesthetics must be administered by only one of the following:
- A qualified anesthesiologist

  or
- A physician qualified to administer anesthesia, a certified registered nurse anesthetist (CRNA) or an anesthesiologist's assistant, or a supervised trainee in an approved educational program. In those cases in which a nonphysician administers the anesthesia, unless exempted,* the anesthetist must be under the supervision of the operating physician, and in the case of an anesthesiologist's assistant, under the supervision of an anesthesiologist.

Standard PC.13.30

Patients are monitored during the procedure and/or administration of moderate or deep sedation or anesthesia.

Elements of Performance for PC.13.30

A 1. Appropriate methods are used to continuously monitor oxygenation, ventilation, and circulation during procedures that may affect the patient's physiological status.

C Ⓜ 2. The procedure and/or the administration of moderate or deep sedation or anesthesia for each patient is documented in the medical record.

Standard PC.13.40

Patients are monitored immediately after the procedure and/or administration of moderate or deep sedation or anesthesia.

---

* An ambulatory surgical center (ASC) may be exempted from the requirement for physician supervision of CRNAs as described in paragraph (b)(2) of 42 CFR 416.42 if the state in which the ASC is located submits a letter to CMS signed by the governor, following consultation with the state's boards of medicine and nursing, requesting exemption from physician supervision of CRNAs. The letter from the governor must attest that he or she has consulted with the state boards of medicine and nursing about issues related to access to and the quality of anesthesia services in the state and has concluded that it is in the best interests of the state's citizens to opt out of the current physician supervision requirement and that the opt-out is consistent with state law. The request for exemption and recognition of state laws and the withdrawal of the request may be submitted at any time and are effective upon submission.

Elements of Performance for PC.13.40

A 1. The patient's status is assessed immediately after the procedure and/or administration of moderate or deep sedation or anesthesia.

C Ⓜ 2. Each patient's physiological status, mental status, and pain level are monitored.

B 3. Monitoring is at a level consistent with the potential effect of the procedure and/or sedation or anesthesia.

B 4. Patients are discharged from the recovery area and the organization by a qualified licensed independent practitioner or according to rigorously applied criteria approved by the clinical leaders.

C Ⓜ 5. Patients who have received sedation or anesthesia are discharged in the company of a responsible, designated adult.

For Medicare-Certified Ambulatory Surgical Centers (EP 6)

A 6. Each patient is evaluated by a licensed independent practitioner for proper recovery before discharge from the ambulatory surgical center.

Standards PC.13.50 Through PC.14.30

Not applicable

Discharge or Transfer from The Organization

Introduction

Patients may be discharged from the organization entirely or discharged or transferred to another level of care, treatment, and services, to different health professionals, or to settings for continued services. The organization's processes for transfer or discharge are based on the patient's assessed needs. To facilitate discharge or transfer, the organization assesses the patient's needs, plans for discharge or transfer, facilitates the discharge or transfer process, and helps to ensure that continuity of care, treatment, and services is maintained.

Standard PC.15.10

A process addresses the needs for continuing care, treatment, and services after discharge or transfer.

Elements of Performance for PC.15.10

B 1. The process addresses the following:
- The reason(s) for transfer or discharge
- The conditions under which transfer or discharge can occur
- Shifting responsibility for a patient's care from one clinician, organization, organizational program, or service to another (which could

include transferring complete responsibility for the patient and his or her care, treatment, and services to others or referring the patient to others, such as one or more agencies or professionals, to provide one or more specific services)

- Mechanisms for internal and external transfer
- The accountability and responsibility for the patient's safety during transfer of both the organization initiating the transfer and the organization receiving the patient

2. Through 15. Not applicable

For Medicare-Certified Ambulatory Surgical Centers (EPs 16–19)

A 16. The ambulatory surgical center has procedures for immediately transferring patients who require emergency care beyond the ambulatory surgical center's capability.

A 17. Transfers are made only to hospitals that meet requirements for payment of emergency services.

A 18. The ambulatory surgical center has a written transfer agreement with the hospital.

A 19. If there is no written agreement, all ambulatory surgical center physicians performing surgery must have admitting privileges at the hospital.

Standard PC.15.20

The transfer or discharge of a patient to another level of care, treatment, and services, different professionals, or different settings is based on the patient's assessed needs and the organization's capabilities.

Rationale for PC.15.20

For some patients, effective planning addresses how needs will be met as they move to the next level of care, treatment, and services. For other patients, planning will consist of a clear understanding of how to access services in the future should the need arise.

Elements of Performance for PC.15.20

C Ⓜ 1. The patient's needs for continuing care to meet physical and psychosocial needs are identified.

C Ⓜ 2. Patients are told in a timely manner of the need to plan for discharge or transfer to another organization or level of care.

C Ⓜ 3. Planning for transfer or discharge involves the patient and all appropriate licensed independent practitioners, staff, and family members involved in the patient's care, treatment, and services.

4. Not applicable

5. Not applicable

6. Not applicable

C Ⓜ 7. When indicated, the patient is educated about how to obtain further care, treatment, and services to meet his or her identified needs.

C Ⓜ 8. When indicated and before discharge, the organization arranges for or helps the family arrange for services needed to meet the patient's needs after discharge.

C Ⓜ 9. Written discharge instructions in a form the patient can understand are given to the patient and/or those responsible for providing continuing care.

Standard PC.15.30

When patients are transferred or discharged, appropriate information related to the care, treatment, and services provided is exchanged with other service providers.

Rationale for PC.15.30

A patient may receive care, treatment, and services in many settings and may move from one organization or provider to another. To facilitate the continuity of care, treatment, and services, information is provided to any organization or provider to which the patient is accepted, transferred, or discharged.

Elements of Performance for PC.15.30

C Ⓜ 1. The organization communicates appropriate information to any organization or provider to which the patient is transferred or discharged.

C Ⓜ 2. The information shared includes the following, as appropriate to the care, treatment, and services provided:
- The reason for transfer or discharge
- The patient's physical and psychosocial status
- A summary of care, treatment, and services provided and progress toward goals
- Community resources or referrals provided to the patient
- A list of current medications, including allergies and other pertinent information

Standard PC.15.40

Not applicable

Standard PC.15.50

Not applicable

Waived Testing

The federal regulation governing laboratory testing, known as the Clinical Laboratories Improvement Amendments of 1988 (CLIA '88), classifies testing into four complexity levels: high complexity, moderate complexity, Provider Performed Microscopy (PPM, a sub-set of moderate complexity), and waived testing. The high, moderate, and PPM levels, otherwise called non-waived testing, have specific and detailed requirements regarding personnel qualifications, quality assurance, quality control, and other systems. Waived testing, on the other hand, has few requirements and is less stringent then the requirements for non-waived testing.

The same laboratory test can be available by more than one method within an organization, and those methods can be of different complexity levels. Waived testing is the most common complexity level performed by caregivers at the patient bedside or point of care (POC). The list of methods that are approved as waived is under constant revision, so it is advisable to check the Food and Drug Administration (FDA), Centers for Disease Control and Prevention (CDC), or Centers for Medicare & Medicaid Services (CMS) Web sites for the most up-to-date information regarding test categorization and complete CLIA requirements. Those Web sites are as follows:

- http://www.fda.gov/cdrh/clia/index.html
- http://www.phppo.cdc.gov/clia
- http://www.cms.hhs.gov/clia

A laboratory test is an activity that evaluates substances removed from a human body and translates the evaluation into a result. A result can be stated as a number, presence or absence of a cell or reaction, or an interpretation, such as what occurs when recording a urine color. Test results that are used to assess a patient condition or make a clinical decision about a patient are governed by CLIA '88.

Tests that produce a result measured as a discrete number are termed "quantitative." Tests that produce a negative or positive result, such as occult bloods and urine pregnancy screens, are termed "qualitative." A test that is more precise than a qualitative test (pos/neg), but less precise than a quantitative test (numerical), usually scored on a graded scale (1+, 2+, 3+) is termed "semi-quantitative." Tests with analysis steps that rely on the use of an instrument to produce a result are instrument-based tests. These can be qualitative, semi-quantitative, or quantitative.

When a patient performs a test on himself or herself (for example, whole blood glucose testing by a patient on his or her own meter cleared by the FDA for home use), the action is not regulated. Testing performed by one individual on another individual while carrying out professional responsibilities is an activity regulated by CLIA '88. This distinction is important when caring for patients who monitor their own health care (such as testing of glucose or prothrombin times with home devices).

Standard PC.16.10

The director named on the CLIA certificate establishes policies and procedures that define the context in which waived test results are used in patient care, treatment, and services.

Elements of Performance for PC.16.10

B 1. The director named on the CLIA certificate determines the context in which waived tests are used.

C Ⓜ 2. Clinical use of results is consistent with the organization's policies and the manufacturer's recommendations for waived tests.

B 3. Quantitative test result reports in the clinical record are accompanied by reference ranges specific to the test method used and population served.

Note: *Semi-quantitative results, such as urine macroscopic and urine dipsticks, are not required to comply with this EP.*

A 4. For qualitative and quantitative tests, criteria for confirmatory testing is specified in the written procedures.

B 5. These written procedures are based on clinical usage and limitations of the test methodology.

C Ⓜ 6. The criteria for confirmatory testing is followed as specified in the written procedures.

Standard PC.16.20

The director named on the CLIA certificate identifies the staff responsible for performing and supervising waived testing.

Elements of Performance for PC.16.20

B 1. The identity of staff members who perform testing is documented.

B 2. The identity of staff members who direct or supervise testing is documented.

Note: *These individuals may be employees of the organization, contracted staff, or employees of a contracted service.*

Standard PC.16.30

Staff receive specific training and orientation for the tests they perform, and demonstrate satisfactory levels of competence.

Rationale for PC.16.30

For waived tests to be performed properly, the staff performing them must be qualified to do so. Staff members who perform waived testing have specific training for each test performed. This training can be acquired through organization or other training programs, such as those provided by another health care organization or manufacturer.

Elements of Performance for PC.16.30

B 1. Staff members who perform testing have been oriented according to the organization's specific services.

B 2. Staff members who perform testing have been trained for each test he or she is authorized to perform.

B 3. Staff members who perform testing that requires the use of an instrument have been trained on the use and maintenance of that instrument.

B 4. Competence is assessed according to organization policy at defined intervals, but at least at the time of orientation and annually thereafter.

B 5. Current competency is assessed using at least two of the following methods per person per test:
- Performing a test on a blind specimen*
- Having the supervisor or qualified delegate periodically observe routine work
- Monitoring each user's quality control performance
- Having written testing that is specific to the method assessed

B 6. The director named on the CLIA certificate or qualified designee evaluates and documents evidence of orientation, training, and competency.

Note: *Staff who perform instrument-based testing, including, but not limited to, physicians, licensed independent practitioners, contracted staff, and R.N.s, participate in training and competence demonstrations.*

PC

Standard PC.16.40

Policies and procedures governing specific testing-related processes are current, approved, and readily available.

Rationale for PC.16.40

Current and up-to-date policies and procedures are an important reference tool in managing laboratory testing activities. Testing policies and procedures include requirements that are in compliance with the manufacturer's recommendations regarding all of the following, as applicable:
- Specimen type (for example, a method for whole blood is not used for spinal fluid)
- Storage considerations for test components (for example, compliance with directions such as store away from direct light, temperature requirements, open container expiration dates, and so forth)
- Instrument maintenance and function checks, such as calibration
- Quality control frequency and type

* **Blind specimen** A sample with known value tested by personnel who do not know the expected result.

- Result follow-up recommendations (for example, a recommendation to repeat the test when results are higher or lower than the reportable range of the test*)
- Tests approved by the FDA for home use only are not used for professional purposes (for example, glucose meters cleared for home use only are not used in a hospital setting by nursing staff except as patient education)

Elements of Performance for PC.16.40

A 1. The director named on the CLIA certificate or a qualified designee approves policies and procedures at the following times:
- Before initial use of the test for patient testing
- Periodically thereafter, defined by the director but at least once every three years
- When there are changes in procedures†

B 2. Written policies and procedures address the following items:
- Specimen type, collection, identification, and required labeling
- Specimen preservation, as appropriate
- Instrument maintenance and function checks, such as calibration
- Storage conditions for test components
  Note: *No reagent is used after its expiration date.*
- Quality control (including frequency and type) and remedial action
- Result reporting
  Note: *Individual patient results are not reported unless the quality control is acceptable.*
- Equipment performance evaluation
- Test performance

B 3. If manufacturers' manuals or package inserts are used as the policies or procedures for each test, they must be enhanced to include specific operational policies (for example, detailed quality control protocols and any other institution-specific procedures regarding the test or instrument).

B 4. Current and complete policies and procedures are readily available to the person performing the test.

B 5. Written policies, procedures, and manufacturers' instructions are followed.

Standard PC.16.50

Quality control checks are conducted on each procedure.

* **Reportable range** The span of test result values over which the laboratory can verify the accuracy of the instrument or test system measurement response.

† **Changes in procedures** Manufacturer updates to package inserts can include procedural changes, or a different manufacturer is used.

Elements of Performance for PC.16.50

B 1. The director named on the CLIA certificate establishes a written quality control plan that specifies how procedures will be controlled for quality, establishes timetables, and explains the rationale for choice of procedures and timetables.

B 2. The documented quality control rationale is based on the following:
- How the test is used
- Reagent stability
- Manufacturers' recommendations
- The organization's experience with the test
- Currently accepted guidelines

B 3. Quality control procedures are performed at least as frequently as recommended by the manufacturer or defined by the organization's policies.

Note: *If frequency of quality control is not defined by the manufacturer, the organization defines frequency of quality control.*

C Ⓜ 4. For instrument-based waived testing, quality control requirements include two levels of control, if commercially available.

C Ⓜ 5. For instrument-based waived testing, quality control procedures are performed at least once each day on each instrument used that day for patient testing.

Standard PC.16.60

Quality control and test result records are maintained.

Elements of Performance for PC.16.60

C Ⓜ 1. Quality control results are documented, including internal and external (liquid and electronic).

Note: *Quality control results may be located in the medical record.*

C Ⓜ 2. Test results are documented in the medical record.

B 3. Individual test results are associated with quality control and instrument records.

Note: *A formal log is not required, but a functional audit trail is maintained that allows retrieval of individual test results and their association with quality control and instrument records.*

A 4. Quality control and test result records are retained for at least two years.

Tissue Storage and Issuance

Note: *The following standards apply to organizations that store or issue tissue, which may include areas outside of the clinical laboratory, for example, surgery and outpatient centers and tissue banks. (Examples of tissue specimens that might be found in an organization can be found in Table 1, Examples of Tissue and Cell Products, below.)*

Table 1. Examples of Tissue and Cell Products* (*See* standards PC.17.10–PC.17.30)

Achilles Tendon	Homograft
ACL (Anterior Cruciate Ligament)	Iliac Crest
Amnion/Amniotic	Leukocytes
Aortic Valve	Limbal Graft
Artery (ies)	Limbal Stem Cells
Autologous Cells	Lymphocytes
Autologous Tissue	Marrow
Bladder Sling	Membrane
Bone	Meniscus
Bone Marrow	Nerve
Bone Paste	Oocyte/Ovarian Cells
Bone Powder	Ovarian Tissue
Bone Putty	Pancreatic Islet Cells
Bone Slurry	Parathyroid(s)
Cadaver/Cadaveric Graft	Patellar Tendon
Cancellous Chips	PCL (Posterior Cruciate Ligament)
Cartilage	Pericardium
Cells	Periostium
Chondrocytes	Peripheral Blood Stem Cells
Conduits	Placenta/Placenta Cells
Conjunctivae	Progenitor Cells
Cornea	Pulmonary Valve
Demineralized Bone	Saphenous Vein
Dendrite Cells	Sclera
Dermis	Semen
Dura Mater	Skin
Embryo	Skin Matrix
Fascia/Fascia Lata	Somatic Cells
Femoral Vein	Sperm
Femur	Tarsal Plate
Graft	Tendon
Heart Valves	Testicular Tissue
Hematopoietic Stem	Therapeutic Cells (T-Cell Pheresis)/T-Cells

* The Tissue and Issuance Standards and accompanying elements of performance would be required to the extent that they are applicable.

Table 1. Examples of Tissue and Cell Products* (See standards PC.17.10–PC.17.30) *(continued)*

Tibialis Tendon
Tissue (also Synthetic Tissue)
Trachea
Umbilical Cord Blood Stem Cells
Vascular Graft
Vein

Other tissues that are classified as tissues by federal law and regulation.

Other tissues that are classified as tissues by state law and regulation (for example, in the state of California, breast milk is classified as tissue).

Standard PC.17.10

The organization uses standardized procedures to acquire, receive, store, and issue tissues.

Elements of Performance for PC.17.10

The organization develops, maintains, and follows procedures to do the following (EPs 1–8):

A 1. Assign responsibility for overseeing the tissue program throughout the organization, including storage and issuance activity

A 2. Validate that source facilities who supply tissues are licensed by state agencies, and/or registered as a tissue establishment with the Food and Drug Administration (FDA)

B 3. Coordinate tissue ordering, receipt, storage, and issuance throughout the organization

C Ⓜ 4. Transport, handle, store, and use tissue according to the source facilities' or manufacturers' (for example, synthetic tissue) written directions

C Ⓜ 5. Log in all incoming tissue.

B 6. Maintain continuous temperature monitoring for storage refrigerators and freezers

C Ⓜ 7. Maintain daily records to show that tissues were stored at the required temperatures.

Note: *Main types of tissue storage used are: "ambient" or room temperature (for example: freeze-dried bone), refrigerated, frozen (for example: deep freezing colder than –40°C), and liquid nitrogen.*

B 8. Storage equipment has functional alarms and emergency back-up.

A 9. The organization complies with state and/or federal regulations when acting as a source facility that supplies tissues.

PC

C Ⓜ 10. The organization develops, maintains and follows procedures to do the following: Verify at receipt that package integrity is met and transport temperature range was controlled and acceptable.

Standard PC.17.20

The organization's record keeping permits bi-directional traceability of all tissues.

Elements of Performance for PC.17.20

A 1. The organization's records permit tracing of any tissue from the donor or source facility to all recipients or other final dispositions, including discarding of tissue, and from the final disposition or recipient back to the donor or source facility.

C Ⓜ 2. The organization's records track and identify materials used to prepare or process tissues and instructions used for preparation.

A 3. The organization's records identify the following:
- Identity of staff involved in preparing or issuing tissue
- Identity of staff who accepts the tissue
- Dates and times of the preceding activities

A 4. The organization's records include documentation in the recipient's clinical record of tissue use, including documentation of the unique identifier of the tissue.

C Ⓜ 5. The organization's records, including storage temperatures and all superseded procedures, manuals, and publications, are retained for a minimum of ten years, or longer if required by state and/or federal laws.

A 6. The organization's records, including the source facility, the original numeric or alphanumeric donor and lot identification, all recipients or other final dispositions of each tissue, and expiration dates are retained for a minimum of ten years beyond the date of distribution, transplantation, disposition or expiration of tissue (whichever is latest), or longer if required by state and/or federal laws.

B 7. The organization that receives tissue provides a system that fully complies with the completion and return of tissue usage information cards requested by source facilities.

Note: *Regarding protected health information, the HIPAA Privacy Rule provides at 45 CFR §164.512: "Uses and disclosures for which consent, an authorization, or opportunity to agree or object is not required.... (h) Standard: uses and disclosures for cadaveric organ, eye or tissue donation purposes."*

Standard PC.17.30

The organization has a defined process to investigate adverse events to tissue or donor infections.

Rationale for PC.17.30

Instances of tissue-borne infection in recipients of donor tissues are well-documented. Organisms that have been documented to be transmitted from infected donors subsequent to tissue transplant include HIV, Hepatitis B and C, and Creutzfeldt-Jakob disease (CJD). Recipients may also contract bacterial or fungal infections through contamination of tissue products during transportation, storage, or handling.

Effective communication of an adverse event directly related to tissue use is critical to patient safety. An organization may become aware of an adverse event directly related to tissue use through external notification or internal detection. Prompt investigation of each event provides response and treatment to recipients affected by the infected tissue and prevents further implantation of the infected tissue(s).

Elements of Performance for PC.17.30

B 1. Procedures are in place to investigate recipient adverse events, including disease transmission or other complication(s), suspected of being directly related to tissue use.

A 2. Cases of post-transplant infections or adverse events are promptly reported to the source facility.

A 3. Tissue reported by the source facility as the cause of possible infection or tissue involved in an event that may have contaminated the product are sequestered.

A 4. Recipients of tissue from donors who are subsequently found to have HIV, HTLV-I/II, viral hepatitis, or other infectious agents known to be transmissible by tissue, are identified and informed of infection risk.

B 5. Procedures have been followed when adverse or suspected events have occurred.

PC

Medication* Management

Overview

Medication management is often an important component in the palliative, symptomatic, and curative treatment of many diseases and conditions. A safe medication management system addresses an organization's medication processes, including the following (as applicable):

- Selection and procurement
- Storage
- Ordering and transcribing
- Preparing and dispensing
- Administration
- Monitoring

Effective and safe medication management involves multiple services and disciplines working closely together. These standards address activities involving various individuals within an organization's medication management system, such as licensed independent practitioners and other health care staff involved in medication management processes.

A well-planned and implemented medication management system supports patient safety and improves the quality of care by doing the following:

- Reducing practice variation, errors, and misuse
- Monitoring medication management processes with regard to efficiency, quality, and safety
- Standardizing equipment and processes across the organization to improve the medication management system
- Using evidence-based good practices to develop medication management processes
- Managing critical processes associated with medication management to promote safe medication management throughout the organization
- Handling all medications in the same manner, including sample medications

An effective medication management system includes mechanisms for reporting potential and actual medication-related errors and a process to improve medication management processes and patient safety based on this information. The most effective feedback and improvement systems usually operate in organizations that have a nonpunitive culture.

---

* For the purpose of these standards, *medication* includes prescription medications, sample medications, herbal remedies, vitamins, nutraceuticals, over-the-counter drugs, vaccines, diagnostic and contrast agents used on or administered to persons to diagnose, treat, or prevent disease or other abnormal conditions; radioactive medications; respiratory therapy treatments; parenteral nutrition; blood derivatives; intravenous solutions (plain, with electrolytes and/or drugs); and any product designated by the Food and Drug Administration (FDA) as a drug. The definition of *medication* does not include enteral nutrition solutions (which are considered food products), oxygen, and other medical gases.

The medication management chapter (MM.1.10 through MM.8.10) addresses critical medication management processes, including those undertaken by the organization and those provided through contracted pharmacy services. When pharmacy services are provided on a contracted basis, the contract addresses responsibility for these standards and performance expectations. An organization that contracts with a pharmacy for services must monitor the performance of contracted services.

Standards

The following is a list of all standards for this chapter. They are presented here for your convenience without footnotes or other explanatory text. If you have a question about a term used here, please check the Glossary.

Note: *A revised standard numbering system is being used with the reformatted standards. This revised numbering system will allow for more flexibility to add standards while maintaining the current label for each standard.*

Patient-Specific Information

MM.1.10 Patient-specific information is readily accessible to those involved in the medication management system.

Selection and Procurement

MM.2.10 Medications available for dispensing or administration (including stock medications) are selected, listed, and procured based on criteria.

Storage

MM.2.20 Medications are properly and safely stored.

MM.2.30 Emergency medications and/or supplies, if any, are consistently available, controlled, and secured.

MM.2.40 A process is established to safely manage medications brought into the organization by patients or their families.

Ordering and Transcribing

MM.3.10 Not applicable

MM.3.20 Medication orders are written clearly and transcribed accurately.

Preparing and Dispensing

MM.4.10 All prescriptions or medication orders are reviewed for appropriateness.

MM.4.20 Medications are prepared safely.

MM.4.30 Medications are labeled.

MM.4.40 Medications are dispensed safely.

MM.4.50 The organization has a system for safely providing medications to meet patient needs when the pharmacy is closed.

MM.4.60 If the organization does not operate a pharmacy but routinely administers medications, the organization has a process for obtaining medications from a pharmacy.

MM.4.70 Medications dispensed by the organization are retrieved when recalled or discontinued by the manufacturer or the Food and Drug Administration for safety reasons.

MM.4.80 The organization has a process to address medications that are returned to the pharmacy or the organization.

Administration

MM.5.10 Medications are safely and accurately administered.

MM.5.20 Not applicable

MM.5.30 Not applicable

Monitoring

MM.6.10 The effects of medication(s) on patients are monitored.

MM.6.20 The organization responds to actual or potential adverse drug events and medication errors.

High-Risk Medications

MM.7.10 The organization develops processes for managing high-risk or high-alert medications.

MM.7.20 Not applicable

MM.7.30 Not applicable

MM.7.40 Investigational medications are safely controlled and administered.

Evaluation

MM.8.10 The organization evaluates its medication management system.

Standards, Rationales, Elements of Performance, and Scoring

Patient-Specific Information

Standard MM.1.10

Patient-specific information is readily accessible to those involved in the medication management system.

Rationale for MM.1.10

A major cause of medication-related sentinel events and medication errors is a lack of information. Licensed independent practitioners and health care staff who participate in the medication management system need access to important information about each patient in order to do the following:

- Facilitate continuity of care, treatment, and services
- Create an accurate medication history and a current list of medications (also known as a drug profile)
- Safely order, prepare, dispense, administer, and monitor medications, as appropriate

Elements of Performance for MM.1.10

B 1. A written policy describes the minimum amount of information about the patient that is to be available to those involved in medication management.

Note: *The organization defines who has access to this information;* see *standard IM.2.10.*

A 2. At a minimum, the information includes the following:

- The patient's age
- The patient's sex
- The patient's current medications
- The patient's diagnoses, comorbidities, and concurrently occurring conditions
- The patient's relevant laboratory values
- The patient's allergies and past sensitivities

As appropriate to the patient, the organization also includes information regarding the following:

- Weight and height
- Pregnancy and lactation status
- Any other information required by the organization for safe medication management

C Ⓜ 3. The information is accessible when needed (except in emergency situations when time does not permit) to licensed independent practitioners and other health care staff.

Selection and Procurement

Standard MM.2.10

Medications available for dispensing or administration (including stock medications) are selected, listed, and procured based on criteria.

Note: *This standard is applicable only to organizations that dispense or administer medications.*

Elements of Performance for MM.2.10

B 1. Licensed independent practitioners and health care staff involved in ordering, dispensing, administering, and/or monitoring effects of medications develop criteria for determining what medications are available for dispensing or administration.

A 2. At a minimum, the criteria include the indication for use, effectiveness, risks (including propensity for medication errors, abuse potential, and sentinel events), and costs.

MM

A 3. A list of medications for dispensing or administration (including strength and dosage form) is maintained and readily available.

Note: *Sample medications are not required to be on this list.*

B 4. Processes and mechanisms are established to monitor patient responses to a newly added medication before the medication is made available for dispensing or administration within the organization.

B 5. Medications designated as available for dispensing or administration are reviewed at least annually based on emerging safety and efficacy information.

B 6. The organization has processes to approve and procure medications that are not on the organization's medication list.

B 7. The organization has processes to address medication shortages and outages, including the following:

- Communicating with prescribers and staff who participate in the medication management system
- Developing approved substitution protocols

- Educating licensed independent practitioners and health care staff who participate in medication management system about these protocols
- Obtaining medications in the event of a disaster

Storage

Standard MM.2.20

Medications are properly and safely stored.

Rationale for MM.2.20

Appropriate medication storage increases patient safety. Medication storage is designed to assist in maintaining medication integrity, promote the availability of medications when needed, minimize the risk of medication diversion, and reduce potential dispensing errors.

Note 1: *This standard is applicable only to organizations that store medications at their sites.*

Note 2: *The following elements of performance also apply to emergency medications. Additional requirements for emergency medications are addressed at standard MM.2.30.*

Elements of Performance for MM.2.20

A Ⓜ 1. Only approved medications are routinely stocked or stored.*

A Ⓜ 2. Medications are stored under conditions suitable for product stability.

A 3. There is a written policy addressing the storage of medication between receipt of a medication by an individual health care provider and medication administration. At a minimum, the policy addresses the following:
- Safe storage
- Safe handling
- Security
- Disposition of these medications (including return to the medication storage area) at the end of the individual's shift

C Ⓜ 4. The policy addressing the storage of medication between receipt of a medication by an individual health care provider and medication administration is implemented.

A 5. Unauthorized persons, in accordance with the organization's policy and law or regulation, cannot obtain access to medications.

---

* *See* standard MM.2.40 for the exception to this standard: The organization has a process to safely manage medications brought in by the patient or the patient's family.

A 6. Controlled substances are stored to prevent diversion and according to state and federal laws and regulations.

A 7. All expired, damaged, and/or contaminated medications are segregated until they are removed from the organization.

8. Identify and, at a minimum, annually review a list of look-alike/sound-alike drugs used in the organization, and take action to prevent errors involving the interchange of these drugs.

Note: *The preceding requirement is not scored here. It is scored at Goal 3, Requirement 3C.*

A 9. Medications and chemicals used to prepare medications are accurately labeled with contents, expiration dates, and warnings.

A 10. Standardize and limit the number of drug concentrations available in the organization.

A Ⓜ 11. Concentrated electrolytes are removed from care units or areas (unless patient safety is at risk if the concentrated electrolyte is not immediately available on a specific care unit or area; in such situations, specific precautions are taken to prevent inadvertent administration).

12. Not applicable

13. Not applicable

14. Not applicable

C Ⓜ 15. All medication storage areas are periodically inspected according to the organization's policy to make sure medications are stored properly.

Standard MM.2.30

Emergency medications and/or supplies, if any, are consistently available, controlled, and secured.

Note: *The following requirements for emergency medications are in addition to the requirements at Standard MM.2.20, which are also applicable to emergency medications.*

Elements of Performance for MM.2.30

B 1. Organization leadership, in conjunction with licensed independent practitioners and other health care staff whose scope of practice includes the dispensing or administration of emergency medications, decides which emergency medications and/or supplies, if any, will be readily available in care areas.

2. Not applicable

B 3. Emergency medications are available in unit-dose, age-specific, and ready-to-administer forms whenever possible.

A Ⓜ 4. Emergency medications are sealed or stored in containers (for example, crash carts, tackle boxes, emergency drug kits, closed bags that are clearly labeled, and so forth) in such a way that staff can readily determine that the contents are complete and have not expired.

5. Not applicable

6. Not applicable

B 7. Emergency medications and supplies are replaced as soon as possible after their use in accordance with the organization's policies and procedures.

Standard MM.2.40

A process is established to safely manage medications brought into the organization by patients or their families.

Rationale for MM.2.40

A number of valid reasons exist for allowing patients to use their own medications in a health care organization, including the need for continuous therapy; a patient's use of a nonformulary medication; or a lack of alternatives to a patient's personal medication. The organization defines its responsibilities for the safe use of these medications.

Elements of Performance for MM.2.40

B 1. The organization addresses the use of medications brought into the organization by patients or their families, including defining when such medications can be used or administered.

B 2. The organization addresses the use of medications brought into the organization by patients or their families, including identifying the medication and visually evaluating its integrity, when medications brought in by the patient or family are allowed.

A 3. The organization addresses the use of medications brought into the organization by patients or their families, including informing the prescriber and patient if medications brought into the organization by patients or their families are not permitted.

Ordering and Transcribing

Standard MM.3.10

Not applicable

Standard MM.3.20

Medication orders are written clearly and transcribed accurately.

Note: *This standard is applicable only to organizations where medications are ordered, dispensed, or administered.*

Rationale for MM.3.20

Many medication errors occur while communicating or transcribing medication orders. The organization is responsible for taking steps to reduce the potential for error or misinterpretation when orders are written or verbally communicated. The required elements of all orders must be specified. To reinforce the skills and judgments needed for safe medication ordering, the organization offers education to care providers. Clear understanding and communication between staff involved in the medication process is essential. Best practices, external and internal data, and medication risks are considered when the organization develops medication policies and procedures.

Elements of Performance for MM.3.20

B 1. Written policy(ies) address the following: the required elements of a complete medication order.

A 2. Written policy(ies) address the following: when generic or brand names are acceptable or required as part of a medication order.

A 3. Written policy(ies) address the following: whether or when indication for use is required on a medication order.

B 4. Written policy(ies) address the following: special precautions or procedures for ordering drugs with look-alike or sound-alike names.

B 5. Written policy(ies) address the following: actions to take when medication orders are incomplete, illegible, or unclear.

B 6. The organization specifies the required elements of the following types of orders that it deems acceptable for use:

- "As needed" (PRN) orders—orders acted upon based on the occurrence of a specific indication or symptom
- Standing orders—written instruction to administer a medication to a person in circumstances specified in instructions without a prescription
- Hold orders—instruction to temporarily suspend (place medication orders on hold) under specified conditions and to alert users at specified times while a medication is on hold
- Automatic stop orders—a date or time to discontinue a medication
- Resume orders—restart an order which was previously held
- Titrating orders—orders in which the dose is either progressively increased or decreased in response to the patient's status
- Taper orders—orders in which the dose is decreased by a particular amount with each dosing interval

- Range orders—orders in which the dose or dosing interval varies over a prescribed range, depending on the situation or patient's status
- Orders for compounded drugs or drug mixtures not commercially available
- Orders for medication-related devices (for example, nebulizers and catheters)
- Orders for investigational medications
- Orders for herbal products
- Orders for medications at discharge or transfer

7. Not applicable

B 8. In addition, the organization reviews and updates preprinted order sheets as needed to support clarity, accuracy, and safety.

A 9. In addition, the organization specifies that blanket reinstatement of previous orders—a summary order to resume all previous orders—for medications are not acceptable.

10. Not applicable

11. Not applicable

For Medicare-Certified Ambulatory Surgical Centers (EP 12 only)

A 12. Orders given verbally for drugs and biologicals are followed by a written order, signed by the prescribing physician.

MM

C Ⓜ 13. Policies and procedures regarding medication orders are implemented. (Applicable to all ambulatory care organizations.)

A 14. Influenza or pneumoccal polysaccharide vaccines are administered according to a physician order, or, as permitted by law and regulation, according to physician-approved, organization-specific protocol(s).

Preparing and Dispensing

Standard MM.4.10

All prescriptions or medication orders are reviewed for appropriateness.

Note: *This standard is applicable only to organizations that dispense medications.*

Elements of Performance for MM.4.10

1. Not applicable

C Ⓜ 2. Before dispensing, a pharmacist reviews all prescription or medication orders unless a licensed independent practitioner controls the ordering, preparing, and dispensing of the medication or in urgent situations when the resulting delay would harm the patient, including situations in which the patient experiences a sudden change in clinical status (for example, new onset of nausea).

3. Not applicable

4. Not applicable

B 5. The organization has a process to review all prescriptions for the following:
- The appropriateness of the drug, dose, frequency, and route of administration
- Therapeutic duplication
- Real or potential allergies or sensitivities
- Real or potential interactions between the prescription and other medications or food
- Current or potential impact as evidenced by laboratory values
- Other contraindications
- Variation from organizational criteria for use
- Other relevant medication-related issues or concerns

B 6. All concerns, issues, or questions are clarified with the individual prescriber before dispensing the medication.

Standard MM.4.20

Medications are prepared safely.

Note: *This standard is applicable to all organizations that dispense or prepare medications for administration.*

Elements of Performance for MM.4.20

B 1. When an on-site, licensed pharmacy is available, only the pharmacy compounds or admixes all sterile medications, intravenous admixtures, or other drugs except in emergencies or when not feasible (for example, when the product's stability is short).

A 2. The organization has a written policy that addresses the safety and use of medications acquired by a practitioner from sources other than the organization for use in patient care in that organization. The policy addresses the following:
- Whether such medications are allowed to be used
- If allowed, a process to evaluate the integrity of medications brought in by a practitioner prior to use in patient care

A 3. The written policy that addresses the safety and use of medications acquired by a practitioner from sources other than the organization for use in patient care is implemented.

C Ⓜ 4. Wherever medications are prepared, staff uses safety materials and equipment while preparing hazardous medications.

C Ⓜ 5. Wherever medications are prepared, staff uses techniques to assure accuracy in medication preparation.

C Ⓜ 6. Wherever medications are prepared, staff follow techniques to avoid contamination during medication preparation including, but not limited to, the following:
- Using clean or sterile techniques
- Maintaining clean, uncluttered, and functionally separate areas for product preparation to minimize the possibility of contamination
- Using a laminar airflow hood or other class 100 environment while preparing any intravenous (IV) admixture in the pharmacy, any sterile product made from nonsterile ingredients, or any sterile product that will not be used within 24 hours
- Visually inspecting the integrity of the medications

Standard MM.4.30

Medications are labeled.

Rationale for MM.4.30

A standardized method for labeling all medications will minimize errors.

Elements of Performance for MM.4.30

B 1. Medications are labeled in a standardized manner according to law or regulation and standards of practice.

B 2. Any time one or more medications or solutions are prepared but are not administered immediately, the medication container* must be labeled.

Note: *An organization that exclusively uses a single medication in an area can draw up or prepare multiple doses for later use as long as the medication is segregated and secured from all other medications in the organization (for example, a vaccine or flu shot) and the container enclosing the individual doses is labeled.*

A 3. At a minimum, all medications prepared in the organization are labeled with the following:
- Drug name, strength, amount (if not apparent from the container)
- Expiration date† when not used within 24 hours
- Expiration time when expiration occurs in less than 24 hours
- The date prepared and the diluent for all compounded IV admixtures and parenteral nutrition solutions

---

* A container can be any storage device such as a plastic bag, syringe, bottle, box, medicine cup, or basin.

† Expiration date, also called the "beyond use date," refers to the last date that the product should be used by the patient.

A 4. When preparing individualized medications for multiple specific patients, or when the person preparing the individualized medications is not the person administering the medication, the label also includes the following:
- Patient name
- Patient location
- Directions for use and any applicable cautionary statements either on the label or attached as an accessory label (for example, "requires refrigeration," "for IM use only")

Standard MM.4.40

Medications are dispensed safely.

Note: *This standard is applicable to all organizations that dispense medications.*

Elements of Performance for MM.4.40

B 1. Quantities of medications are dispensed and minimize diversion yet are still consistent with the patient's needs.

B 2. Dispensing adheres to law, regulation, licensure, and professional standards of practice, including record keeping.

C Ⓜ 3. Medications are dispensed in a timely* manner to meet patient needs.

C Ⓜ 4. Medications are dispensed in the most ready-to-administer forms available from the manufacturer or if feasible, in unit-doses that have been repackaged by the pharmacy or licensed repackager.

Standard MM.4.50

The organization has a system for safely providing medications to meet patient needs when the pharmacy is closed.

Note: *This standard only applies when an organization has an on-site pharmacy and patients present in the organization.*

Rationale for MM.4.50

If an urgent or emergent patient need occurs, the organization is able to provide medications to the patients in its facility.

Element of Performance for MM.4.50

B 1. The organization has a process for providing medications to meet patient needs when the pharmacy is closed.

---

* **Timely** Defined by organization policy and based on the intended use of the information.

Standard MM.4.60

If the organization does not operate a pharmacy but routinely administers medications, the organization has a process for obtaining medications from a pharmacy.

Elements of Performance for MM.4.60

A 1. If the organization does not operate a pharmacy, the organization has a process for obtaining medications from a pharmacy for patients.

A 2. If the organization obtains medications from a pharmacy that is not open 24 hours a day, 7 days a week, the organization has a process for obtaining medications from another source for urgent or emergent conditions when the pharmacy is closed.

Standard MM.4.70

Medications dispensed by the organization are retrieved when recalled or discontinued by the manufacturer or the Food and Drug Administration for safety reasons.

Note: *This standard is applicable to all organizations that dispense medications, including those organizations that dispense sample medications.*

Elements of Performance for MM.4.70

A 1. When the organization has been informed of a medication recall or discontinuation by the manufacturer or the Food and Drug Administration (FDA) for safety reasons, medications within the organization are retrieved* and handled per organization policy and law or regulation.

A 2. The organization notifies all those ordering, dispensing, and/or administering active† medications of any manufacturer or FDA recall or discontinuance.

A 3. When the organization has been informed of a medication recall or discontinuation by the manufacturer or the FDA for safety reasons, patients who are actively receiving the medication are identified and informed of the recall or discontinuation.

MM

Standard MM.4.80

The organization has a process to address medications that are returned to the pharmacy or the organization.

Rationale for MM.4.80

Medications may be returned when allowed under law or regulation and organization policy. Previously dispensed but unused, expired, or returned medications in

* Although recalls are generally by lot number, an organization may retrieve all lots of a recalled medication instead of recording and identifying medications by their lot number.

† Dispensed medications that have not passed expiration date and prescriptions that can be refilled without an additional physician order.

the organization must be accounted for, controlled, and disposed of. The pharmacy is responsible for controlling and accounting for all unused medications returned to the pharmacy.

Note: *When allowed under law or regulations, all unused, expired, or returned medications in the control of the organization are managed and accounted for either by the organization that uses the medications or the pharmacy services used by the organization.*

Elements of Performance for MM.4.80

B 1. The organization has a process in place that addresses if and when unused, expired, or returned medications will be managed by the pharmacy or by the organization.

B 2. The organization has a process in place that addresses how medications are returned to the pharmacy's or organization's control, including procedures that address preventing diversion of medications and account for all unused, expired, or returned medications.

B 3. The organization has a process in place that addresses how outside sources, if any, are used for destruction of medications.

C Ⓜ 4. These processes for addressing medications returned to the pharmacy or organization are implemented.

Administration

Standard MM.5.10

Medications are safely and accurately administered.

Elements of Performance for MM.5.10

B 1. Policies and procedures address health care staff who are allowed to administer medications, with or without supervision, consistent with law or regulation and organization policy.

C Ⓜ 2. Before administering a medication, the licensed independent practitioner or qualified individual administering the medication does the following: verifies that the medication selected for administration is the correct one based on the medication order and product label.

C Ⓜ 3. Before administering a medication, the licensed independent practitioner or qualified individual administering the medication does the following: verifies that the medication is stable based on visual examination for particulates or discoloration and that the medication has not expired.

C Ⓜ 4. Before administering a medication, the licensed independent practitioner or qualified individual administering the medication does the following: verifies that there is no contraindication for administering the medication.

C Ⓜ 5. Before administering a medication, the licensed independent practitioner or qualified individual administering the medication does the following: verifies that the medication is being administered at the proper time, in the prescribed dose, and by the correct route.

C Ⓜ 6. Before administering a medication, the licensed independent practitioner or qualified individual administering the medication does the following: advises the patient or if appropriate, the patient's family about any potential clinically significant adverse reaction or other concerns about administering a new medication.*

C Ⓜ 7. Before administering a medication, the licensed independent practitioner or qualified individual administering the medication does the following: discusses any unresolved, significant concerns about the medication with the patient's physician, prescriber (if different from the physician), and/or relevant staff involved with the patient's care, treatment, and service.

B 8. Policies and procedures address guidelines for prescriber notification in the event of an adverse drug reaction or medication error.

Standard MM.5.20

Not applicable

Standard MM.5.30

Not applicable

Monitoring

Standard MM.6.10

The effects of medication(s) on patients are monitored.

Rationale for MM.6.10

Monitoring the effects of medications on patients helps to assure that medication therapy is appropriate and minimizes the occurrence of adverse events.

* Please refer to PC.6.10, EP 3 for additional information addressing the education of patients regarding medication use.

Elements of Performance for MM.6.10

C Ⓜ 1. Each patient's response to his or her medication is monitored according to the clinical needs of the patient and addresses the patient's response to the prescribed medication and actual or potential medication-related problems.

C Ⓜ 2. Monitoring a medication's effect on a patient includes the following:
- Gathering the patient's own perceptions about side effects, and when appropriate, perceived efficacy
- Referring to information from the patient's medical record, relevant laboratory results, clinical response, and medication profile

B 3. The organization has a process for monitoring the patient's response to the first dose(s) of a medication new to a patient when he or she is under the direct care of the organization.

Standard MM.6.20

The organization responds to actual or potential adverse drug events and medication errors.

Elements of Performance for MM.6.20

B 1. The organization has a process to respond to actual or potential adverse drug events and medication errors.

C Ⓜ 2. Action is taken when an actual or potential adverse drug event is identified (depending on the organization's services, this may be limited to calling for outside assistance, for example, community-sponsored 911 service).

C Ⓜ 3. The organization or responsible individual complies with internal and external reporting requirements for actual or potential adverse drug events (for example, to the United States Pharmacopoeia [USP], the FDA, and the Institute for Safe Medication Practices [ISMP]).

4. Not applicable

For Medicare-Certified Ambulatory Surgical Centers

A Ⓜ 5. All adverse drug reactions are reported to the physician responsible for the patient and are documented in the medical record.

High-Risk Medications

High-risk or high-alert drugs are those drugs involved in a high percentage of medication errors and/or sentinel events and medications that carry a higher risk for abuse, errors, or other adverse outcomes. Lists of high-risk or high-alert drugs are available from such organizations as the ISMP, the USP, and so forth, based on national data about medication use. However, the organization needs to develop its own list of high-risk or high-alert drugs based on its unique utilization patterns or drugs and its own internal data about medication errors and sentinel events. Examples of high-risk drugs include investigational drugs, controlled medications, medications not on the approved FDA list, medications with a narrow therapeutic range, psychotherapeutic medications, and look-alike/sound-alike medications. Organizations determine whether medications that are new to the market or new to the organization are high risk.

Standard MM.7.10

The organization develops processes for managing high-risk or high-alert medications.

Elements of Performance for MM.7.10

A 1. The organization identifies the high-risk or high-alert medications used within the organization, if any.

B 2. Based on the services provided, the organization develops processes for procuring, storing, ordering, transcribing, preparing, dispensing, administering, and/or monitoring high-risk or high-alert medications.

C Ⓜ 3. The processes for managing high-risk or high-alert medications are implemented.

Standard MM.7.20

Not applicable

Standard MM.7.30

Not applicable

Standard MM.7.40

Investigational medications are safely controlled and administered.

Rationale for MM.7.40

The organization protects the safety of patients participating in investigational or clinical medication studies by controlling and monitoring the use of these medications. In addition, the organization addresses the use of specific populations for experimentation and research and reviews all investigational medications to evaluate safety (*see* standard RI.2.180).

Elements of Performance for MM.7.40

B 1. Procedures for the use of investigational medications specify a written process for reviewing, approving, supervising, and monitoring investigational medications use.

B 2. When the organization operates a pharmacy, procedures specify the pharmacy controls the storage, dispensing, labeling, and distribution of the investigational medication.

B 3. Procedures specify that when a patient is involved in an investigational protocol that is independent of the organization, the organization will review and accommodate the patient's continued participation in the protocol (*see* standard RI.2.180).

B 4. The procedures for the use of investigational medications are implemented.

Evaluation

Standard MM.8.10

The organization evaluates its medication management system.

Elements of Performance for MM.8.10

B 1. The organization evaluates its medication management system for risk points and identifies areas to improve safety.

B 2. The organization identifies opportunities for improvement by routinely evaluating the literature for new technologies or successful practices that have been demonstrated to enhance safety in other organizations to determine if it can improve its own medication management system.

B 3. The organization reviews internally generated reports to identify trends or issues in its medication management system (*see* standards PI.2.10 and PI.2.20).

B 4. The organization acts to implement improvements based on the following:
- Evaluation of its medication management system
- Review of new technologies
- External data
- Successful practices that have been demonstrated to enhance safety

B 5. The performance of new and modified medication management processes is measured.

B 6. The organization uses information from data analysis to identify subsequent changes to improve its medication management system.

Surveillance, Prevention, and Control of Infection

Overview

Health care–associated infections (HAIs) are a national problem not limited to hospitals. Infections can be acquired within any care, treatment, and service setting and transferred between settings or brought in from the community. Therefore, prevention of HAIs represents one of the major safety initiatives that an ambulatory care organization can undertake.

Ambulatory care services are delivered in diverse settings such as ambulatory surgical centers, jails and prisons, sleep labs, and imaging centers. As such, these settings have different levels of risk for transmission of infection. The design and scope of the infection prevention and control program (hereafter referred to as the "IC program") are based on the risk(s) that the organization faces for the transmission of infectious disease. Therefore, the organization must assess its risk(s) and design the IC program based on this assessment. Activities that address the identified risks should be included in the IC program.

The goal of an effective IC program is to reduce the risk of acquisition and transmission of HAIs. Ambulatory care organizations must do the following to achieve this goal:

- The organization incorporates its infection control program as a major component of its safety and performance improvement programs.
- The organization performs an ongoing assessment to identify its risks for the acquisition and transmission of infectious agents.
- The organization effectively conducts surveillance, collects data, and interprets the data.
- The organization effectively implements infection prevention and control processes.
- The organization educates and collaborates with leaders across the organization to effectively participate in the design and implementation of the IC program.
- The organization integrates its efforts with health care and community leaders to the extent practicable, recognizing that infection prevention and control is a communitywide effort.
- The organization plans for responding to infections that may potentially overwhelm its resources.

A program with aims of such broad scope and depth requires the direct involvement of organization leaders. Only with the ongoing attention and direction of organization leaders can the appropriate scope of the IC program be determined and adequately resourced.

The standards in this chapter, which focus on development and implementation of plans to prevent and control infections, are supported by standards in other chapters, such as "Management of the Environment of Care" (EC), "Management of Human Resources" (HR), "Improving Organization Performance" (PI), and "Leadership" (LD), to produce a comprehensive approach to infection control.

Standards

The following is a list of all standards for this function. They are presented here for your convenience without footnotes or other explanatory text. If you have a question about a term used here, please check the Glossary.

Note: *A revised standard numbering system is being used with the reformatted standards. The revised numbering system will allow for more flexibility to add standards while maintaining the current number for each standard.*

The IC Program and Its Components

IC.1.10 The risk of development of a health care–associated infection is minimized through an organizationwide infection control program.

IC.2.10 The infection control program identifies risks for the acquisition and transmission of infectious agents on an ongoing basis.

IC.3.10 Based on risks, the organization establishes priorities and sets goals for preventing the development of health care–associated infections within the organization.

IC.4.10 Once the organization has prioritized its goals, strategies must be implemented to achieve those goals.

IC.4.15 Not applicable

IC.5.10 The infection control program evaluates the effectiveness of the infection control interventions and, as necessary, redesigns the infection control interventions.

IC.6.10 As part of its emergency management activities, the organization prepares to respond to an influx, or the risk of an influx, of infectious patients.

Structure and Resources for the IC Program

IC.7.10 The infection control program is managed effectively.

IC.8.10 Relevant components/functions within the organization collaborate to implement the infection control program.

IC.9.10 Organization leaders allocate adequate resources for the infection control program.

Standards, Rationales, Elements of Performance, and Scoring

The IC Program and Its Components

Standard IC.1.10

The risk of development of a health care–associated infection is minimized through an organizationwide infection control program.

Rationale for IC.1.10

The risk of HAIs exists throughout the organization. An effective IC program that can systematically identify risks and respond appropriately must involve all relevant programs and settings within the organization.

Elements of Performance for IC.1.10

B 1. An organizationwide IC program is implemented.

B 2. Individuals and/or positions with the authority to take steps to prevent or control the acquisition and transmission of infectious agents are identified.

B 3. All applicable organizational components and functions are integrated into the IC program.

B 4. Systems are in place to communicate with licensed independent practitioners, staff, students/trainees, volunteers, and, as appropriate, visitors, patients, and families about infection prevention and control issues, including their responsibilities in preventing the spread of infection within the organization.

B 5. The organization has systems for reporting infection surveillance, prevention, and control information to the following:

- The appropriate staff within the organization
- Federal, state, and local public health authorities in accordance with law and regulation
- Accrediting bodies (*see* Sentinel Event Reporting, page 102, and National Patient Safety Goals, page 121)
- The referring or receiving organization when a patient was transferred or referred and the presence of an infection was not known at the time of transfer or referral

Note: *When a referring organization becomes aware that a patient it has transferred has an active infection for which treatment should start or change, the referring organization communicates this to the receiving organization. If a receiving organization identifies an infection not identi-*

fied by the referring organization (such as an infected wound), the receiving organization should communicate the omission to the referring organization. This action will aid the referring organization's improvement efforts.

B 6. Systems for the investigation of outbreaks of infectious diseases are in place.

B 7. Applicable policies and procedures are in place throughout the organization.

8. Not applicable

B 9. The organization has a written IC plan* that includes the following:
- A description of prioritized risks
- A statement of the goals of the IC program
- A description of the organization's strategies to minimize, reduce, or eliminate the prioritized risks
- A description of how the strategies will be evaluated

Standard IC.2.10

The infection control program identifies risks for the acquisition and transmission of infectious agents on an ongoing basis.

Rationale for IC.2.10

An organization's risks of infection will vary based on the organization's geographic location, the community environment, the types of programs/services provided, and the characteristics and behaviors of the population served. Because these risks change over time—sometimes rapidly—risk assessment must be an ongoing process.

Elements of Performance for IC.2.10

B 1. The organization identifies risks for the transmission and acquisition of infectious agents throughout the organization based on the following factors:
- The geographic location and community environment of the organization, program/services provided, and the characteristics of the population served
- The results of the analysis of the organization's infection prevention and control data
- The care, treatment, and services provided

A 2. The risk analysis is formally reviewed at least annually and whenever significant changes occur in any of the above factors.

---

* **Written plan** A succinct, useful document, formulated beforehand, that identifies needs, lists strategies to meet those needs, and sets goals and objectives. The format of the "plan" may include narratives, policies and procedures, protocols, practice guidelines, clinical paths, care maps, or a combination of these.

B 3. Surveillance activities, including data collection and analysis, are used to identify infection prevention and control risks pertaining to the following:
- Patients
- Licensed independent practitioners, staff, volunteers, and students/trainees
- Visitors and families, as warranted

Standard IC.3.10

Based on risks, the organization establishes priorities and sets goals for preventing the development of health care–associated infections within the organization.

Rationale for IC.3.10

The risks of HAIs within an organization are many while resources are limited. An effective IC program requires a thoughtful prioritization of the most important risks to be addressed. Priorities and goals related to the identified risks guide the choice and design of strategies for infection prevention and control in an organization. These priorities and goals provide a framework for evaluating the strategies.

Elements of Performance for IC.3.10

B 1. Priorities are established and goals related to preventing the acquisition and transmission of potentially infectious agents are developed based on the risks identified.

These goals include, but are not limited to, the following (EPs 2–5):

A 2. Limiting unprotected exposure to pathogens throughout the organization

A 3. Enhancing hand hygiene

4. Not applicable

A 5. Minimizing the risk of transmitting infections associated with the use of procedures, medical equipment, and medical devices

Standard IC.4.10

Once the organization has prioritized its goals, strategies must be implemented to achieve those goals.

Rationale for IC.4.10

The organization plans and implements interventions to address the IC issues that it finds important based on prioritized risks and associated surveillance data.

Elements of Performance for IC.4.10

B 1. Interventions are designed to incorporate relevant guidelines* for infection prevention and control activities.

Interventions are implemented which include the following (EPs 2 and 3):

A 2. An organizationwide hand hygiene program that complies with World Health Organization (WHO) Hand Hygiene Guidelines or current Centers for Disease Control and Prevention (CDC) hand hygiene guidelines (National Patient Safety Goal 7, requirement 7.a)†

Note: *The preceding requirement is not scored here. It is scored at National Patient Safety Goal 7, Requirement 7A.*

B 3. Methods to reduce the risks associated with procedures, medical equipment,‡ and medical devices, including the following:
- Appropriate storage, cleaning, disinfection, sterilization, and/or disposal of supplies and equipment
- Reuse of equipment designated by the manufacturer as disposable in a manner that is consistent with regulatory and professional standards
- The appropriate use of personal protective equipment

B 4. Implementation of applicable precautions, as appropriate, is based on the following:
- The potential for transmission
- The mechanism of transmission
- The care, treatment, and service setting
- The emergence and reemergence of pathogens in the community that could affect the organization

Interventions are implemented which include the following (EPs 5–8):

C Ⓜ 5. Screening for exposure (for example, tuberculosis testing) and/or immunity to infectious diseases that licensed independent practitioners, staff, students/trainees, and volunteers may come in contact with in their work is available as warranted

C Ⓜ 6. Referral for assessment, potential testing, immunization and/or prophylaxis/treatment, and counseling, as appropriate, of licensed independent practitioners, staff, students/trainees, and volunteers who are identified as potentially having an infectious disease or risk of infectious disease that may put the population they serve at risk

---

* Examples of guidelines include those offered by the CDC, Healthcare Infection Control Practices Advisory Committee (HICPAC), and National Quality Forum (NQF).

† Organizations are required to comply with all IA, IB, and IC CDC recommendations.

‡ **Medical equipment** Fixed and portable equipment used for the diagnosis, treatment, monitoring, and direct care of individuals.

C Ⓜ 7. Referral for assessment, potential testing, immunization and/or prophylaxis/treatment, and counseling, as appropriate, of patients, students/trainees, and volunteers who have been exposed to infectious disease(s) at the organization and licensed independent practitioners or staff who are occupationally exposed

B 8. Reduction of risks associated with animals brought into the organization (such as management of animal waste)

Standard IC.4.15

Not applicable

Standard IC.5.10

The infection control program evaluates the effectiveness of the infection control interventions and, as necessary, redesigns the infection control interventions.

Rationale for IC.5.10

The evaluation of the effectiveness of interventions helps to identify which activities of the IC program are effective and which activities need to be changed to improve outcomes.

Elements of Performance for IC.5.10

A 1. The organization formally evaluates and revises the goals and program (or portions of the program) at least annually and whenever risks significantly change.

B 2. The evaluation addresses changes in the scope of the IC program (for example, resulting from the introduction of new services or new sites of care).

B 3. The evaluation addresses changes in the results of the IC program risk analysis.

B 4. The evaluation addresses emerging and reemerging problems in the health care community that potentially affect the organization (for example, highly infectious agents).

B 5. The evaluation addresses the assessment of the success or failure of interventions for preventing and controlling infection.

B 6. The evaluation addresses responses to concerns raised by leadership and others within the organization.

B 7. The evaluation addresses the evolution of relevant infection prevention and control guidelines that are based on evidence or, in the absence of evidence, expert consensus.

Standard IC.6.10

As part of its emergency management activities, the organization prepares to respond to an influx, or the risk of an influx, of infectious patients.

Rationale for IC.6.10

The health care organization is an important resource for the continued functioning of a community. An organization's ability to deliver care, treatment, or services is threatened when it is ill-prepared to respond to an epidemic or infections likely to require expanded or extended care capabilities over a prolonged period. Therefore, it is important for an organization to plan how to prevent the introduction of the infection into the organization, how to quickly recognize that existing patients have become infected, and/or how to contain the risk or spread of the infection.

This planned response may include a broad range of options, including the temporary halting of services and/or admissions, delaying transfer or discharge, limiting visitors within an organization, or fully activating the organization's emergency management plan. The actual response depends on issues such as the extent to which the community is affected by the epidemic or infection, the types of services the organization offers, and the organization's capabilities.

The concepts included in these standards are supported by standards found elsewhere in the book, including standard EC.4.10.

Elements of Performance for IC.6.10

B 1. The organization determines its response to an influx or risk of an influx of infectious patients.

B 2. If the organization will continue to accept or treat patients, then the organization has a plan for managing an ongoing influx of potentially infectious patients over an extended period.

B 3. The organization does the following:
- Determines how it will keep abreast of current information about the emergence of epidemics or new infections which may result in the organization activating its response
- Determines how it will disseminate critical information to staff and other key practitioners
- Identifies resources in the community (through local, state, and/or federal public health systems) for obtaining additional information

Structure and Resources for the IC Program

Standard IC.7.10

The infection control program is managed effectively.

Rationale for IC.7.10

The IC program requires management by an individual (or individuals) with knowledge that is appropriate to the level of risks identified by the organization, as well as knowledge of the analysis of infection risks, principles of infection prevention and control, and data analysis. The individual gathering data for the IC program does not have to be the person analyzing the data and managing the program. The individual may be employed by the organization or the organization may contract with this individual. The number of individuals and their qualifications are based on the organization's size, complexity, and needs.

Elements of Performance for IC.7.10

A 1. The organization assigns responsibility for managing IC program activities to one or more individuals whose number, competency, and skill mix are determined by the goals and objectives of the IC activities.

B 2. Qualifications of the individual(s) responsible for managing the IC program are determined by the risks entailed in the care, treatment, and services provided; the organization's patient population(s); and the complexity of the activities that will be carried out.

Note: *Qualifications may be met through ongoing education, training, experience, and/or certification (such as that offered by the Certification Board for Infection Control [CBIC]) in the prevention and control of infections).*

B 3. This individual(s) coordinates all infection prevention and control activities within the organization.

IC

B 4. This individual(s) facilitates ongoing monitoring of the effectiveness of prevention and/or control activities and interventions.

Standard IC.8.10

Relevant components/functions within the organization collaborate to implement the infection control program.

Rationale for IC.8.10

The successful creation of an organizationwide IC program requires collaboration with all relevant components/functions. This collaboration is vital to successful data gathering and interpretation, design of interventions, and effective implementation of interventions. Individuals within the organization who have the power to implement plans and make decisions about interventions related to infection prevention and control participate in the IC program. In smaller organizations, this may only represent one or two people, while in larger organizations this may require representation by multiple divisions. Whatever the number of components/functions represented, it is important that the components/functions that have a direct impact on infection control are represented. While a formal committee consisting of leadership and other components is not required as evidence of this collaboration, the organization may want to consider this option.

Elements of Performance for IC.8.10

B 1. Organization leaders, with licensed independent practitioners and other direct and indirect patient care staff (including, when applicable, administration, building maintenance/engineering, food services, housekeeping, laboratory, pharmacy, and sterilization services), collaborate on an ongoing basis with the qualified individual(s) managing the IC program.

B 2. These representatives participate in the following:
- Development of strategies for each component/function's role in the IC program
- Assessment of the adequacy of the human, information, physical, and financial resources allocated to support infection prevention and control activities
- Assessment of the overall failure or success of key processes for preventing and controlling infection
- The review and revision of the IC program as warranted to improve outcomes

Standard IC.9.10

Organization leaders allocate adequate resources for the infection control program.

Rationale for IC.9.10

Adequate resources are needed to effectively plan and successfully implement a program of this scope.

Elements of Performance for IC.9.10

A 1. The effectiveness of the organization's infection prevention and control activities is reviewed on an ongoing basis, and findings are reported to the integrated patient safety program at least annually.

B 2. Adequate systems to access information are provided to support infection prevention and control activities.

B 3. When applicable, adequate laboratory support is provided to support infection prevention and control activities.

B 4. Adequate equipment and supplies are provided to support infection prevention and control activities.

Improving Organization Performance

Overview

Performance improvement (PI) is a continuous process. It involves measuring the functioning of important processes and services, and, when indicated, identifying changes that enhance performance. These changes are incorporated into new or existing work processes, products, or services, and performance is monitored to ensure that the improvements are sustained.

PI focuses on outcomes of care, treatment, and services. Leaders establish a planned, systematic, and organizationwide approach(es) to performance improvement. They set priorities for PI and ensure that the disciplines representing the scope of care, treatment, and services across the organization work collaboratively to plan and implement improvement activities. The leaders' responsibilities are described in the "Leadership" chapter (standards LD.4.10 through LD.4.70) of this book.

An important aspect of improving organization performance is effectively reducing factors that contribute to unanticipated adverse events and/or outcomes. Unanticipated adverse events and/or outcomes may be caused by poorly designed systems, system failures, or errors. Reducing unanticipated adverse events and/or unanticipated outcomes requires an environment in which patients, their families, and organization staff and leaders can identify and manage actual and potential risks to safety. Such an environment encourages the following:

- Recognizing and acknowledging risks and unanticipated adverse events
- Initiating actions to reduce these risks and unanticipated adverse events
- Reporting internally on risk reduction initiatives and their effectiveness
- Focusing on processes and systems
- Minimizing individual blame or retribution for involvement in an unanticipated adverse event
- Investigating factors that contribute to unanticipated adverse events and sharing that acquired knowledge both internally and with other organizations

The leaders are responsible for fostering such an environment through their personal example and by supporting effective responses to actual occurrences of unanticipated adverse events; ongoing proactive reduction of safety risks to patients; and integration of safety priorities into the design and redesign of all relevant organization processes, functions, and services. (*See* standard LD.4.50.)

This chapter focuses on the following fundamental components of performance improvement:

- Measuring performance through data collection
- Assessing current performance
- Improving performance

Standards

The following is a list of all standards for this function. They are presented here for your convenience without footnotes or other explanatory text. If you have a question about a term used here, please check the Glossary.

Note: *A revised standard numbering system is being used with the reformatted standards. This revised numbering system will allow for more flexibility to add standards while maintaining the current label for each standard.*

PI.1.10 The organization collects data to monitor its performance.

PI.1.20 Not applicable

Aggregating and Analyzing Data to Support Performance Improvement

PI.2.10 Data are systematically aggregated and analyzed.

PI.2.20 Undesirable patterns or trends in performance are analyzed.

PI.2.30 Processes for identifying and managing sentinel events are defined and implemented.

PI.3.10 Information from data analysis is used to make changes that improve performance and patient safety and reduce the risk of sentinel events.

PI.3.20 An ongoing, proactive program for identifying and reducing unanticipated adverse events and safety risks to patients is defined and implemented.

Standards, Rationales, Elements of Performance, and Scoring

Standard PI.1.10

The organization collects data to monitor its performance.

Rationale for PI.1.10

Data help determine PI priorities. The data collected for high priority and required areas are used to monitor the stability of existing processes, identify opportunities for improvement, identify changes that lead to improvement, or sustain improvement. Data collection helps identify specific areas that require further study. These areas are determined by considering the information provided by the data about process stability, risks, and sentinel events and priorities set by the leaders. Data may come from internal sources such as staff or external sources such as patients, referral sources, and so on. In addition, the organization identifies those areas needing improvement and identifies desired changes. Performance measures are used to determine whether the changes result in desired outcomes. The organization identifies the frequency and detail of data collection.

Note: *The organization also collects data on evaluation and improvement of conditions in the environment* (see *the "Management of the Environment of Care" [EC] chapter, where it is scored).*

Elements of Performance for PI.1.10

B 1. The organization collects data for priorities identified by leaders (*see* standard LD.4.50).

B 2. The organization considers collecting data in the following areas:
- Staff opinions and needs
- Staff perceptions of risks to individuals and suggestions for improving patient safety
- Staff willingness to report unanticipated adverse events

B 3. The organization collects data on the perceptions of care, treatment, and services* of patients, including the following:
- Their specific needs and expectations
- How well the organization meets these needs and expectations
- How the organization can improve patient safety
- The effectiveness of pain management, when applicable

PI

* The Joint Commission is moving from the phrase *satisfaction with care, treatment, and services* toward the more inclusive phrase *perception of care, treatment, and services* to better measure the performance of organizations meeting the needs, expectations, and concerns of patients. By using this term, the organization will be prompted to assess not only patients' and/or families' satisfaction with care, treatment, or services, but also whether the organization meets their needs and expectations.

The organization collects data that measure the performance of each of the following potentially high-risk processes, when provided (EPs 4–12):

A 4. Medication management

A 5. Blood and blood product use

A 6. Restraint use

7. Through 10. Not applicable

A 11. Operative and other procedures that place patients at risk

12. Not applicable

Relevant information developed from the following activities is integrated into PI initiatives. This occurs in a way consistent with any organization policies or procedures intended to preserve any confidentiality or privilege of information established by applicable law (EPs 13–17):

B 13. Risk management

B 14. Utilization management

B 15. Quality control

B 16. Infection control surveillance and reporting

B 17. Research, as applicable

18. Through 22. Not applicable

For Medicare-Certified Ambulatory Surgical Centers

A 23. The ambulatory surgical center, with the medical staff's active participation, collects data on an ongoing basis about the medical necessity of procedures.

A 24. The ambulatory surgical center, with the medical staff's active participation, collects data on an ongoing basis about the appropriateness of care.

Standard PI.1.20

Not applicable

Aggregating and Analyzing Data to Support Performance Improvement

Standard PI.2.10

Data are systematically aggregated and analyzed.

Rationale for PI.2.10

Aggregating and analyzing data means transforming data into information. Aggregating data at points in time enables the organization to judge a particular process' stability or a particular outcome's predictability in relation to performance expectations. Accumulated data are analyzed in such a way that current performance levels, patterns, or trends can be identified.

Elements of Performance for PI.2.10

B 1. Collected data are aggregated and analyzed.

B 2. Data are aggregated at the frequency appropriate to the activity or process being studied.

B 3. Statistical tools and techniques are used to analyze and display data.

B 4. Data are analyzed and compared internally over time and externally* with other sources of information when available.

B 5. Comparative data are used to determine if there is excessive variability or unacceptable levels of performance when available.

Standard PI.2.20

Undesirable patterns or trends in performance are analyzed.

Elements of Performance for PI.2.20

B 1. Analysis is performed when data comparisons indicate that levels of performance, patterns, or trends vary substantially from those expected.

B 2. Analysis occurs for those topics chosen by leaders as PI priorities.

B 3. Analysis is performed when undesirable variation occurs which changes priorities.

An analysis is performed for the following (EPs 4–9):

A 4. All confirmed transfusion reactions, if applicable to the organization

A 5. All serious adverse drug events, if applicable and as defined by the organization

A 6. All significant medication errors, if applicable and as defined by the organization

A 7. All major discrepancies between preoperative and postoperative (including pathologic) diagnoses

* External sources of information include recent scientific, clinical, and management literature, including *Sentinel Event Alerts;* well-formulated practice guidelines or parameters; performance measures; reference databases; other organizations with similar processes; and standards that are periodically reviewed and revised.

A 8. Adverse events or patterns of adverse events during moderate or deep sedation and anesthesia use

A 9. Hazardous conditions*

Standard PI.2.30

Processes for identifying and managing sentinel events are defined and implemented.

Rationale for PI.2.30

Identifying, reporting, analyzing, and managing sentinel events can help the organization to prevent such incidents. Leaders define and implement such a program as part of the process to measure, assess, and improve the organization's performance.

Elements of Performance for PI.2.30

Processes for identifying and managing sentinel events include the following (EPs 1–4):

A 1. Defining "sentinel event" and communicating this definition throughout the organization (At a minimum, the organization's definition includes those events subject to review under the Joint Commission's Sentinel Event Policy as published in this book and may include any process variation which does not affect the outcome or result in an adverse event, but for which a recurrence carries significant chance of a serious adverse outcome or result in an adverse event, often referred to as a "near miss.")

A 2. Reporting sentinel events through established channels in the organization and, as appropriate, to external agencies in accordance with law and regulation

B 3. Conducting thorough and credible root cause analyses that focus on process and system factors

B 4. Creating, documenting, and implementing a risk-reduction strategy and action plan that includes measuring the effectiveness of process and system improvements to reduce risk

B 5. The processes are implemented.

Standard PI.3.10

Information from data analysis is used to make changes that improve performance and patient safety and reduce the risk of sentinel events.

---

* Any set of circumstances, defined by the organization (exclusive of the disease or condition for which the individual is being treated) which significantly increases the likelihood of a serious adverse outcome.

Elements of Performance for PI.3.10

B 1. The organization uses the information from data analysis to identify and implement changes that will improve the quality of care, treatment, and services.

B 2. The organization identifies and implements changes that will reduce the risk of sentinel events.

B 3. The organization uses the information from data analysis to identify changes that will improve patient safety.

B 4. Changes made to improve processes or outcomes are evaluated to ensure that they achieve the expected results.

B 5. Appropriate actions are undertaken when planned improvements are not achieved or sustained.

Standard PI.3.20

An ongoing, proactive program for identifying and reducing unanticipated adverse events and safety risks to patients is defined and implemented.

Rationale for PI.3.20

Organizations should proactively seek to identify and reduce risks to the safety of patients. Such initiatives have the obvious advantage of *preventing* adverse events rather than simply *reacting* when they occur. This approach also avoids the barriers to understanding created by hindsight bias and the fear of disclosure, embarrassment, blame, and punishment that can happen after an event.

Elements of Performance for PI.3.20

The following proactive activities to reduce risks to patients are conducted (EPs 1–9):

A 1. Selecting a high-risk process* to be analyzed (at least one high-risk process is chosen annually†—the choice should be based in part on information published periodically by the Joint Commission about the most frequent sentinel events and risks)

---

* **High-risk process** A process that if not planned and/or implemented correctly, has a significant potential for impacting the safety of the patient.

† On rare occasions, the organization may determine that it has no high-risk processes to be analyzed due to the nature of the care, treatment, and services provided (for example, a home medical equipment service provider that only delivers commodes). If this situation occurs, the organization must document on an annual basis that it has determined there are no high-risk processes as well as the reasons for the determination.

Additionally, there may be rare occasions when the organization has a limited number of high-risk processes due to the nature of the care, treatment, or services provided. In those instances, the organization can re-analyze a high-risk process, provided that all identified high-risk processes related to the care, treatment, and services provided have been reviewed.

B 2. Describing the chosen process (for example, through the use of a flowchart)

B 3. Identifying the ways in which the process could break down* or fail to perform its desired function

B 4. Identifying the possible effects that a breakdown or failure of the process could have on patients and the seriousness of the possible effects

B 5. Prioritizing the potential process breakdowns or failures

B 6. Determining why the prioritized breakdowns or failures could occur, which may include performing a hypothetical root cause analysis

B 7. Redesigning the process and/or underlying systems to minimize the risk of the effects on patients

B 8. Testing and implementing the redesigned process

B 9. Monitoring the effectiveness of the redesigned process

PI

* The ways in which a process could break down or fail to perform its desired function are many times referred to as "the failure modes".

Leadership

Overview

An organization's leaders provide the framework for planning, directing, coordinating, providing, and improving care, treatment, and services to respond to community and patient needs and improve health care outcomes.

Effective leadership depends on the following processes and tools:

- **Governance.** The governance of an organization sets the framework for supporting quality patient care, treatment, and services.
- **Management.** Leaders create an environment that enables an organization to fulfill its mission and meet or exceed its goals. They provide for a well-managed organization with clear lines of responsibility and accountability.
- **Planning, designing, and providing services.** Leaders develop a mission that is reflected in long-range, strategic, and operational plans; service design; resource allocation; and organizational policies. They provide organization, direction, and staffing for care, treatment, and services. Leaders also communicate objectives and coordinate efforts to integrate care, treatment, and services throughout the organization.
- **Improving safety and quality of care.** Leaders plan and implement a safety management program. They are ultimately responsible for the safety of all patients and staff. Leaders also establish expectations, plans, and priorities and manage the performance improvement process. They ensure that a process is in place to measure, assess, and improve the organization's governance, management, clinical, and support functions.
- **Use of clinical practice guidelines.** A guideline provides an effective way to improve processes by reducing variance. An organization's success in implementing and using clinical practice guidelines on an ongoing basis depends on the processes for reviewing, revising, and implementing the guidelines.
- **Teaching and coaching staff.** To realize the organization's vision and values, leaders are involved in teaching and coaching staff; thus, staff education is an essential leadership function.

Standards

The following is a list of all standards for this function. They are presented here for your convenience without footnotes or other explanatory text. If you have a question about a term used here, please check the Glossary.

Note: *A revised standard numbering system is being used with the reformatted standards. This revised numbering system will allow for more flexibility to add standards while maintaining the current label for each standard.*

LD.1.10 The organization identifies how it is governed.

LD.1.20 Governance responsibilities are defined in writing, as applicable.

LD.1.30 The organization complies with applicable law and regulation.

LD.2.10 An individual(s) or designee(s) is responsible for operating the organization according to the authority conferred by governance.

LD.2.20 Each organizational program, service, site, or department has effective leadership.

LD.2.30 Not applicable

LD.2.40 Not applicable

LD.2.50 The leaders develop and monitor an annual operating budget and, as appropriate, a long-term capital expenditure plan.

LD.2.60 Through LD.2.200 Not applicable

LD.3.10 The leaders engage in both short-term and long-term planning.

LD.3.15 Not applicable

LD.3.20 Patients with comparable needs receive the same standard of care, treatment, and services throughout the organization.

LD.3.30 Not applicable

LD.3.40 Not applicable

LD.3.50 Care, treatment, and services provided through contractual agreement are provided safely and efffectively.

LD.3.60 Communication is effective throughout the organization.

LD.3.70 The leaders define the required qualifications and competence of those staff who provide care, treatment, and services, and recommend a sufficient number of qualified and competent staff to provide care, treatment, and services.

LD.3.80 The leaders provide for adequate space, equipment, and other resources.

LD.3.90 The leaders develop and implement policies and procedures for care, treatment, and services.

LD.3.100 Not applicable

LD.3.110 Not applicable

LD.3.120 The leaders plan for and support the provision and coordination of patient education activities.

LD.3.130 Not applicable

LD.3.140 Not applicable

LD.3.150 Not applicable

LD.4.10 The leaders set expectations, plan, and manage processes to measure, assess, and improve the organization's governance, management, clinical, and support activities.

LD.4.20 New or modified services or processes are designed well.

LD.4.30 Not applicable

LD.4.40 The leaders ensure that an integrated patient safety program is implemented throughout the organization.

LD.4.50 The leaders set performance improvement priorities and identify how the organization adjusts priorities in response to unusual or urgent events.

LD.4.60 The leaders allocate adequate resources for measuring, assessing, and improving the organization's performance and improving patient safety.

LD.4.70 The leaders measure and assess the effectiveness of the performance improvement and safety improvement activities.

LD.5.10 Through LD.5.40 Not applicable

LD.5.50 Clinical practice guidelines are used in designing or improving processes that evaluate and treat specific diagnoses, conditions, and/or symptoms.

LD.5.60 The leaders identify criteria for selecting and implementing clinical practice guidelines.

LD.5.70 Appropriate leaders, practitioners, and health care professionals in the organization review and approve clinical practice guidelines selected for implementation.

LD.5.80 The leaders evaluate the outcomes related to clinical practice guidelines and refine the guidelines to improve processes.

Standards, Rationales, Elements of Performance, and Scoring

Standard LD.1.10

The organization identifies how it is governed.

Rationale for LD.1.10

The organization has governance with ultimate responsibility and legal authority for the safety and quality of care, treatment, and services. Governance establishes policy, promotes performance improvement, and provides for organizational management and planning.

Elements of Performance for LD.1.10

A 1. The organization identifies how it is governed.

A 2. The organization identifies lines of authority for key planning, management, and operations activities.

A 3. The organization identifies those responsible for governance.

Standard LD.1.20

Governance responsibilities are defined in writing, as applicable.

Elements of Performance for LD.1.20

A 1. Governance defines its responsibilities in writing, as applicable.

A 2. If the organization is part of a larger corporate structure, the scope and degree of leaders' involvement, authority, and responsibility in corporate policy decisions are described in writing.

B 3. Governance provides for organizational management and planning.

A 4. The organization's scope of services is defined in writing and approved by the governance.

A 5. Governance either selects the individual(s) responsible for operating the organization or approves one selected by corporate management or another group.

B 6. Governance provides for coordination and integration among the organization's leaders to establish policy, maintain quality care and patient safety, and provide for necessary resources.

A 7. Governance annually evaluates the organization's performance in relation to its vision, mission, and goals.

Standard LD.1.30

The organization complies with applicable law and regulation.

Elements of Performance for LD.1.30

A 1. The organization provides all care, treatment, and services in accordance with applicable licensure requirements, law, rules, and regulation.

A 2. The organization acts upon any reports and/or recommendations from authorized agencies, as appropriate.

A 3. The organization possesses a license, certificate, or permit, as required by applicable law and regulation, to provide the health care services for which the organization is seeking accreditation.

Standard LD.2.10

An individual(s) or designee(s) is responsible for operating the organization according to the authority conferred by governance.

Elements of Performance for LD.2.10

B 1. The individual(s) designated by governance is responsible for establishing internal controls to effectively operate the organization, including the following:
- Establishing and maintaining information and support systems
- Recruiting and retaining staff
- Conserving physical and financial assets

A 2. When this individual(s) is absent from the organization, an appropriately qualified individual(s) is designated to perform the duties of that position.

3. Not applicable

B 4. As appropriate, reports are provided to governance.

Standard LD.2.20

Each organizational program, service, site, or department has effective leadership.

Rationale for LD.2.20

Effective leaders at the site or department level help to create an environment or culture that enables an organization to fulfill its mission and meet or exceed its goals. They support staff and instill in them a sense of ownership of their work processes. Although it may be appropriate for leaders to delegate work to qualified staff, the leaders are ultimately responsible for care, treatment, or services provided in their area.

Elements of Performance for LD.2.20

B 1. The program, service, site, or department leaders ensure that operations are effective and efficient.

B 2. Leaders hold staff accountable for their responsibilities.

B 3. Programs, services, sites, or departments providing patient care are directed by one or more qualified professionals with appropriate training and experience or by a qualified licensed independent practitioner with appropriate clinical privileges.

B 4. Responsibility for administrative and clinical direction of these programs, services, sites, or departments is defined in writing.

B 5. Leaders ensure that a process is in place to coordinate care, treatment, and service processes among programs, services, sites, or departments.

Standard LD.2.30

Not applicable

Standard LD.2.40

Not applicable

Standard LD.2.50

The leaders develop and monitor an annual operating budget and, as appropriate, a long-term capital expenditure plan.

Elements of Performance for LD.2.50

A 1. An operating budget is developed annually and approved by the governance.

A 2. The budget reflects the organization's goals and objectives and, at a minimum, meets applicable law and regulation.

B 3. The leaders include staff input when developing the budget.

A 4. The governing body or authority approves a long-term capital expenditure plan, as appropriate.

5. Not applicable

6. Not applicable

B 7. Implementation of the budget and, as appropriate, the long-term capital expenditure plan is monitored.

Standards LD.2.60 Through LD.2.200
Not applicable

Standard LD.3.10
The leaders engage in both short-term and long-term planning.

Elements of Performance for LD.3.10
A 1. Leaders create vision, mission, and goal statements.

A 2. The organization's plan for services specifies which care, treatment, or services are provided directly and which through consultation, contract, or other agreement.

3. Through 25. Not applicable

B 26. Planning for care, treatment, and services addresses the following:
- The needs and expectations of patients and, as appropriate, families and referral sources
- Staff needs
- The scope of care, treatment, and services needed by patients at all of the organization's locations
- Resources (financial and human) for providing care and support services
- Recruitment, retention, development, and continuing education needs of all staff
- Data for measuring the performance of processes and outcomes of care

Standard LD.3.15

Not applicable

Standard LD.3.20
Patients with comparable needs receive the same standard of care, treatment, and services throughout the organization.

Rationale for LD.3.20
The leaders must make sure that factors such as different individuals providing care, treatment, and services; different payment sources; or different settings of care do not intentionally negatively influence the outcome.

Elements of Performance for LD.3.20
B 1. Patients with comparable needs receive the same standard of care, treatment, and services throughout the organization.

B 2. The organization plans, designs, and monitors care, treatment, and services so they are consistent with the mission, vision, and goals.

Standard LD.3.30

Not applicable

Standard LD.3.40

Not applicable

Standard for Oversight of Care, Treatment, and Services Provided Through Contractual Agreement*

Introduction

The same level of high-quality care should be delivered to patients regardless of whether services are provided directly by the organization or through contractual agreement. Leaders provide oversight to make sure that care, treatment, and services provided directly are safe and effective. Likewise, leaders must also oversee contracted services to make sure that they are provided safely and effectively. Standard LD.3.50 outlines the requirements for leadership oversight of care, treatment, and services provided through contractual agreement.

The only contractual agreements subject to the requirements in Standard LD.3.50 are those for the provision of care, treatment, and services provided to the organization's patients. Any contract not for care, treatment, and services is not subject to this standard. For example, contracts for consultation or referrals are not subject to the requirements in LD.3.50. However, regardless of whether or not a contract is subject to LD.3.50, the actual performance of any contracted service is evaluated at the other standards in this book appropriate to the nature of the contracted service.

Monitoring Contracted Services

The elements of performance require contracted services to be monitored, but they do not prescribe a specific monitoring strategy. While monitoring activities should focus on the safety and quality of the contracted service, the organization is free to select monitoring activities appropriate to the risk posed to patients by the contracted care, treatment, and services.

The expectations that leaders set for the performance of contracted services should reflect basic principles of risk reduction, safety, staff competence, and performance

* **Contractual agreement** An agreement with any organization, group, agency, or individual for services or personnel to be provided by, to, or on behalf of the organization. Such agreements are defined in a contract or in some other form of written agreement such as a letter of agreement or memorandum of understanding (also referred to as *contract, contracted services, contractual services, memorandum of understanding, letter of agreement,* or *written agreement*).

improvement. The requirements outlined in Standards EC.1.10, EC.1.20, PI.1.10, and HR.3.10 can provide ideas for setting expectations related to these topics. Additional ideas for expectations can also come from the elements of performance found in specific standards applicable to the contracted service. Although leaders have the same responsibility for oversight of contracted services outside the organization's expertise as they do for contracted services within the organization's expertise, it is more difficult to determine how to monitor such services. In these cases, information from relevant professional organizations can provide guidance for setting expectations.

The elements of performance do not prescribe the methods for evaluating contracted services; leaders are expected to select the best methods for their organization to oversee the quality and safety of services provided through contractual agreement. Examples of sources of information that may be used for evaluating contracted services include the following:

- Review of information about the contractor's Joint Commission accreditation or certification status
- Direct observation of the provision of care
- Audit of documentation, including medical records
- Review of incident reports
- Review of periodic reports submitted by the individual or organization providing services under contractual agreement
- Collection of data that address the efficacy of the contracted service
- Review of performance reports based on indicators required in the contractual agreement
- Input from staff and from patients
- Review of patient satisfaction studies
- Review of results of risk management activities

In the event that contracted services do not meet expectations, leaders are expected to take steps to improve care, treatment, and services. In some cases, it may be best to work with the contractor to make improvements, whereas in other cases it may be best to renegotiate or terminate the contractual relationship. When the leaders anticipate the renegotiation or termination of a contractual agreement, planning needs to occur so that the continuity of care, treatment, and services is not disrupted.

Credentialing and Privileging

In most cases, each licensed independent practitioner providing services through a contractual agreement must be credentialed and privileged by the organization using their services following the process described in the "Management of Human Resources" chapter. However, there is one special circumstance:

- Off-site services provided by a Joint Commission–accredited contractor: A footnote to EP 4 of Standard LD.3.50 outlines how an organization can expect a Joint Commission–accredited or –certified contractor to demonstrate the appropriate privileges of the licensed independent practitioners who will be providing patient care, treatment, and services have appropriate privileges. The options outlined in the footnote apply when patients are sent off-site for services.

Standard LD.3.50

Care, treatment, and services provided through contractual agreement are provided safely and effectively.

Rationale for LD.3.50

The guiding principle behind the requirements for contracted services is that the same level of high-quality care should be delivered regardless of whether services are provided directly by the organization or through contractual agreement. Just as leadership oversight is necessary to make sure that services provided directly are safe and effective, leadership oversight of services provided through contractual agreement is required in order to assure that those services are provided safely and effectively.

Elements of Performance for LD.3.50

B 1. Clinical leaders have an opportunity to provide advice about the sources of clinical services that are to be provided through contractual agreement.

A 2. The nature and scope of services provided through contractual agreements are described in writing

A 3. Designated leaders approve the contractual agreements.

B 4. Leaders monitor contracted services by establishing expectations for the performance of the contracted services*

B 5. Leaders monitor contracted services by communicating the expectations in writing† to the provider of the contracted services.

B 6. Leaders monitor contracted services by evaluating the contracted services in relation to the expectations.

LD

---

* When the organization contracts with another accredited organization for patient care, treatment, and services to be provided off-site, it can do the following:

- Verify that all licensed independent practitioners who will be providing patient care, treatment, and services have appropriate privileges by obtaining, for example, a copy of the list of privileges

  or
- Specify in the written agreement that the contracted organization will ensure that all contracted services provided by licensed independent practitioners will be within the scope of their privileges.

† A written description of the expectations can be provided either as part of the written agreement or in addition to it.

B 7. The leaders take steps to improve contracted services that do not meet expectations.*

A 8. When contractual agreements are renegotiated or terminated, the continuity of patient care is maintained.

9. Not applicable

A 10. Reference and contract lab services meet the applicable federal regulations for clinical laboratories and maintain evidence of the same.

Standard LD.3.60

Communication is effective throughout the organization.

Elements of Performance for LD.3.60

B 1. The leaders ensure processes are in place for communicating relevant information throughout the organization in a timely manner.

B 2. Effective communication occurs in the organization, among the organization's programs, among related organizations, with outside organizations, and with patients and families, as appropriate.

B 3. The leaders communicate the organization's mission and appropriate policies, plans, and goals to all staff.

Standard LD.3.70

The leaders define the required qualifications and competence of those staff who provide care, treatment, and services and recommend a sufficient number of qualified and competent staff to provide care, treatment, and services.

LD

Rationale for LD.3.70

The determination of competence and qualifications of staff is based on the following:

- The organization's mission
- The organization's care, treatment, and services
- The complexity of care, treatment, and services needed by patients
- The technology used
- The health status of staff, as required by law and regulation

A single set of criteria must be used to judge the competency of all clinicians who provide care, treatment, and services within the organization, regardless of whether they are employees of the organization or of licensed independent practitioners.

---

* This EP does not prescribe the steps to take when contracted services do not meet expectations. Some examples to consider include the following:

- Increase monitoring of the contracted services
- Provide consultation or training to the contractor
- Renegotiate the contract terms
- Apply defined penalties
- Terminate the contract

Note: *The qualification requirements pertaining to students and volunteers who work in the same capacity as staff when they provide care, treatment, and services are addressed in Standard HR.1.20.*

Element of Performance for LD.3.70

B 1. The leaders provide for the allocation of competent qualified staff.

Standard LD.3.80

The leaders provide for adequate space, equipment, and other resources.

Elements of Performance for LD.3.80

B 1. The leaders provide for the arrangement and allocation of space to facilitate efficient, effective delivery of care, treatment, and services.

B 2. The leaders provide for the appropriateness of interior and exterior space for the care, treatment, and services offered and for the ages and other characteristics of the patients.

B 3. The leaders provide for the safe use, maintenance, accessibility, and supervision of grounds, equipment, and special activity areas.

B 4. The leaders provide for adequate equipment and other resources.

Standard LD.3.90

The leaders develop and implement policies and procedures for care, treatment, and services.

Elements of Performance for LD.3.90

B 1. The leaders develop policies and procedures that guide and support patient care, treatment, and services.

C Ⓜ 2. Policies and procedures are consistently implemented.

Standard LD.3.100

Not applicable

Standard LD.3.110

Not applicable

Standard LD.3.120

The leaders plan for and support the provision and coordination of patient education activities.

Elements of Performance for LD.3.120

B 1. The leaders plan and support patient education activities appropriate to the organization's mission and scope of services.

B 2. The leaders identify and provide the resources necessary for achieving educational objectives.

Standard LD.3.130

Not applicable

Standard LD.3.140

Not applicable

Standard LD.3.150

Not applicable

Standard LD.4.10

The leaders set expectations, plan, and manage processes to measure, assess, and improve the organization's governance, management, clinical, and support activities.

Elements of Performance for LD.4.10

B 1. The leaders set expectations for performance improvement.

B 2. The leaders develop plans for performance improvement.

B 3. The leaders manage processes to improve organization performance.

B 4. The leaders participate in performance improvement activities.

B 5. Appropriate individuals and professions from each relevant program, service, site, or department participate collaboratively in organizationwide performance improvement activities.

Standard LD.4.20

New or modified services or processes are designed well.

Elements of Performance for LD.4.20

The design of new or modified services or processes incorporates the following (EPs 1–6):

B 1. The needs and expectations of patients, staff, and others

B 2. The results of performance improvement activities, when available

B 3. Information about potential risks to patients, when available

B 4. Current knowledge, when available and relevant (for example, practice guidelines, successful practices, information from relevant literature and clinical standards)

B 5. Information about sentinel events, when available and relevant

B 6. Testing and analysis to determine whether the proposed design or redesign is an improvement

B 7. The leaders collaborate with staff and appropriate stakeholders to design services.

Standard LD.4.30

Not applicable

Standard LD.4.40

The leaders ensure that an integrated patient safety program is implemented throughout the organization.

Rationale for LD.4.40

The leaders should work to foster a safe environment throughout the organization by integrating safety priorities into all relevant organization processes, functions, and services. In pursuit of this effort, a patient safety program can work to improve safety by reducing the risk of system or process failures. As part of its responsibility to communicate objectives and coordinate efforts to integrate patient care and support services throughout the organization and with contracted services, leadership takes the lead in developing, implementing, and overseeing a patient safety program.

The standard does not require the creation of new structures or "offices" in the organization; rather, the standard emphasizes the need to integrate all patient-safety activities, both existing and newly created, with the organization's leadership identified as accountable for this integration.

Elements of Performance for LD.4.40

The patient safety program includes the following (EPs 1–8):

A 1. One or more qualified individuals or an interdisciplinary group assigned to manage the organizationwide safety program

B 2. Definition of the scope of the program's oversight, typically ranging from no-harm, frequently occurring "slips" to sentinel events with serious adverse outcomes

B 3. Integration into and participation of all components of the organization into the organizationwide program

B 4. Procedures for immediately responding to system or process failures, including care, treatment, or services for the affected individual(s), containing risk to others, and preserving factual information for subsequent analysis

B 5. Clear systems for internal and external reporting of information about system or process failures

B 6. Defined responses to various types of unanticipated adverse events and processes for conducting proactive risk assessment/risk reduction activities

B 7. Defined support systems* for staff members who have been involved in a sentinel event

A 8. Reports, at least annually, to the organization's governance or authority on system or process failures and actions taken to improve safety, both proactively and in response to actual occurrences

Standard LD.4.50

The leaders set performance improvement priorities and identify how the organization adjusts priorities in response to unusual or urgent events.

Elements of Performance for LD.4.50

B 1. The leaders set priorities for performance improvement for organizationwide activities and patient health outcomes.

B 2. The leaders give high priority to high-volume, high-risk, or problem-prone processes.

B 3. Performance improvement activities are reprioritized in response to significant changes in the internal or external environment.

Standard LD.4.60

The leaders allocate adequate resources for measuring, assessing, and improving the organization's performance and improving patient safety.

Elements of Performance for LD.4.60

B 1. Sufficient staff is assigned to conduct activities for performance improvement and safety improvement.

B 2. Adequate time is provided for staff to participate in activities for performance improvement and safety improvement.

* Support systems provide individuals with additional help and support as well as additional resources through the human resources function or an employee assistance program. Support systems recognize that conscientious health care workers who are involved in sentinel events are themselves victims of the event and require support. Support systems also focus on the process rather than blaming the involved individuals.

B 3. Adequate information systems are provided to support activities for performance improvement and safety improvement.

B 4. Staff is trained in performance improvement and safety improvement approaches and methods.

Standard LD.4.70

The leaders measure and assess the effectiveness of the performance improvement and safety improvement activities.

Elements of Performance for LD.4.70

B 1. Leaders continually monitor the effectiveness of the performance improvement and safety improvement activities.

B 2. The leaders develop and implement improvements for these activities.

B 3. The leaders assess the adequacy of the human, information, physical, and financial resources allocated to support performance improvement and safety improvement activities.

Standards LD.5.10 Through LD.5.40

Not applicable

Standard LD.5.50

Clinical practice guidelines are used in designing or improving processes that evaluate and treat specific diagnoses, conditions, and/or symptoms.

Rationale for LD.5.50

Clinical practice guidelines can improve quality, appropriate utilization of health care services, and the value of health care services. Clinical practice guidelines help practitioners in making decisions about preventing, diagnosing, treating, and managing selected conditions. Clinical practice guidelines can also be used in designing processes or checking the design of existing processes. The leaders identify and consider for implementation clinical practice guidelines from such sources as the Agency for Healthcare Research and Quality, National Guideline Clearinghouse, and professional organizations.

Element of Performance for LD.5.50

B 1. The leaders have used clinical practice guidelines in designing or improving processes.

Standard LD.5.60

The leaders identify criteria for selecting and implementing clinical practice guidelines.

Rationale for LD.5.60

Selecting and implementing critical practice guidelines that are appropriate to the organization are critical. Therefore, the leaders set criteria to guide the selection and implementation of guidelines that are consistent with the organization's mission and priorities. The leaders also consider the steps and changes or variations needed to encourage use, dissemination, and implementation of chosen guidelines throughout the organization. This includes staff communication, training, implementation, feedback, and evaluation.

Elements of Performance for LD.5.60

B 1. The leaders identify criteria to guide the selection and implementation of guidelines.

B 2. The organization manages, evaluates, and learns from variation.

Standard LD.5.70

Appropriate leaders, practitioners, and health care professionals in the organization review and approve clinical practice guidelines selected for implementation.

Rationale for LD.5.70

To be successfully implemented, clinical practice guidelines should be reviewed, revised or adapted by the providers using them and approved by the organization's leaders.

Element of Performance for LD.5.70

A 1. Appropriate organization leaders review and approve the clinical practice guidelines selected for use.

Standard LD.5.80

The leaders evaluate the outcomes related to clinical practice guidelines and refine the guidelines to improve processes.

Rationale for LD.5.80

To fully benefit from the use of clinical practice guidelines, the outcomes of patients treated using clinical practice guidelines are evaluated, and refinements are made in how the guidelines are used, if necessary.

Element of Performance for LD.5.80

B 1. Clinical practice guidelines are monitored and reviewed for effectiveness and modified as appropriate.

Management of the Environment of Care

Overview

The **goal** of this function is to provide a safe, functional, supportive, and effective environment for patients, staff members, and other individuals in the organization. This is crucial to providing quality patient care, achieving good outcomes, and improving patient safety. Achieving this goal depends on performing the following processes:

- Performing strategic and ongoing master planning by organization leaders for the space, clear circulation of occupants, equipment, supportive environment, and resources needed to safely and effectively support the services provided. Planning and designing of the environment is consistent with the organization's mission and vision and the patient's physical condition/health, cultural background, age, and cognitive abilities.
- Educating staff about the role of the environment in safely, sensitively, and effectively supporting patient care. The organization educates staff about the physical characteristics necessary for attaining such an environment, and the processes for monitoring, maintaining, and reporting on the organization's environment of care.
- Developing standards to measure the performance of staff and organization performance in managing and improving the environment of care.
- Implementing plans to create and manage the organization's environment of care. An Information Collection and Evaluation System (ICES) is developed and used to continuously measure, assess, and improve the status of the environment of care.

"Environment of care" refers to a variety of key elements and issues that contribute to creating the way the space feels and works for patients, families, staff, and others experiencing the health care delivery system. Certain key elements and issues that can be significant in their ability to positively influence patient outcomes and satisfaction and improve patient safety include the following:

- Light (both natural and artificial)
- Privacy (visual and auditory)
- Space size and configuration appropriate and consistent with the clinical philosophy
- Security
- Clarity of access (both exterior and interior circulation)
- Color
- Efficient layouts that support staffing and overall functional operation

When appropriately designed into and managed as part of the physical environment, these elements create safe, welcoming, and comfortable environments that support and maintain patient dignity and personhood, allow ease of interaction, reduce stressors, and encourage family participation in the delivery of care.

These key elements and issues need to be incorporated into outpatient settings such as clinics, counseling centers, preadmission testing offices, infirmaries, same-day surgery centers, dialysis centers, or imaging centers. Such environments are made up of three basic components: building(s), equipment, and people. Effective management of the environment of care includes using processes and activities to do the following:

- Reduce and control environmental hazards and risks
- Prevent accidents and injuries
- Maintain safe conditions for patients, staff, and others coming to the organization's facilities
- Maintain an environment that is sensitive to patient needs for comfort, social interaction, and positive distraction
- Maintain an environment that minimizes unnecessary environmental stresses for patients, staff, and others coming to the organization's facilities

The standards in this chapter focus on how everyone in the organization participates in the processes and activities that make the care environment safe and effective. They also address leaders' responsibility for identifying and responding to the care environment needs and allocating appropriate space, equipment, and resources to safely and effectively support the organization's services.

Some of the standards in this chapter recognize that certain settings where care, treatment, and services are provided have more risk than others. Therefore, some of the requirements are noted as being applicable to only certain "occupancy* types." The following occupancy definitions are used in this chapter:

- **Ambulatory health care occupancy** An occupancy used to provide to four or more patients at the same time either (1) outpatient services or treatment that render them incapable of taking actions for self-preservation under emergency conditions without the assistance of others; or (2) anesthesia that renders them incapable of taking actions for self-preservation under emergency conditions without the assistance of others.
- **Business occupancy** An occupancy used to provide outpatient services or treatment that do not meet the criteria in the ambulatory health care occupancy definition.

Note 1: *The standards in this chapter do not prescribe any particular structure (such as a safety committee), specific individual (such as one employee hired to be a safety officer), or format for the required designs and planning activities.*

Note 2: *The standards do not require the Statement of Conditions™ (SOC) compliance document† to be completed by anyone other than an employee of the organiza-*

* **Occupancy** The purpose for which a building or portion thereof is used or intended to be used.

† **Statement of Conditions™ (SOC) compliance document** A proactive document that helps an organization perform a critical self-assessment of its current level of compliance and describe how to resolve any *LSC* deficiencies. The SOC was created to be a living, ongoing management tool that should be used in a management process that continually identifies, assesses, and resolves *LSC* deficiencies.

tion. This statement is the basis for corrective actions needed to make the environment compliant with the requirements of the Life Safety Code® *(LSC), NFPA 101®.**

Note 3: *The standards in this chapter require each organization to develop a written plan for the following:*
1. *Safety management (EC.1.10)*
2. *Security management (EC.2.10)*
3. *Hazardous materials and waste management (EC.3.10)*
4. *Emergency management (EC.4.10)*
5. *Fire safety (EC.5.10)*
6. *Medical equipment management (EC.6.10)*
7. *Utilities management (EC.7.10)*

If an organization has multiple sites, it may have separate management plans for each of its locations, or it may choose to have one comprehensive set of plans. In either case, the organization must address specific risks and the unique conditions at each of its sites.

* *Life Safety Code®* is a registered trademark of the National Fire Protection Association, Quincy, Massachusetts.

Standards

The following is a list of all standards for this function. They are presented here for your convenience without footnotes or other explanatory text. If you have a question about a term used here, please check the Glossary.

Note: *A revised standard numbering system is being used with the reformatted standards. The revised numbering system will allow for more flexibility to add standards while maintaining the current number for each standard.*

Planning and Implementation Activities

EC.1.10 The organization manages safety risks.

EC.1.20 The organization maintains a safe environment.

EC.1.25 Not applicable

EC.1.27 Not applicable

EC.1.30 The organization develops and implements a policy to prohibit smoking except in specified circumstances.

EC.2.10 The organization identifies and manages its security risks.

EC.3.10 The organization manages its hazardous materials and waste risks.

EC.4.10 The organization addresses emergency management.

EC.4.20 The organization regularly tests its emergency management plan.

EC.5.10 The organization manages fire safety risks.

EC.5.20 Newly constructed and existing environments are designed and maintained to comply with the *Life Safety Code*®.

EC.5.30 The organization conducts fire drills regularly.

EC.5.40 The organization maintains fire-safety equipment and building features.

EC.5.50 The organization develops and implements activities to protect occupants during periods when a building does not meet the applicable provisions of the *Life Safety Code*®.

EC.6.10 The organization manages medical equipment risks.

EC.6.20 Medical equipment is maintained, tested, and inspected.

EC.6.30 Through EC.6.130 Not applicable

EC.7.10 The organization manages its utility risks.

EC.7.20 The organization provides an emergency electrical power source.

EC.7.30 The organization maintains, tests, and inspects its utility systems.

EC.7.40 The organization maintains, tests, and inspects its emergency power systems.

EC.7.50 The organization maintains, tests, and inspects its medical gas and vacuum systems.

EC.8.10 The organization establishes and maintains an appropriate environment.

EC.8.20 Not applicable

EC.8.30 The organization manages the design and building of the environment when it is renovated, altered, or newly created.

Measuring and Improving Activities

EC.9.10 The organization monitors conditions in the environment.

EC.9.20 The organization analyzes identified environment issues and develops recommendations for resolving them.

EC.9.30 The organization improves the environment.

Standards, Rationales, Elements of Performance, and Scoring

Planning and Implementation Activities

No organization can ensure that patients, staff, and others coming to the organization's facilities will never suffer an accidental injury. However, organizations can minimize avoidable risks and injuries through sound planning, resource allocation (*see* the "Leadership" [LD] chapter), effective training (*see* the "Management of Human Resources" [HR] chapter), implementation, and ongoing monitoring and improvement of risk reduction activities. These activities can be accomplished through the management process, staff activities, and/or technology.

Standard EC.1.10

The organization manages safety risks.

Rationale for EC.1.10

Each organization has inherent safety risks associated with providing services for patients, the performance of daily activities by staff, and the physical environment in which services occur. It is important that each organization identifies these risks and plans and implements processes to minimize the likelihood of those risks causing incidents.

Elements of Performance for EC.1.10

B 1. The organization develops and maintains a written management plan describing the processes it implements to effectively manage the environmental safety of patients, staff, and other people coming to the organization's facilities.

EC

A 2. The organization identifies a person(s), as designated by leadership, to coordinate the development, implementation, and monitoring of the safety management activities.

A 3. The organization identifies a person(s) to intervene whenever conditions immediately threaten life or health or threaten damage to equipment or buildings.

B 4. The organization conducts comprehensive, proactive risk assessments that evaluate the potential adverse impact of buildings, grounds, equipment, occupants, and internal physical systems on the safety and health of patients, staff, and other people coming to the organization's facilities.

C Ⓜ 5. The organization uses the risks identified to select and implement procedures and controls to achieve the lowest potential for adverse impact on the safety and health of patients, staff, and other people coming to the organization's facilities.

C Ⓜ 6. The organization establishes safety policies and procedures that are practiced and reviewed as frequently as necessary, but at least every three years.

7. Not applicable

B 8. The organization ensures that a process exists for responding to product safety recalls by appropriate organization staff.

B 9. The organization ensures that all grounds and equipment are maintained appropriately.

Standard EC.1.20

The organization maintains a safe environment.

Rationale for EC.1.20

It is essential that the organization conduct periodic environmental tours to determine if its current processes for managing patient, public, and staff safety risks are being practiced correctly and are effective. These tours can also be used to assess staff knowledge and behaviors, identify new or altered risks in areas where construction or changes in services have occurred, and identify opportunities to improve the environment.

Elements of Performance for EC.1.20

B 1. The organization conducts environmental tours to identify environmental deficiencies, hazards, and unsafe practices.

C Ⓜ 2. The organization conducts environmental tours at least every six months in all areas where individuals are served.

C Ⓜ 3. The organization conducts environmental tours at least annually in areas where individuals are not served.

Standard EC.1.25

Not applicable

Standard EC.1.27

Not applicable

Standard EC.1.30

The organization develops and implements a policy to prohibit smoking except in specifiedcircumstances.

Rationale for EC.1.30

This standard is intended to reduce the following risks:

- To people who smoke, including possible adverse effects on care, treatment, and services
- Of passive smoking for others
- Of fire

Elements of Performance for EC.1.30

B 1. The organization develops a policy regarding smoking in all areas of all building(s) under the organization's control.

2. Through 5. Not applicable

B 6. The organization identifies and implements a process(es) for monitoring compliance with the policy.

B 7. The organization develops strategies to eliminate the incidence of policy violations when identified.

Standard EC.2.10

The organization identifies and manages its security risks.

Rationale for EC.2.10

It is essential that an organization manages the physical and personal security of patients, staff (including addressing the risks of violence in the workplace), and individuals coming to the organization's facilities. In addition, security of the established environment, equipment, supplies, and information is also important.

Elements of Performance for EC.2.10

B 1. The organization develops and maintains a written management plan describing the processes it implements to effectively manage the security of patients, staff, and other people coming to the organization's facilities.

A 2. The organization identifies a person(s), as designated by leadership, to coordinate the development, implementation, and monitoring of the security management activities.

B 3. The organization conducts proactive risk assessments that evaluate the potential adverse impact of the external environment and the services provided on the security of patients, staff, and other people coming to the organization's facilities.*

C Ⓜ 4. The organization uses the risks identified to select and implement procedures and controls to achieve the lowest potential for adverse impact on security.

* The potential for workplace violence is considered during the risk assessment.

B 5. The organization identifies, as appropriate, patients, staff, and other people entering the organization's facilities.

C Ⓜ 6. The organization controls access to and egress from security-sensitive areas, as determined by the organization.

B 7. The organization identifies and implements security procedures that address actions taken in the event of a security incident.

8. Not applicable

B 9. The organization identifies and implements security procedures that address handling of situations involving VIPs or the media.

Standard EC.3.10

The organization manages its hazardous materials and waste* risks.

Rationale for EC.3.10

Organizations must identify materials they use that need special handling and implement processes to minimize the risks of their unsafe use and improper disposal.

Elements of Performance for EC.3.10

B 1. The organization develops and maintains a written management plan describing the processes it implements to effectively manage hazardous materials and wastes.

B 2. The organization creates and maintains an inventory that identifies hazardous materials and waste used, stored, or generated using criteria consistent with applicable law and regulation (for example, the Environmental Protection Agency [EPA] and the Occupational Safety and Health Administration [OSHA]).

The organization establishes and implements processes for selecting, handling, storing, transporting, using, and disposing of hazardous materials and waste from receipt or generation through use and/or final disposal, including managing the following (EPs 3–6):

C Ⓜ 3. Chemicals

A 4. Chemotherapeutic materials

A 5. Radioactive materials

EC

* **Hazardous materials (HAZMAT) and waste** Materials whose handling, use, and storage are guided or regulated by local, state, or federal regulation. Examples include OSHA's Regulations for Bloodborne Pathogens (regarding blood, other infectious materials, contaminated items which would release blood or other infectious materials, or contaminated sharps), the Nuclear Regulatory Commission's regulations for handling and disposal of radioactive waste, management of hazardous vapors (such as glutaraldehyde, ethylene oxide, and nitrous oxide), chemicals regulated by the EPA, Department of Transportation requirements, and hazardous energy sources (for example, ionizing or non-ionizing radiation, lasers, microwaves, ultrasound).

C Ⓜ 6. Infectious and regulated medical wastes, including sharps

B 7. The organization provides adequate and appropriate space and equipment for safely handling and storing hazardous materials and waste.

B 8. The organization monitors and disposes of hazardous gases and vapors.

B 9. The organization identifies and implements emergency procedures that include the specific precautions, procedures, and protective equipment used during hazardous materials and waste spills or exposures.

A 10. The organization maintains documentation, including required permits, licenses, and adherence to other regulations.

C Ⓜ 11. The organization maintains required manifests for handling hazardous materials and waste.

C Ⓜ 12. The organization properly labels hazardous materials and waste.

B 13. The organization effectively separates hazardous materials and waste storage and processing areas from other areas of the facility.

Standard EC.4.10

The organization addresses emergency management.

Rationale for EC.4.10

An emergency* in the organization or its community could suddenly and significantly affect the need for the organization's services or its ability to provide those services. Therefore, an organization needs to have an emergency management plan that comprehensively describes its approach to emergencies in the organization or in its community.

Elements of Performance for EC.4.10

A 1. The organization conducts a hazard vulnerability analysis† to identify potential emergencies that could affect the need for its services or its ability to provide those services.

A 2. The organization establishes the following with the community:
- Priorities among the potential emergencies identified in the hazard vulnerability analysis

---

* **Emergency** A natural or manmade event that significantly disrupts the environment of care (for example, damage to the organization's building[s] and grounds due to severe winds, storms, or earthquakes); that significantly disrupts care, treatment, and services (for example, loss of utilities such as power, water, or telephones due to floods, civil disturbances, accidents, or emergencies within the organization or in its community); or that results in sudden, significantly changed, or increased demands for the organization's services (for example, bioterrorist attack, building collapse, plane crash in the organization's community). Some emergencies are called "disasters" or "potential injury creating events" (PICEs).

† **Hazard vulnerability analysis** The identification of potential emergencies and the direct and indirect effects these emergencies may have on the organization's operations and the demand for its services.

- The organization's role in relation to a communitywide emergency management program
- An "all-hazards" command structure within the organization that links with the community's command structure

B 3. The organization develops and maintains a written emergency management plan describing the process for disaster readiness and emergency management, and implements it when appropriate.

A 4. At a minimum, an emergency management plan is developed with the involvement of the organization's leaders.

B 5. The plan identifies specific procedures that describe mitigation,* preparedness,† response, and recovery strategies, actions, and responsibilities for each priority emergency.

B 6. The plan provides processes for initiating the response and recovery phases of the plan, including a description of how, when, and by whom the phases are to be activated.

B 7. The plan provides processes for notifying staff when emergency response measures are initiated.

B 8. The plan provides processes for notifying external authorities of emergencies, including possible community emergencies identified by the organization.

B 9. The plan provides processes for identifying and assigning staff to cover all essential staff functions under emergency conditions.

B 10. The plan provides processes for managing the following under emergency conditions:
- Activities related to care, treatment, and services (for example, scheduling, modifying, or discontinuing services; controlling information about patients; referrals; transporting patients)
- Logistics relating to critical supplies (for example, supplies, food, linen, water)
- Security (for example, access, crowd control, traffic control)

B 11. When required by the organization's role within their community, the plan provides processes for establishing the means and methods to continue care, treatment, and services during the potential emergencies.

B 12. The plan provides processes for evacuating the entire facility (both horizontally and, when applicable, vertically) when the environment cannot support adequate care, treatment, and services.

---

* **Mitigation activities** Those activities an organization undertakes in attempting to lessen the severity and impact of a potential emergency.

† **Preparedness activities** Those activities an organization undertakes to build capacity and identify resources that may be used if an emergency occurs.

13. Not applicable

B 14. The plan provides processes for identifying care providers and other personnel during emergencies.

15. Not applicable

16. Not applicable

17. Not applicable

B 18. The plan identifies backup internal and external communication systems in the event of failure during emergencies.

B 19. The plan identifies alternate roles and responsibilities of staff during emergencies, including to whom they report in the organization's command structure and, when activated, in the community's command structure.

B 20. The plan identifies an alternative means of meeting essential building utility needs when the organization is designated by its emergency management plan to provide continuous service during an emergency (for example, electricity, water, ventilation, fuel sources, medical gas/vacuum systems).

B 21. The plan identifies means for radioactive, biological, and chemical isolation and decontamination.

Emergency Management Drills

Introduction

Periodic testing of an emergency management plan enables organizations to assess the plan's appropriateness and adequacy and the effectiveness of logistics, human resources, training, policies, procedures, and protocols. Exercises should stress the limits of the organization's emergency management system. The goal of this testing is to assess the organization's preparedness capabilities and performance when systems are stressed during an actual emergency or a simulated situation.

Exercises should be developed using plausible scenarios that are realistic and relevant to the organization. Events should be based on each organization's hazard vulnerability analysis (HVA) and should validate the effectiveness of the plan and identify opportunities to improve.

This standard will help health care organizations test their emergency management plans, identify deficiencies, and take corrective actions to continuously improve the effectiveness of their emergency management plan. Only a thorough and objective evaluation of performance during an emergency management event or a planned exercise will demonstrate how effective the organization's planning efforts have been.

It is important to communicate the strengths and weaknesses of the performance revealed by the exercise to all levels of the organization, including administration, clinical staff, governing body, and those responsible for managing the patient safety program.

Standard EC.4.20

The organization regularly tests its emergency management plan.

Elements of Performance for EC.4.20

Number and Types of Exercises

A 1. The organization tests its emergency management plan twice a year, either in response to an actual emergency or in a planned exercise.

Note 1: *Staff in freestanding buildings classified as a business occupancy (as defined by the* Life Safety Code®*) that does not offer emergency services nor is community-designated as a disaster receiving station need to conduct only one emergency preparedness exercise annually.*

Note 2: *Tabletop sessions, though useful, are not acceptable substitutes for exercises.*

A 2. Organizations that offer emergency services or are community-designated disaster receiving stations conduct at least one exercise a year that includes an influx of actual or simulated patients.

Note: *The following EPs have been renumbered from the previous book.*

3. Not applicable

4. Not applicable

5. Not applicable

Scope of Exercises

B 6. Planned exercise scenarios are realistic and related to the priority emergencies identified in the organization's hazard vulnerability analysis.

7. Through 14. Not applicable

B 15. All exercises are critiqued to identify deficiencies and opportunities for improvement based on all monitoring activities and observations during the exercise.

B 16. Completed exercises are critiqued through a multidisciplinary process that includes administration, clinical, and support staff.

B 17. The organization modifies its emergency management plan in response to critiques of exercises.

B 18. Planned exercises evaluate the effectiveness of improvements that were made in response to critiques of the previous exercise.

Note: *When improvements require substantive resources that cannot be accomplished by the next planned exercise, interim improvements must be put in place until final resolution.*

B 19. The strengths and weaknesses identified during exercises are communicated to the multidisciplinary improvement team responsible for monitoring environment-of-care issues (*see* Standard EC.9.20).

Standard EC.5.10

The organization manages fire safety risks.

Elements of Performance for EC.5.10

B 1. The organization develops and maintains a written management plan describing the processes it implements to effectively manage fire safety.

B 2. The organization identifies proactive processes for protecting patients, staff, and others coming to the organization's facilities, as well as protecting property from fire, smoke, and other products of combustion.

B 3. The organization identifies processes for regularly inspecting, testing, and maintaining fire protection and fire safety systems, equipment, and components.

B 4. The organization develops and implements a fire response plan that addresses the following:
- Facilitywide fire response
- Area-specific needs, including fire evacuation routes
- Specific roles and responsibilities of staff, licensed independent practitioners, and volunteers at a fire's point of origin
- Specific roles and responsibilities of staff, licensed independent practitioners, and volunteers away from a fire's point of origin
- Specific roles and responsibilities of staff, licensed independent practitioners, and volunteers in preparing for building evacuation

EC

B 5. The organization reviews proposed acquisitions of bedding, window draperies, and other curtains, furnishings, decorations, and other equipment for fire safety.

Note: *Applies to ambulatory surgical settings only.*

Standard EC.5.20

Newly constructed and existing environments are designed and maintained to comply with the *Life Safety Code*®.*

* *Life Safety Code*® is a registered trademark of the National Fire Protection Association, Quincy, Massachusetts.

Rationale for EC.5.20

The *Life Safety Code*® (*LSC*) requires that a building is designed, constructed, and maintained with the capability of being fire safe. When undertaking the design of a newly remodeled building, the organization should also satisfy any requirements of others (local, state, or federal) that may be more stringent than the *LSC*.

When evaluating *LSC* compliance within the Statement of Conditions™ (SOC)* assessment process, it is important that health care organizations establish the qualifications of the person(s) they select for performing this assessment. While there is no prescriptive requirement for the education and experience of this person(s), these qualifications should be based upon the scope of the required *LSC* assessment activities and the building complexity and occupancy type(s) being assessed.

Note 1: *This standard does not apply to the following facilities:*
- *Classified as a business occupancy by the* LSC *that are freestanding buildings*
- *Classified as a business occupancy by the* LSC *that are connected to a health care occupancy but are separated by a two-hour–rated fire barrier and do not serve as a required means of egress from the health care occupancy*
- *Housing three or fewer patients*

Note 2: *This standard applies to all ambulatory surgical centers seeking accreditation for Medicare certification purposes. These facilities must meet the Ambulatory Health Care Occupancy requirements of the* LSC.

Elements of Performance for EC.5.20

B 1. Each building in which patients are housed or receive care, treatment, and services complies with the *LSC*, NFPA 101® 2000

or

Each building in which patients are housed or receive care, treatment, and services does not comply with the *LSC*, but the resolution of all deficiencies is evidenced through the following:
- An equivalency approved by the Joint Commission
  or
- Continued progress in completing an acceptable Plan for Improvement (SOC, Part 4)

A 2. A current, organizationwide electronic Statement of Conditions compliance document (e-SOC)† has been prepared.

Note: *You can access the e-Statement of Conditions™—Part 2 & Part 4 compliance documents through your Joint Commission Connect™ extranet Web site. You can also download a paper version of the entire SOC from your Joint Commission Connect extranet Web site or http://www.jointcommission.org.*

EC

---

* **Statement of Conditions™ (SOC) compliance document** A proactive document that helps an organization perform a critical self-assessment of its current level of compliance and describe how to resolve any *LSC* deficiencies. The SOC was created to be a living, ongoing management tool that should be used in a management process that continually identifies, assesses, and resolves *LSC* deficiencies.

3. Not applicable

4. Not applicable

A 5. The organization is making sufficient progress* toward the corrective actions described in an SOC previously accepted by the Joint Commission.

B 6. The organization assigns responsibility for completing the SOC to one or more individuals whose experience and/or education is commensurate with the scope of the required *LSC* assessment activities and the building complexity and occupancy type(s) being assessed.

Standard EC.5.30

The organization conducts fire drills regularly.

Rationale for EC.5.30

The development of a fire response plan is an important part of achieving a fire-safe environment (*see* standard EC.5.10). It is important that this plan be regularly evaluated during implementations (in drill scenarios or actual fire situations) for performance of the fire safety equipment and staff.

Implementation of the plan should be realistic and held at varied times. Actual evacuation of patients during the drills is not required.

Elements of Performance for EC.5.30

C Ⓜ 1. Fire drills are conducted quarterly in each building defined by the *LSC* as the following:
- Ambulatory Health Care Occupancy

A 2. Fire drills are conducted annually in all freestanding buildings classified as a business occupancy as defined by the *LSC* where patients are seen or treated.

Note 1: *In leased or rented facilities, only staff in areas of the building that the organization occupies must participate in such drills.*

Note 2: *All ambulatory surgical centers seeking accreditation for Medicare certification purposes must conduct fire drills quarterly.*

3. Not applicable

C Ⓜ 4. At least 50% of the required drills are unannounced.

5. Not applicable

EC

* **Sufficient progress** Failure to make sufficient progress toward the corrective actions described in an approved SOC Part 4–Plan for Improvement, would result in a recommendation of Conditional Accreditation (see Conditional Accreditation rule CON04 in "The Accreditation Process" chapter).

B 6. All fire drills are critiqued to identify deficiencies and opportunities for improvement.

A 7. The effectiveness of fire response training according to the fire plan is evaluated at least annually.

B 8. During fire drills, staff knowledge is evaluated including the following:
- When and how to sound fire alarms (where such alarms are available)
- When and how to transmit for off-site fire responders
- Containment of smoke and fire
- Transfer of patients to areas of refuge
- Fire extinguishment
- Specific fire response duties
- Preparation for building evacuation

Standard EC.5.40

The organization maintains fire-safety equipment and building features.

Note 1: *This standard does not require organizations to have the types of fire-safety equipment and building features discussed below. However, if these types of equipment or features exist within the organization, then the following maintenance, testing, and inspection requirements apply.*

Note 2: *Organizations that offer care, treatment, and services in leased facilities need to communicate maintenance expectations for building equipment not under their control to their landlord through contractual language, lease agreements, memos, and so forth. These organizations are not required to possess maintenance documentation, but must only have access to such documentation as needed and during survey. It is also important that the landlord communicate to the organization any building equipment problems identified that could negatively affect the safety or health of patients, staff, and other people coming to the organization, as well as the landlord's plan to resolve such issues.*

EC

Elements of Performance for EC.5.40

C Ⓜ 1. Initiating devices and fire detection and alarm equipment are tested as follows:*
- All supervisory signal devices (except valve tamper switches) are tested at least quarterly
- All valve tamper switches and water flow devices are tested at least semiannually
- All duct detectors, electromechanical releasing devices, heat detectors, manual fire alarm boxes, and smoke detectors are tested at least annually

* For additional guidance, see NFPA 72-1999 edition (Table 7-3.2).

C Ⓜ 2. Occupant alarm notification devices, including all audible devices, speakers, and visible devices, are tested at least annually. *

A 3. Off-premises emergency services notification transmission equipment is tested at least quarterly. *

C Ⓜ 4. For water-based automatic fire-extinguishing systems, all fire pumps are tested at least weekly under no-flow condition.†

C Ⓜ 5. For water-based automatic fire-extinguishing systems, all water-storage tank high- and low-water level alarms are tested at least semiannually.

C Ⓜ 6. For water-based automatic fire-extinguishing systems, all water-storage tank low-water temperature alarms (during cold weather only) are tested at least monthly.

C Ⓜ 7. For water-based automatic fire-extinguishing systems, main drain tests are conducted at least annually at all system risers.

C Ⓜ 8. For water-based automatic fire-extinguishing systems, all fire department connections are inspected quarterly.

A 9. For water-based automatic fire-extinguishing systems, all fire pumps are tested at least annually under flow.

A 10. Kitchen automatic fire-extinguishing systems are inspected for proper operation at least semiannually (actual discharge of the fire-extinguishing system is not required).

C Ⓜ 11. Carbon dioxide and other gaseous automatic fire-extinguishing systems are tested for proper operation at least annually (actual discharge of the fire-extinguishing system is not required).

C Ⓜ 12. All portable fire extinguishers‡ are clearly identified, inspected at least monthly, and maintained at least annually.

C Ⓜ 13. All standpipe occupant hoses are hydrostatically tested five years after installation and at least every three years thereafter;§ and systems receive water-flow tests at least every five years.‖

EC

---

* The *Life Safety Code*®, NFPA 101-2000 edition, requires that the municipal fire department (or applicable emergency forces group) is notified and a fire watch is provided whenever an approved fire alarm or automatic sprinkler system is out of service for more than four hours in a 24-hour period in an occupied building.

† For additional guidance, see NFPA 25-1998 edition.

‡ For additional guidance, see NFPA 10-1998 edition (sections 1-6, 4-3, and 4-4).

§ For additional guidance, see NFPA 1962-1998 edition (section 2-3).

‖ For additional guidance, see NFPA 25-1998 edition.

C Ⓜ 14. All fire and smoke dampers are operated at least every four years (with fusible links removed where applicable) to verify that they fully close.*

A 15. All automatic smoke-detection shutdown devices for air-handling equipment are tested at least annually.†

C Ⓜ 16. All horizontal and vertical sliding and rolling fire doors are tested for proper operation and full closure at least annually.‡

Standard EC.5.50

The organization develops and implements activities to protect occupants during periods when a building does not meet the applicable provisions of the *Life Safety Code®*.

Note 1: *This standard does not apply to facilities classified as a business occupancy by the* LSC.

Note 2: *This standard does apply to all facilities classified as an ambulatory health care occupancy by the* LSC *and all ambulatory surgical centers seeking accreditation for Medicare certification purposes.*

Rationale for EC.5.50

When building code deficiencies are identified and cannot be immediately corrected or during renovation or construction activities, the safety of patients, staff, and other people coming to the organization's facilities is diminished. Organizations need to proactively identify administrative actions (for example, additional training, additional inspections, additional fire drills, and so on) to be taken if these scenarios arise.

Elements of Performance for EC.5.50

B 1. Each organization develops a policy for using interim life safety measures (ILSMs).

B 2. The policy includes written criteria for evaluating various deficiencies and construction hazards to determine when and to what extent one or more of the following measures apply:

- Ensuring free and unobstructed exits. Staff receives additional information/communication when alternative exits are designated. Buildings or areas under construction must maintain escape routes for construction workers at all times, and the means of exiting construction areas are inspected daily.
- Ensuring free and unobstructed access to emergency services and for fire, police, and other emergency forces.

EC

* For additional guidance, see NFPA 90A-1999 edition (section 3-4.7).

† For additional guidance, see NFPA 90A-1999 edition (section 4-4.1).

‡ For additional guidancc, see NFPA 80-1999 edition (section 15-2.4).

- Ensuring that fire alarm, detection, and suppression systems are in good working order. A temporary but equivalent system must be provided when any fire system is impaired. Temporary systems must be inspected and tested monthly.*
- Ensuring that temporary construction partitions are smoke tight and built of noncombustible or limited combustible materials that will not contribute to the development or spread of fire.
- Providing additional fire-fighting equipment and training staff in its use.
- Prohibiting smoking throughout the organization's buildings and in and near construction areas.
- Developing and enforcing storage, housekeeping, and debris-removal practices that reduce the building's flammable and combustible fire load to the lowest feasible level.
- Conducting a minimum of two fire drills per quarter.
- Increasing surveillance of buildings, grounds, and equipment, with special attention to excavations, construction areas, construction storage, and field offices.
- Training staff to compensate for impaired structural or compartmentalization† features of fire safety.
- Conducting organizationwide safety education programs to promote awareness of fire-safety building deficiencies, construction hazards, and ILSMs.

A 3. Each organization implements ILSMs as defined in its policy.

Standard EC.6.10

The organization manages medical equipment risks.

Rationale for EC.6.10

Medical equipment is a significant contributor to the quality of care. It is used in treatment, diagnostic activities, and monitoring of the patient. It is essential that the equipment is appropriate for the intended use; that staff, including licensed independent practitioners, be trained to use the equipment safely and effectively; and that the equipment is maintained appropriately by qualified individuals.

EC

---

* *The Life Safety Code*®, NFPA 101-2000 edition, requires that the municipal fire department (or applicable emergency forces group) is notified and a fire watch is provided whenever an approved fire alarm or automatic sprinkler system is out of service for more than four hours in a 24-hour period in an occupied building.

† **Compartmentalization** The concept of using various building components (fire walls and doors, smoke barriers, fire-rated floor slabs, and so forth) to prevent the spread of fire and the production's combustion, and to provide a safe means of egress to an approved exit. The presence of these features varies depending upon the building occupancy classification.

Elements of Performance for EC.6.10

B 1. The organization develops and maintains a written management plan describing the processes it implements to manage the effective, safe, and reliable operation of medical equipment.

B 2. The organization identifies and implements a process(es) for selecting and acquiring medical equipment.*

B 3. The organization establishes and uses risk criteria† for identifying, evaluating, and creating an inventory of equipment to be included in the medical equipment management plan before the equipment is used. These criteria address the following:
- Equipment function (diagnosis, care, treatment, life support, and monitoring)
- Physical risks associated with use
- Equipment incident history

B 4. The organization identifies appropriate inspection and maintenance strategies for all equipment on the inventory for achieving effective, safe, and reliable operation of all equipment in the inventory.‡

B 5. The organization defines intervals for inspecting, testing, and maintaining appropriate equipment on the inventory (that is, those pieces of equipment on the inventory benefiting from scheduled activities to minimize the clinical and physical risks) that are based upon criteria such as manufacturers' recommendations, risk levels, and current organization experience.

B 6. The organization identifies and implements processes for monitoring and acting on equipment hazard notices and recalls.

B 7. The organization identifies and implements processes for monitoring and reporting incidents in which a medical device is suspected or attributed to the death, serious injury, or serious illness of any individual, as required by the Safe Medical Devices Act of 1990.

A 8. The organization identifies and implements processes for emergency procedures that address the following:
- What to do in the event of equipment disruption or failure
- When and how to perform emergency clinical interventions when medical equipment fails

EC

---

* The acquisition process includes initially evaluating the condition and function of the equipment when received and evaluating the training of users before use on patients.

† The organization may choose not to use risk criteria to limit the types of equipment to be included in the medical equipment management plan, but rather include all medical equipment.

‡ Organizations may use different strategies for different items as appropriate. For example, strategies such as predictive maintenance, interval-based inspections, corrective maintenance, or metered maintenance may be selected to ensure reliable performance.

- Availability of backup equipment
- How to obtain repair services

Standard EC.6.20

Medical equipment is maintained, tested, and inspected.

Elements of Performance for EC.6.20

C Ⓜ 1. The organization documents a current, accurate, and separate inventory of all equipment identified in the medical equipment management plan, regardless of ownership.

A 2. The organization documents performance and safety testing of all equipment identified in the medical equipment management program before initial use.

A 3. The organization documents inspection and maintenance of equipment used for life support* that is consistent with maintenance strategies to minimize clinical and physical risks identified in the equipment management plan (*see* standard EC.6.10).

C Ⓜ 4. The organization documents inspection and maintenance of non–life support equipment on the inventory that is consistent with maintenance strategies to minimize clinical and physical risks identified in the equipment management plan (*see* standard EC.6.10).

A Ⓜ 5. The organization documents performance testing of all sterilizers used.

A Ⓜ 6. The organization documents chemical and biological testing of water used in renal dialysis and other applicable tests based upon regulations, manufacturers' recommendations, and organization experience.

Standards EC.6.30 Through EC.6.130

Not applicable

Standard EC.7.10

The organization manages its utility risks.

* **Life support equipment** Any device intended to sustain life and whose failure to perform its primary function, when used according to manufacturer's instructions and clinical protocol, is expected to result in imminent death in the absence of immediate intervention (examples include ventilators, anesthesia machines, and heart-lung bypass machines).

Rationale for EC.7.10

Utility systems* are essential to the proper operation of the environment of care and significantly contribute to effective, safe, and reliable provision of care to patients in health care organizations. It is important that health care organizations establish and maintain a utility systems management program to promote a safe, controlled, and comfortable environment that does the following:

- Ensures operational reliability of utility systems
- Reduces the potential for organization-acquired illness to be transmitted through the utility systems
- Assesses the reliability and minimizes potential risks of utility system failures

Elements of Performance for EC.7.10

1. Through 6. Not applicable

B 7. The organization develops and maintains a written management plan describing the processes it implements to manage the effective, safe, and reliable operation of utility systems.

B 8. The organization designs and installs utility systems that meet the patient care and operational needs of the services in the organization's buildings.

B 9. The organization establishes risk criteria† for identifying, evaluating, and creating an inventory of operating components of systems before the equipment is used. These criteria address the following:

- Life support
- Infection control
- Support of the environment
- Equipment support
- Communication

B 10. The organization develops appropriate strategies for all utility systems equipment on the inventory for ensuring effective, safe, and reliable operation of all equipment in the inventory.‡

B 11. The organization defines intervals for inspecting, testing, and maintaining appropriate utility systems equipment on the inventory (that is, those pieces of equipment on the inventory benefiting from scheduled activities to minimize the clinical and physical risks) that are based

EC

---

* **Utility systems** May include electrical distribution; emergency power; vertical and horizontal transport; heating, ventilating, and air conditioning; plumbing, boiler, and steam; piped gases; vacuum systems; or communication systems including data-exchange systems.

† The organization may choose not to use risk criteria to limit the types of utility systems to be included in the utility management plan, but rather include all utility systems.

‡ Organizations may use different strategies as appropriate. For example, strategies such as predictive maintenance, interval-based inspections, corrective maintenance, or metered maintenance may be selected to ensure reliable performance.

upon criteria such as manufacturers' recommendations, risk levels, and current organization experience.

A 12. The organization identifies and implements emergency procedures for responding to utility system disruptions or failures that address the following:
- What to do if utility systems malfunction
- Identification of an alternative source of organization-defined essential utilities
- Shutting off the malfunctioning systems and notifying staff in affected areas
- How and when to perform emergency clinical interventions when utility systems fail
- Obtaining repair services

B 13. The organization maps the distribution of utility systems.

C Ⓜ 14. The organization labels controls for a partial or complete emergency shutdown.

B 15. The organization identifies and implements processes to minimize pathogenic biological agents in cooling towers, domestic hot/cold water systems, and other aerosolizing water systems.

A 16. The organization designs, installs, and maintains ventilation equipment to provide appropriate pressure relationships, air-exchange rates, and filtration efficiencies for ventilation systems serving areas specially designed* to control air-borne contaminants (such as biological agents, gases, fumes, and dust).

Standard EC.7.20

The organization provides an emergency electrical power source.

EC

Rationale for EC.7.20

The organization properly installs an emergency power source that is adequately sized, designed, and fueled, as required by the *LSC* occupancy requirements and the services provided.

Elements of Performance for EC.7.20

The organization provides a reliable emergency power system†, as required by the *LSC* occupancy requirements, that supplies electricity to the following areas when normal electricity is interrupted (EPs 1–4):

* **Areas specially designed** Include spaces such as operating rooms, special procedure rooms, delivery rooms for patients diagnosed or suspected of having airborne communicable diseases (for example, pulmonary or laryngeal tuberculosis), patients in "protective environment" rooms (for example, those receiving bone marrow transplants), laboratories, pharmacies, and sterile supply rooms.

† **Reliable emergency power system** For guidance in establishing a reliable emergency power system (that is, an Essential Electrical Distribution System), see NFPA 99-2002 edition (chapters 13 and 14).

A 1. Alarm systems

C Ⓜ 2. Exit route illumination

A 3. Emergency communication systems

C Ⓜ 4. Illumination of exit signs

Additional Elements of Performance for EC.7.20

The organization provides a reliable emergency power system, as required by the services provided and patients served, that supplies electricity to the following areas when normal electricity is interrupted (EPs 5–15):

A 5. Blood, bone, and tissue storage units

6. Not applicable

A 7. Emergency/urgent care areas

A 8. Elevators (at least one for nonambulatory patients)

A 9. Medical air compressors

A 10. Medical and surgical vacuum systems

A 11. Areas where electrically powered life-support equipment is used

12. Not applicable

13. Not applicable

A 14. Operating rooms

A 15. Postoperative recovery rooms

Standard EC.7.30

The organization maintains, tests, and inspects its utility systems.

Note: *Organizations that offer care, treatment, and services in leased facilities need to communicate maintenance expectations for building equipment not under their control to their landlord through contractual language, lease agreements, memos, and so forth. These organizations are not required to possess maintenance documentation, but must only have access to such documentation as needed and during survey. It is also important that the landlord communicate to the organization any building equipment problems identified that could negatively affect the safety or health of patients, staff, and other people coming to the organization, as well as the landlord's plan to resolve such issues.*

EC

Elements of Performance for EC.7.30

C Ⓜ 1. The organization maintains documentation of a current, accurate, and separate inventory of utility components identified in the utility management plan.

A Ⓜ 2. The organization maintains documentation of performance and safety testing of each critical component identified in the plan before initial use.

A Ⓜ 3. The organization maintains documentation of maintenance of critical components of life support utility systems/equipment consistent with maintenance strategies identified in the utility management plan (*see* standard EC.7.10).

A Ⓜ 4. The organization maintains documentation of maintenance of critical components of infection control utility systems/equipment for high-risk patients consistent with maintenance strategies identified in the utility management plan (*see* standard EC.7.10).

C Ⓜ 5. The organization maintains documentation of maintenance of critical components of non–life support utility systems/equipment on the inventory consistent with maintenance strategies identified in the utility management plan (*see* standard EC.7.10).

Standard EC.7.40

The organization maintains, tests, and inspects its emergency power systems.

Rationale for EC.7.40

Emergency electrical power supply systems may fail during a power disruption leaving an organization unable to deliver safe care to individuals for whom it is responsible. Testing these systems for sufficient lengths of time at regular frequencies increases the likelihood of detecting reliability problems and reduces the risk of losing this critical resource when it is most needed.

While not all organizations are required to have the types of emergency power systems described below, an organization that has these types of systems must comply with the maintenance, testing, and inspection requirements of this standard.

EC

Elements of Performance for EC.7.40

C Ⓜ 1. The organization tests each generator 12 times a year, with testing intervals not less than 20 days and not more than 40 days apart. These tests shall be conducted for at least 30 continuous minutes under a dynamic load that is at least 30% of the nameplate rating of the generator.

Note: *Organizations may choose to test to less than 30% of the emergency generator's nameplate. However, these organizations shall (in addition to performing a test for 30 continuous minutes under operating temperature at the intervals described above) revise their existing documented management plan to conform to NFPA 110 (2005 edition) testing and maintenance activities. These activities shall include inspection procedures for assessing the prime movers' exhaust gas temperature against the minimum temperature recommended by the manufacturer.*

If diesel-powered generators do not meet the minimum exhaust gas temperatures as determined during these tests, they shall be exercised for 30 continuous minutes at the intervals described above with available Emergency Power Supply Systems (EPSS) load, and exercised annually with supplemental loads of

- *25% of nameplate rating for 30 minutes, followed by*
- *50% of nameplate rating for 30 minutes, followed by*
- *75% of nameplate rating for 60 minutes for a total of two continuous hours.*

C Ⓜ 2. The organization tests all automatic transfer switches 12 times a year, with testing intervals not less than 20 days and not more than 40 days apart.

C Ⓜ 3. The organization tests all battery-powered lights required for egress. Testing includes (a) a functional test at 30-day intervals for a minimum of 30 seconds and (b) an annual test for a duration of 1.5 hours.

C Ⓜ 4. The organization tests Stored Emergency Power Supply Systems (SEPSS) whose malfunction may severely jeopardize the occupants' life and safety.* Testing includes (a) a quarterly functional test for 5 minutes or as specified for its class,† whichever is less, and (b) an annual test at full load for 60% of the full duration of its class.

A 5. Facilities that have a generator providing emergency power for the services listed in Elements of Performance 5–15 of standard EC.7.20: The organization tests each emergency generator at least once every 36 months for a minimum of four continuous hours. This test shall be conducted under a load (dynamic or static) that is at least 30% of the nameplate rating of the generator.‡§

Note 1: *To be in initial compliance with this EP, organizations must have performed this test by July 1, 2007. Organizations that have successfully operated their generator(s) since July 1, 2004, according to the test criteria described above, will be considered to be in initial compliance with this EP and are required to retest before the three-year anniversary date of such occurrence.*

* **Stored Emergency Power Supply Systems (SEPSS)** Are intended to automatically supply illumination or power to critical areas and equipment essential for safety to human life. Included are systems that supply emergency power for such functions as illumination for safe exiting, ventilation where it is essential to maintain life, fire detection and alarm systems, public safety communications systems, and processes where the current interruption would produce serious life safety or health hazards to patients, the public, or staff. *Other non-SEPSS battery back-up emergency power systems that an organization has determined to be critical for operations during a power failure (for example, laboratory equipment, electronic medical records) should be properly tested and maintained in accordance with manufacturer's recommendations.*

† **Class** Defines the minimum time for which the SEPSS is designed to operate at its rated load without being recharged (for additional guidance, see NFPA 111 (1996 edition) *Standard on Stored Electrical Energy Emergency and Standby Power Systems*).

‡ This test may satisfy one of the tests required by EP 1.

§ After the test, the fuel supply should be replenished. Any problems identified during the test shall be resolved promptly. For additional guidance, see *NFPA 110 (2005 edition) Standard for Emergency & Standby Power Systems.*

Note 2: *Organizations that cannot achieve a minimum load of 30% of the emergency generator's nameplate rating must assess the prime movers' exhaust gas temperature and meet the minimum temperature recommended by the manufacturer.*

B 6. If a test(s) required by EC.7.40 fails, the organization implements interim measures to compensate for the risk to patients, visitors, and staff until necessary repairs or corrections are completed.

A 7. If a test(s) required by EC.7.40 fails, the organization performs a retest after making the necessary repairs or corrections.

Standard EC.7.50

The organization maintains, tests, and inspects its medical gas and vacuum systems.

Note: *This standard does not require organizations to have the medical gas and vacuum systems discussed below. However, if an organization has these types of systems, then the following maintenance, testing, and inspection requirements apply.*

Elements of Performance for EC.7.50

A 1. The organization inspects, tests, and maintains critical components of piped medical gas systems including master signal panels, area alarms, automatic pressure switches, shutoff valves, flexible connectors, and outlets.

A 2. The organization tests piped medical gas and vacuum systems when the systems are installed, modified, or repaired, including cross-connection testing, piping purity testing, and pressure testing.

A 3. The organization maintains the main supply valve and area shut-off valves of piped medical gas and vacuum systems to be accessible and clearly labeled.

Standard EC.8.10

The organization establishes and maintains an appropriate environment.

Elements of Performance for EC.8.10

B 1. Interior spaces should be the following:

- Appropriate to the care, treatment, and services provided and to the needs of the patients related to age and other characteristics

2. Not applicable

3. Not applicable

C Ⓜ 4. Areas used by the patient are safe, clean, functional, and comfortable.

B 5. Lighting is suitable for care, treatment, and services and the specific activities being conducted.

6. Not applicable

B 7. Ventilation provides for acceptable levels of temperature and humidity and eliminates odors.

8. Not applicable

9. Not applicable

10. Not applicable

A 11. Door locks and other structural restraints used are consistent with the needs of patients, program policy, law, and regulation.

A 12. Emergency access provision is provided to all locked, occupied spaces.

13. Not applicable

For Medicare-Certified Ambulatory Surgical Centers

A 14. Separate waiting and postanesthesia recovery areas are provided.

Standard EC.8.20

Not applicable

Standard EC.8.30

The organization manages the design and building of the environment when it is renovated, altered, or newly created (*see also* standard EC.5.50).

Elements of Performance for EC.8.30

B 1. When planning for the size, configuration, and equipping of the space of renovated, altered, or new construction, the organization uses one of the following: applicable state rules and regulations; *Guidelines for Design and Construction of Hospitals and Health Care Facilities,* 2001 edition, published by the American Institute of Architects; or standards or guidelines that provide equivalent design criteria.

B 2. When planning demolition, construction, or renovation, the organization conducts a proactive risk assessment using risk criteria to identify hazards that could potentially compromise care, treatment, and services in occupied areas of the organization's buildings. The scope and nature of the activities should determine the extent of risk assessment.

B 3. When planning demolition, construction, or renovation, the organization uses risk criteria that address the impact of demolition, renovation, or new construction on air quality requirements, infection control, utility requirements, noise, vibration, and emergency procedures.

B 4. When planning demolition, construction, or renovation, the organization selects and implements proper controls, as required, to reduce risk and minimize impact of these activities.

Measuring and Improving Activities

Standard EC.9.10

The organization monitors conditions in the environment.

Elements of Performance for EC.9.10

B 1. The organization establishes and implements process(es) for reporting and investigating the following:*
- Injuries to patients or others coming to the organization's facilities, as well as incidents of property damage
- Occupational illnesses and injuries to staff
- Security incidents involving patients, staff, or others coming to the organization's facilities or property
- Hazardous materials and waste spills, exposures, and other related incidents
- Fire-safety management problems, deficiencies, and failures
- Equipment management problems, failures, and user errors
- Utility-systems management problems, failures, or user errors

B 2. The organization's leaders assign a person(s) (hereafter referred to as the "assigned person[s]") to monitor and respond to conditions in the organization's environment. The assigned individual performs the following tasks:
- Coordinates the ongoing, organizationwide collection of information about deficiencies and opportunities for improvement in the environment of care
- Coordinates the ongoing collection and dissemination of other sources of information, such as published hazard notices or recall reports
- Coordinates the preparation of summaries of deficiencies, problems, failures, and user errors related to managing the environment of care†

EC

* Organizations have the flexibility to develop a single reporting method that addresses one or more of the items listed.

† Incidents involving patients may be reported to appropriate staff such as staff in quality assessment, improvement, or other functions. However, at least a summary of incidents is shared with the person designated to coordinate safety management activities (*see* standard EC.1.10). Review of incident reports often requires that various legal processes be followed to preserve confidentiality. Opportunities to improve care, treatment, and services or to prevent future similar incidents are not lost as a result of the legal process followed.

- Coordinates the preparation of summaries on findings, recommendations, actions taken, and results of performance improvement (PI) activities
- Participates in hazard surveillance and incident reporting
- Participates in developing safety policies and procedures

B 3. The organization establishes and implements a process(es) for ongoing monitoring of performance regarding actual or potential risk(s) in each of the environment of care management plans.*

A 4. Each of the environment of care management plans is evaluated at least annually.

B 5. The objectives, scope, performance, and effectiveness of each of the environment of care management plans are evaluated at least annually.

6. Through 9. Not applicable

B 10. Environmental safety monitoring and response activities are communicated to the patient safety program required in the "Leadership" (LD) chapter of this book.

Standard EC.9.20

The organization analyzes identified environment issues and develops recommendations for resolving them.

Elements of Performance for EC.9.20

B 1. The organization establishes an ongoing process for resolving environment of care issues that involves representatives from clinical, administrative, and support services.

2. Not applicable

B 3. The organization analyzes environment of care issues in a timely manner.

B 4. Recommendations are developed and approved as appropriate.

B 5. Appropriate staff establishes measurement guidelines.

B 6. Environment of care issues are communicated to the organization's leaders and person(s) responsible for PI activities.

7. Not applicable

A 8. A recommendation for one or more PI activities is communicated at least annually to the organization's leaders based on the ongoing performance monitoring of the environment of care management plans.

---

* The environment of care plans are for managing safety, security, hazardous materials and waste, emergency management, fire safety, medical equipment, and utilities.

B 9. Recommendations for resolving environmental safety issues are communicated, when appropriate, to those responsible for managing the patient safety program required in the "Leadership" (LD) chapter of this book.

Standard EC.9.30

The organization improves the environment.

Elements of Performance for EC.9.30

B 1. Appropriate staff participates in implementing recommendations.

B 2. Appropriate staff monitors the effectiveness of the recommendation's implementation.

B 3. Monitoring results are reported through appropriate channels, including the organization's leaders.

4. Not applicable

B 5. Results of monitoring are reported (when appropriate) to those responsible for managing the patient safety program required in the "Leadership" (LD) chapter of this book.

Management of Human Resources

Overview

The goal of the human resources function is to ensure that the organization determines the qualifications and competencies for staff* positions based on its mission, population(s), and care, treatment, and services. Organizations must also provide the right number of competent staff to meet patients' needs. To meet this goal, the organization carries out the following processes and activities:

- **Planning.** The planning process defines the qualifications, competencies, and staffing necessary to provide for the organization's care, treatment, and services.
- **Providing competent staff.** The organization provides for competent staff either through traditional employer–employee arrangements or through contractual arrangements with other entities or persons.
- **Orienting, training, and educating staff.** The organization provides ongoing in-service and other education and training to increase staff knowledge of specific work-related issues.
- **Assessing, maintaining, and improving staff competence.** Ongoing, periodic competence assessment evaluates staff members' continuing abilities to perform throughout their association with the organization.
- **Promoting self-development and learning.** Staff is encouraged to pursue ongoing professional development goals and provide feedback about the work environment.

HR

* **Staff** As appropriate to their roles and responsibilities, all people who provide care, treatment, and services in the organization, including those receiving pay (for example, permanent, temporary, and part-time personnel, as well as contract employees), volunteers, and health profession students. The definition of staff does not include licensed independent practitioners who are not paid staff or who are not contract employees.

Standards

The following is a list of all standards for this function. They are presented here for your convenience without footnotes or other explanatory text. If you have a question about a term used here, please check the Glossary.

Note: *A revised standard numbering system is being used with the reformatted standards. The revised numbering system will allow for more flexibility to add standards while maintaining the current number for each standard.*

Planning

HR.1.10 The organization provides an adequate number and mix of staff and licensed independent practitioners consistent with the organization's staffing plan.

HR.1.15 Not applicable

HR.1.20 Staff qualifications are consistent with his or her job responsibilities.

HR.1.25 The organization may assign disaster responsibilities to volunteer practitioners.

HR.1.30 Not applicable

Orientation, Training, and Education

HR.2.10 The organization provides initial orientation.

HR.2.20 Staff and licensed independent practitioners, as appropriate, can describe or demonstrate their roles and responsibilities relative to safety.

HR.2.30 Ongoing education, including in-services, training, and other activities, maintains and improves staff competence.

Assessing Competence

HR.3.10 Staff competence to perform job responsibilities is assessed, demonstrated, and maintained.

HR.3.20 The organization periodically conducts performance evaluations.

HR.3.25 Through HR.3.60 Not applicable

Credentialing and Assignment of Clinical Responsibilities of Licensed Independent Practitioners

HR.4.10 There is a process for ensuring the competence of all practitioners permitted by law and the organization to practice independently.

HR.4.20 Individuals permitted by law and the organization to practice independently are granted clinical privileges.

HR.4.30 The organization has a process for granting temporary clinical privileges, when appropriate.

HR.4.32 Deliberations by organization leaders in developing recommendations for initial granting of clinical privileges and revision or revocation of clinical privileges includes information provided by peers of the applicant.

HR.4.33 The leadership implements a process to identify and manage matters of individual health for licensed independent practitioners which is separate from actions taken for disciplinary purposes.

HR.4.34 There is a process that defines circumstances requiring a focused review of a practitioner's performance and evaluation of a practitioner's performance by peers.

Disaster Privileges

HR.4.35 The organization may grant disaster privileges to volunteers eligible to be licensed independent practitioners.

HR.4.40 There are mechanisms, including a fair hearing and appeal process, for addressing adverse decisions regarding reappointment denial, reduction, suspension, or revocation of clinical privileges that may relate to quality of care, treatment, and service issues.

HR.4.50 Clinical privileges and appointments/reappointments are reviewed and revised at least every two years.

HR.4.60 Through HR.5.40 Not applicable

Standards, Rationales, Elements of Performance, and Scoring

Planning

Standard HR.1.10

The organization provides an adequate number and mix of staff and licensed independent practitioners consistent with the organization's staffing plan.

Rationale for HR.1.10

An organization must provide appropriate types and numbers of qualified staff necessary to furnish the care, treatment, and services offered by the organization. This can be done either through traditional employer–employee arrangements or through contractual arrangements.

Elements of Performance for HR.1.10

B 1. The organization has an adequate number and mix of staff and licensed independent practitioners to meet the care, treatment, and service needs of the patients.

2. Not applicable

3. Not applicable

4. Not applicable

For Medicare-Certified Ambulatory Surgical Centers (EP 5):

A Ⓜ 5. Staff trained in emergency equipment use and cardiopulmonary resuscitation through an evidence-based* training program is available whenever a patient is in the ambulatory surgery center.

6. Through 11. Not applicable

For Medicare-Certified Ambulatory Surgical Centers (EPs 12–15):

A 12. The nursing services of the ambulatory surgical center (ASC) must be directed and staffed to assure that the nursing needs of all patients are met.

A 13. Patient care responsibilities are delineated for all nursing service personnel.

A 14. Nursing services are provided in accordance with recognized standards of practice.

---

* **Evidence-based** Based on empirical evidence or in the absence of empirical evidence, expert consensus (such as consensus statements promoted by professional societies).

A 15. There must be a registered nurse available for emergency treatment whenever there is a patient in the ambulatory surgical center.

Standard HR.1.15

Not applicable

Standard HR.1.20

Staff qualifications are consistent with his or her job responsibilities.

Elements of Performance for HR.1.20

B 1. The organization defines the required competence and qualifications of staff in each program(s) or service(s).

C Ⓜ 2. When the organization requires current licensure, certification, or registration, but these credentials are not required by law or regulation, the organization verifies these credentials at the time of hire and upon expiration of the credentials.

B 3. When current licensure, certification, or registration are required by law or regulation to practice a profession,* the organization verifies these credentials with the primary source at the time of hire and upon expiration of the credentials.

Note: *It is acceptable to verify current licensure, certification, or registration with the primary source via a secure electronic communication or by telephone, if this verification is documented. For additional information,* see *"primary source verification" in the Glossary.*

Note: *A primary source of information may designate another agency to communicate credentials information. The designated agency then can be used as a primary source.*

Note: *An external organization (for example, a credentials verification organization [CVO]) may be used to collect credentials information. A CVO must meet the CVO guidelines listed in the Glossary.*

C Ⓜ 4. The organization also verifies the education, experience, and competence appropriate for assigned responsibilities.

C Ⓜ 5. The organization also verifies information on criminal background if required by law and regulation or organization policy.

* **Profession** is a specialized work function within society, generally performed by a professional. It often refers specifically to fields that require extensive study and mastery of specialized knowledge and skills. Examples of a profession include but are not limited to a nurse, pharmacist, medical technologist, respiratory care practitioner, radiology technician, and social worker.

C Ⓜ 6. The organization also verifies compliance with applicable health screening requirements if required by law and regulation or established by the organization.*

A 7. The information obtained from EPs 2–6 is used in making decisions regarding staff job responsibilities.

A 8. All staff that provide patient care, treatment, and services possess a license, certification, or registration as required by law and regulation.

9. Not applicable

10. Not applicable

C Ⓜ 11. Prior to the provision of care, treatment or services, the qualifications and competence of a non-employee individual, brought into the organization by a licensed independent practitioner to provide care, treatment or services within the scope of the organization's services are assessed by the organization and determined to be commensurate with the qualifications and competence required if the individual were to be employed by the organization to perform the same or similar services.

Note: *When the service to be provided by the individual is not currently performed by anyone employed by the organization, it is leadership's responsibility to consult the appropriate professional organization guidelines with respect to expectations for credentials and competence.*

C Ⓜ 12. The organization reviews the qualifications, performance, and competence of each non-employee individual brought into the organization by a licensed independent practitioner to provide care, treatment, or services at the same frequency as individuals employed by the organization.

13. Not applicable

B 14. Staff supervises students when they provide patient care, treatment, and services as part of their training.

Disaster Responsibilities

Standard HR.1.25

The organization may assign disaster responsibilities to volunteer practitioners.

Rationale for HR.1.25

When the disaster plan has been implemented (*see* standard EC.4.10 for a description of emergency management planning requirements) and the immediate needs

* Organizations should consider the applicability of the Americans with Disabilities Act (ADA) and, if applicable, review policies and procedures. Federal entities are required to comply with the Rehabilitation Act of 1974.

of the patients cannot be met, the organization may implement a modified process for determining qualifications and competence of volunteer practitioners* (*see* EPs 5–8). The volunteer practitioners that are addressed by this standard only include those practitioners that are required by law and regulation to have a license, certification, or registration to practice their profession. The usual process to determine the qualifications and competence of these practitioners would not allow a volunteer practitioner to provide immediate care, treatment, and services in the event of a disaster (refer to the Glossary for definitions of *disaster* and *emergency*) due to the length of time it would take to complete the process. A similar modified process for the assignment of disaster privileges for volunteer licensed independent practitioners exists at standard HR.4.35.

While this standard allows for a method to streamline the process for determining qualifications and competence, safeguards must be in place to assure that the volunteer practitioners are competent to provide safe and adequate care, treatment, and services. Even in a disaster, the integrity of the following two parts of the usual process for determining qualifications and competence must be maintained:

1. Verification of licensure, certification, or registration required to practice a profession
2. Oversight of the care, treatment, and services provided

This option to assign disaster responsibilities to volunteer practitioners is made on a case-by-case basis in accordance with the needs of the organization and its patients, and on the qualifications of its volunteer practitioners.

There are a number of state and federal systems engaged in pre-event verification of qualifications that may facilitate the assigning of disaster responsibilities to volunteer practitioners at the time of a disaster. Examples of such systems include the Medical Reserve Corps (MRC[†]) and the Emergency System for Advance Registration of Volunteer Health Professionals (ESAR-VHP[‡]). It is expected that additional programs will emerge and evolve.

* Individuals who are qualified to practice a health care profession (for example, a nurse) and are engaged in the provision of care and services. Practitioners are often required to be licensed as defined by law.

† **MRC** Medical Reserve Corps units are comprised of locally-based medical and public health volunteers who can assist their communities during emergencies, such as an influenza epidemic, a chemical spill, or an act of terrorism. The MRC Program was formed in 2002, in cooperation with the White House's USA Freedom Corps, as one of the charter programs of Citizen Corps. Pre-identifying, training and organizing medical and public health professionals to strengthen their communities through volunteerism is at the core of the MRC concept. MRC volunteers offer their expertise throughout the year by supporting local public health initiatives, such as immunization and prevention activities. When an emergency community need occurs, MRC volunteers can work in coordination with existing local emergency response programs.

‡ **ESAR-VHP** The Emergency System for Advance Registration of Volunteer Health Professionals (ESAR-VHP) program, created by the Health Resources and Services Administration (HRSA), allows for the advance registration and credentialing of health care professionals needed to augment a hospital or other medical facility to meet increased patient/victim care and increased surge capacity needs.

Elements of Performance for HR.1.25

A 1. Disaster responsibilities are assigned only when the following two conditions are present: the emergency management plan has been activated, and the organization is unable to meet immediate patient needs.

A 2. The organization identifies in writing the individual(s) responsible for assigning disaster responsibilities.

B 3. The organization describes in writing a mechanism (for example, direct observation, mentoring, and clinical record review) to oversee the professional performance of volunteer practitioners who are assigned disaster responsibilities.

B 4. The organization has a mechanism to identify volunteer practitioners that have been assigned disaster responsibilities.

A 5. For volunteer practitioners to be assigned disaster responsibilities, the organization obtains for each volunteer practitioner, at a minimum, a valid government-issued photo identification issued by a state or federal agency (for example, driver's license or passport) and at least one of the following:

- A current health care organization (such as a long term care, ambulatory care, laboratory, or hospital) picture identification card that clearly identifies professional designation
- A current license, certification, or registration
- Primary source verification of licensure, certification, or registration (if required by law and regulation to practice a profession)
- Identification indicating that the individual is a member of a Disaster Medical Assistance Team (DMAT*), or MRC, ESAR-VHP, or other recognized state or federal organizations or groups
- Identification indicating that the individual has been granted authority to render patient care, treatment, and services in disaster circumstances (such authority having been granted by a federal, state, or municipal entity)
- Identification by current organization member(s) who possesses personal knowledge regarding the volunteer practitioner's qualifications

HR

A 6. Primary source verification of licensure, certification, or registration (if required by law and regulation to practice a profession) begins as soon as the immediate situation is under control and is completed within 72 hours from the time the volunteer practitioner presents to the organization.

Note: *In the extraordinary circumstance that primary source verification of licensure, certification, or registration* (if required by law and regulation to practice a profession) *cannot be completed in 72 hours (for exam-*

* **DMAT** A group of medical and support personnel designed to provide emergency medical care during a disaster or other unusual event. The DMAT is a component of the National Disaster Medical System (NDMS). The Department of Health and Human Services, in partnership with other federal agencies such as Department of Defense, Department of Veterans Affairs, and the Federal Emergency Management Agency, administers the program.

ple, no means of communication or a lack of resources), it is expected that it be done as soon as possible. In this extraordinary circumstance, there must be documentation of the following: why primary source verification could not be performed in the required time frame; evidence of a demonstrated ability to continue to provide adequate care, treatment, and services; and an attempt to rectify the situation as soon as possible. Primary source verification of licensure, certification, or registration (if required by law and regulation to practice a profession) *would not be required if the volunteer practitioner has not provided care, treatment, and services under the disaster responsibilities.*

B 7. The organization oversees the professional practice of volunteer practitioners.

A 8. The organization makes a decision (based on information obtained regarding the professional practice of the volunteer practitioner) within 72 hours related to the continuation of the disaster responsibilities initially assigned.

Standard HR.1.30

Not applicable

Orientation, Training, and Education

Standard HR.2.10

The organization provides initial orientation.

Rationale for HR.2.10

Orientation is a process in which initial job training and information is provided to staff and licensed independent practitioners. Staff and licensed independent practitioner orientation promotes safe and effective job performance. Some elements of orientation need to occur before staff and licensed independent practitioners provide care, treatment, and services. Other elements of orientation can occur when staff and licensed independent practitioners are providing care, treatment, and services.

HR

Elements of Performance for HR.2.10

B 1. The organization determines what key elements of orientation should occur before staff and licensed independent practitioners provide care, treatment, and services.

C Ⓜ 2. The organization orients staff and licensed independent practitioners to the identified key elements prior to the provision of care, treatment, and services.

C Ⓜ 3. As appropriate, staff and licensed independent practitioner orientation addresses the organization's mission and goals.

C Ⓜ 4. As appropriate, staff and licensed independent practitioner orientation addresses organizationwide policies and procedures (including safety and infection control) and relevant unit, setting, or program-specific policies and procedures.

C Ⓜ 5. As appropriate, staff and licensed independent practitioner orientation addresses specific job duties and responsibilities and service, setting, or program-specific job duties and responsibilities related to safety and infection control.

6. Not applicable

C Ⓜ 7. As appropriate, staff and licensed independent practitioner orientation addresses cultural diversity and sensitivity.

C Ⓜ 8. Staff orientation includes education about the rights of patients and ethical aspects of care, treatment, and services and the process used to address ethical issues.

Standard HR.2.20

Staff and licensed independent practitioners, as appropriate, can describe or demonstrate their roles and responsibilities relative to safety.

Rationale for HR.2.20

The human element is the most critical factor in any process, determining whether the right things are done correctly. The best policies and procedures for minimizing risks in the environment where care, treatment, and services are provided are meaningless if staff, licensed independent practitioners if applicable, do not know and understand them well enough to perform them properly.

It is important that everyday precautions identified by the health care organization for minimizing various risks, including those related to patient safety and environmental safety,* are properly implemented. It is also important that the appropriate emergency procedures be instituted should an incident or failure occur in the environment.

Elements of Performance for HR.2.20

C Ⓜ 1. Staff and licensed independent practitioners, as appropriate, can describe or demonstrate risks within the organization's environment.

C Ⓜ 2. Staff and licensed independent practitioners, as appropriate, can describe or demonstrate actions to eliminate, minimize, or report risks.

* The "Management of the Environment of Care" chapter of this book identifies risks associated with the following categories: safety, security, hazardous materials and wastes, emergency management, medical equipment, and utility management.

C Ⓜ 3. Staff and licensed independent practitioners, as appropriate, can describe or demonstrate procedures to follow in the event of an incident.

C Ⓜ 4. Staff and licensed independent practitioners, as appropriate, can describe or demonstrate reporting processes for common problems, failures, and user errors.

Standard HR.2.30

Ongoing education, including in-services, training, and other activities, maintains and improves staff competence.

Elements of Performance for HR.2.30

B 1. Staff training occurs when job responsibilities or duties change.

C Ⓜ 2. Staff participate in ongoing in-services, training, or other activities to increase knowledge of work-related issues.

C Ⓜ 3. Ongoing in-services and other education and training of staff are appropriate to the needs of the population(s) served and comply with law and regulation.

C Ⓜ 4. Ongoing in-services, training, or other staff activities emphasize specific job-related aspects of safety and infection prevention and control.

C Ⓜ 5. Ongoing in-services, training, or other staff education incorporate methods of team training, when appropriate.

C Ⓜ 6. Ongoing in-services, training, or other staff education reinforce the need and ways to report unanticipated adverse events.

C Ⓜ 7. Ongoing in-services or other staff education are offered in response to learning needs identified through performance improvement findings and other data analysis (that is, data from staff surveys, performance evaluations, or other needs assessments).

C Ⓜ 8. Ongoing staff education is documented.

Assessing Competence

Standard HR.3.10

Staff competence to perform job responsibilities is assessed, demonstrated, and maintained.

Rationale for HR.3.10

Competence assessment is systematic and allows for a measurable assessment of the person's ability to perform required activities. Information used as part of competence assessment may include data from performance evaluations, performance improvement, and aggregate data on competence, as well as the assessment of learning needs.

Elements of Performance for HR.3.10

B 1. The competence assessment process for staff is based on the population(s) served

B 2. The competence assessment process for staff is based on the defined competencies to be required.

B 3. The competence assessment process for staff is based on the defined competencies to be assessed during orientation.

B 4. The competence assessment process for staff is based on the defined competencies that need to be assessed and reassessed on an ongoing basis, based on techniques, procedures, technology, equipment, or skills needed to provide care, treatment, and services.

B 5. The competence assessment process for staff is based on a defined time frame for how often competence assessments are performed for each person, minimally, once in the three-year accreditation cycle and in accordance with law and regulation.

B 6. The competence assessment process for staff is based on the assessment methods (appropriate to determine the skill being assessed).

B 7. The competence assessment process for staff is based on the use of qualified individuals to assess competence.

Note: *When there is no qualified individual in the organization that performs comparable care, treatment, and services, the organization may*
- *Utilize qualified staff from other organizations to assist with the assessment of competence*
  or
- *Consult the appropriate professional organization guidelines with respect to expectations for competence and use these guidelines to assess competence*

C Ⓜ 8. The organization assesses and documents staff's ability to carry out assigned responsibilities safely, competently, and in a timely manner upon completion of orientation.

C Ⓜ 9. The organization assesses staff according to its competence assessment process.

B 10. When improvement activities lead to a determination that a person with performance problems is unable or unwilling to improve, the organization takes appropriate action (which may include modifying the person's job assignment).

Standard HR.3.20

The organization periodically conducts performance evaluations.

Rationale for HR.3.20

Performance is evaluated as an ongoing process for providing positive and negative feedback to staff. Formal performance evaluations can be conducted concurrently with competence assessments or can be completed at a separate time.

Elements of Performance for HR.3.20

C Ⓜ 1. The organization conducts performance evaluations periodically at time frames identified by the organization (at a minimum, at least once in the three-year accreditation cycle).

C Ⓜ 2. Performance is evaluated based on the performance expectations described in job descriptions or through the privileging process.

3. Not applicable

C Ⓜ 4. Performance evaluations are documented.

Standards HR.3.25 through HR.3.60

Not applicable

Credentialing and Privileging of Licensed Independent Practitioners

Introduction

Credentialing

Credentialing involves the collection, verification, and assessment of information regarding four critical parameters: current licensure, relevant training, current competence, and the ability to perform the clinical privileges requested.

The verification of current licensure informs the organization that the individual is appropriately licensed to practice as required by state and/or federal law. The license verification process is conducted prior to initial granting of clinical privileges, at the time of renewal of clinical privileges, and at the time of expiration of the license.

The verification of relevant training informs the organization of the licensed independent practitioner's clinical knowledge and skill set. Verification must be obtained from the primary source of the specific credential. Primary sources include the specialty certifying boards approved by the American Dental Association for a dentist's board certification, letters from professional schools (for example, medical and dental) and from residency or postdoctoral programs for completion of training. When it is not possible to obtain information from the primary source, reliable secondary sources* may be used.

* A reliable secondary source can be another health care organization that has documented primary source verification of the applicant's credentials.

Designated equivalent sources may be used to verify certain credentials in lieu of using the primary source. *See* the Glossary for the list of designated equivalent sources.

Current competence in performing clinical privileges is verified by peers knowledgeable about the applicant's professional performance.

Standard HR.4.10

There is a process for ensuring the competence of all practitioners permitted by law and the organization to practice independently.

Elements of Performance for HR.4.10

1. Through 4. Not applicable

B 5. The organization has a defined process approved by the leaders for appointing and reappointing licensed independent practitioners.

A 6. At the time of initial granting of privileges, the organization verifies, by viewing a valid government-issued photo identification issued by a state or federal agency (for example, driver's license or passport), that the individual being granted (clinical privileges) is the same individual identified in the credentialing documents.

A 7. The credentialing process requires that the organization does the following:

- Verifies in writing current licensure, from the primary source at time of initial granting, renewal and revision of clinical privileges, and prior to licensure expiration
- Verifies in writing training (required by the organization to perform the clinical privileges) from the primary source at the time of initial granting and renewal and revision of clinical privileges
- Verifies in writing current competence from the primary source at time of initial granting of clinical privileges
- Obtains a statement from the applicant at the time of initial granting, renewal, or revision of clinical privileges that no health problems exist that could effect his or her ability to perform the privileges requested.*

Note: *Verification of current licensure with the primary source through a secure electronic communication or by telephone is acceptable, if this verification is documented. For additional information,* see *"primary source verification" in the Glossary.*

Note: *An external organization (for example, a credentials verification organization [CVO] or a Joint Commission–accredited health care orga-*

HR

* Organizations should consider the applicability of the Americans with Disabilities Act (ADA) to their credentialing and privileging activities, and, if applicable, review their policies and procedures. Federal entities are required to comply with the Rehabilitation Act of 1974.

nization functioning as a CVO) may be used to collect credentialing information. Both of these organizations must meet the CVO guidelines listed in the Glossary section of the accreditation manual.

Note: *A primary source of verified information may designate to an agency the role of communicating credentials information. The delegated agency then becomes acceptable to be used as a primary source.*

A 8. All licensed independent practitioners that provide patient care possess a license, certification, or registration as required by law and regulation.

For Medicare-Certified Ambulatory Surgical Centers (EPs 9–10):

A 9. Medical staff members are legally and professionally qualified for the positions to which they are appointed.

A 10. Medical staff members are legally and professionally qualified to perform the privileges granted.

Standard HR.4.20

Individuals permitted by law and the organization to practice independently are granted clinical privileges.

Elements of Performance for HR.4.20

B 1. Based on the scope of services provided, the organization establishes criteria for each privilege. These criteria include the following:
- Current licensure and/or certification as appropriate, verified with the primary source
- Successful completion of training specific to each requested privilege, verified with the primary source
- Peer* and or faculty recommendation
- Evidence of the ability to perform the requested privilege

A 2. Before granting, renewing, or revising privileges, the clinical leadership evaluates the following:
- Challenges to any licensure or registration
- Voluntary and involuntary relinquishment of any license or registration
- Voluntary and involuntary termination of medical staff membership at another organization
- Voluntary and involuntary limitation, reduction, or loss of clinical privileges
- Any evidence of an unusual pattern or an excessive number of professional liability actions resulting in a final judgment against the applicant
- Documentation as to the applicant's health status

HR

* *See* Glossary for definition of peer recommendation.

A 3. The organization queries the National Practitioner Data Bank (NPDB) at the time of initial granting of privileges, as well as at least every two years thereafter, for information on physicians and dentists granted clinical privileges.

C Ⓜ 4. Clinical privileges for licensed independent practitioners are delineated according to organization policy and based on the licensed independent practitioner's current credentials and competence, as well as the population(s) served and the types of care, treatment, and services provided in the organization.

A 5. The decision by leaders to appoint licensed independent practitioners is based on the credentials information obtained.

C Ⓜ 6. The licensed independent practitioner is notified in writing of the leaders' decision.

A 7. Individuals with clinical privileges practice within the scope of their privileges.

8. Through 14. Not applicable

For Medicare-Certified Ambulatory Surgical Centers (EP 15 only):

A 15. Physicians performing surgery in the ambulatory surgical center have been granted clinical privileges to do so by the ambulatory surgical center's governing body.

16. Not applicable

Organizations offering the services of licensed independent practitioners through a telemedical link for either direct care or interpretive services must also meet the following requirements:

A 17. The organization has a clearly defined procedure for the processing of applications for the granting, renewal, or revision of clinical privileges.

The process for awarding privileges also includes the following (EPs 18–20):

C Ⓜ 18. Completed applications for privileges are acted on within the time period specified by the organization.

C Ⓜ 19. Information regarding each practitioner's scope of privileges is updated as changes in clinical privileges for each practitioner are made.

C Ⓜ 20. Decisions on granting of privileges must consider criteria that are directly related to the quality of health care, treatment, and services. If privileging criteria are used that are unrelated to quality of care, treatment, and services or professional competence, evidence exists that the impact of resulting decisions on the quality of care, treatment, and services is evaluated.

A 21. The organization queries the National Practitioner Data Bank (NPDB) when clinical privileges are initially granted, at the time of renewal of privileges, and when a new privilege(s) is requested.

B 22. Before granting privileges, designated clinical leaders* evaluate the following:
- Challenges to any licensure or registration
- Voluntary and involuntary relinquishment of any license or registration
- Voluntary and involuntary termination of medical staff membership
- Voluntary and involuntary limitation, reduction, or loss of clinical privileges
- Any evidence of an unusual pattern or an excessive number of professional liability actions resulting in a final judgment against the applicant
- Documentation as to the applicant's health status
- Relevant practitioner-specific data are compared to aggregate data, when available
- Morbidity and mortality data, when available

Standard HR.4.30

The organization has a process for granting temporary clinical privileges, when appropriate.

Rationale for HR.4.30

There are two circumstances in which temporary clinical privileges may be granted. Each circumstance has different criteria for granting clinical privileges. The two circumstances are to meet the important needs of patients and for new applicants.

Elements of Performance for HR.4.30

B 1. Policies and procedures, rules, or regulations describe the process for granting temporary privileges for meeting the important needs of patients or for new applicants.

A 2. To grant temporary privileges to meet the important needs of patients, there must be verification (which can be done by telephone) of current licensure and current competence.

A 3. To grant temporary privileges for new applicants, there must be verification (which may be done by telephone) of the following:
- Current licensure
- Relevant education training or experience
- Current competence

HR

* Clinical leaders chosen to evaluate credentialing and privileging information should, whenever possible, represent disciplines and expertise consistent with the privileges being sought.

- Ability to perform the privileges requested
- A query and evaluation of the NPDB for physicians or dentists
- Other criteria required by policies and procedures, rules, or regulations.

A 4. To grant temporary privileges for new applicants, the applicant has the following:
- A complete application
- No current or previously successful challenge to licensure or registration
- Not been subject to involuntary termination of professional or medical staff membership at another organization, when applicable to the discipline
- Not been subject to involuntary limitation, reduction, denial, or loss of privileges, when applicable to the discipline

A 5. The administrator or designee grants temporary privileges for meeting important patient needs and for new applicants upon recommendation of clinical leadership or the medical director.

A 6. Temporary privileges for new applicants are granted for no more than 120 days.

Organizations offering the services of licensed independent practitioners through a telemedical link for either direct care or interpretive services must also meet standards HR.4.32 through HR.4.34 (*see* pages 308–310).

Standard HR.4.32

Deliberations by organization leaders in developing recommendations for initial granting of clinical privileges and revision or revocation of clinical privileges includes information provided by peers of the applicant.

Elements of Performance for HR.4.32

C Ⓜ 1. Recommendations from peers are obtained and evaluated for all new applicants for privileges.

HR

C Ⓜ 2. Upon renewal of privileges, when insufficient practitioner-specific data are available, the leadership obtains and evaluates peer recommendations.

C Ⓜ 3. Peer recommendations include the following information:
- Relevant training and experience
- Current competence
- Any effects of health status on privileges being requested

C Ⓜ 4. Peer recommendations are obtained from a practitioner in the same professional discipline as the applicant with personal knowledge of the applicant's ability to practice.

Standard HR.4.33

The leadership implements a process to identify and manage matters of individual health for licensed independent practitioners which is separate from actions taken for disciplinary purposes.

Elements of Performance for HR.4.33

Process design addresses the following issues (EPs 1–9):

B 1. Education of licensed independent practitioners and other organization staff about illness and impairment recognition issues specific to licensed independent practitioners (at-risk criteria)

A 2. Self referral by a licensed independent practitioner

A 3. Referral by others and maintaining informant confidentiality

A 4. Referral of the licensed independent practitioner to appropriate professional internal or external resources for evaluation, diagnosis, and treatment of the condition or concern

A 5. Maintenance of confidentiality of the licensed independent practitioner seeking referral or referred for assistance, except as limited by applicable law, ethical obligation, or when the health and safety of a patient is threatened

A 6. Evaluation of the credibility of a complaint, allegation, or concern

A 7. Monitoring the licensed independent practitioner and the safety of patients until the rehabilitation is complete and periodically thereafter, if required

A 8. Reporting to leadership instances in which a licensed independent practitioner is providing unsafe treatment

A 9. Initiating appropriate actions when a licensed independent practitioner fails to complete the required rehabilitation program

Standard HR.4.34

There is a process that defines circumstances requiring a focused review of a practitioner's performance and evaluation of a practitioner's performance by peers.

Elements of Performance for HR.4.34

The focused review process includes the following (EPs 1–6):

A 1. Definition of the special circumstances requiring focused review

A 2. Method for selecting focused review panels for specific circumstances

A 3. Time frames in which focused review activities are reasonably adhered to

A 4. Circumstances under which external peer review is required

A 5. Provision of participation in the review process by the individual whose performance is being reviewed

C Ⓜ 6. The focused review is conducted in accordance with circumstances requiring a focused review, as defined by the organization

Leadership is involved in the following (EPs 7–9):

C Ⓜ 7. Evaluation of individuals with clinical privileges whose performance is questioned as a result of the measurement and assessment activities

C Ⓜ 8. Communication to the appropriate parties of the findings, conclusions, recommendations, and actions taken to improve practitioner performance

C Ⓜ 9. Implementation of changes to improve performance

Disaster Privileges

Standard HR.4.35

The organization may grant disaster privileges to volunteers eligible to be licensed independent practitioners.

Rationale for HR.4.35

When the disaster plan has been implemented (*see* standard EC.4.10 for a description of emergency management planning requirements) and the immediate needs of the patients cannot be met, the organization may implement a modified credentialing and privileging process for eligible volunteer practitioners (*see* EPs 5–8). The usual process to credential and privilege practitioners would not allow a volunteer practitioner to provide immediate care, treatment, and services in the event of a disaster (refer to the Glossary for definitions of *disaster* and *emergency*) due to the length of time it would take to complete the process. A similar modified process for the assignment of disaster responsibilities for volunteers that are not licensed independent practitioners exists at standard HR.1.25.

While this standard allows for a method to streamline the credentialing and privileging process, safeguards must be in place to assure that volunteer practitioners are competent to provide safe and adequate care, treatment, and services. Even in a disaster, the integrity of two parts of the usual credentialing and privileging process must be maintained:

1. Verification of licensure
2. Oversight of the care, treatment, and services provided

This option to grant disaster privileges to volunteer practitioners is made on a case-by-case basis in accordance with the needs of the organization and its patients, and on the qualifications of its volunteer practitioners.

There are a number of state and federal systems engaged in pre-event credentialing that may facilitate the implementation of disaster privileging of volunteers at the time of a disaster. Examples of such systems include the Medical Reserve Corps (MRC*) and the Emergency System for Advance Registration of Volunteer Health Professionals (ESAR-VHP†). It is expected that additional programs will emerge and evolve.

Elements of Performance for HR.4.35

A 1. Disaster privileges are granted only when the following two conditions are present: the emergency management plan has been activated, and the organization is unable to meet immediate patient needs.

A 2. The organization identifies in writing the individual(s) responsible for granting disaster privileges.

B 3. The organization describes in writing a mechanism (for example, direct observation, mentoring, and clinical record review) to oversee the professional performance of volunteer practitioners who receive disaster privileges.

B 4. The organization has a mechanism to identify the volunteer practitioners who have been granted disaster privileges.

A 5. In order for volunteers to be considered eligible to act as licensed independent practitioners, the organization obtains for each volunteer practitioner at a minimum, a valid government-issued photo identification issued by a state or federal agency (for example, driver's license or passport) and at least one of the following:
- A current health care organization (such as a long term care, ambulatory care, or hospital) picture identification card that clearly identifies professional designation
- A current license to practice
- Primary source verification of the license

HR

* **MRC** Medical Reserve Corps units are comprised of locally-based medical and public health volunteers who can assist their communities during emergencies, such as an influenza epidemic, a chemical spill, or an act of terrorism. The MRC Program was formed in 2002, in cooperation with the White House's USA Freedom Corps, as one of the charter programs of Citizen Corps. Pre-identifying, training and organizing medical and public health professionals to strengthen their communities through volunteerism is at the core of the MRC concept. MRC volunteers offer their expertise throughout the year by supporting local public health initiatives, such as immunization and prevention activities. When an emergency community need occurs, MRC volunteers can work in coordination with existing local emergency response programs.

† **ESAR-VHP** The Emergency System for Advance Registration of Volunteer Health Professionals (ESAR-VHP) program, created by the Health Resources and Services Administration (HRSA), allows for the advance registration and credentialing of health care professionals needed to augment a hospital or other medical facility to meet increased patient/victim care and increased surge capacity needs.

- Identification indicating that the individual is a member of a Disaster Medical Assistance Team (DMAT*), or MRC, ESAR-VHP, or other recognized state or federal organizations or groups
- Identification indicating that the individual has been granted authority to render patient care, treatment, and services in disaster circumstances (such authority having been granted by a federal, state, or municipal entity)
- Identification by current organization member(s) who possesses personal knowledge regarding the volunteer's ability to act as a licensed independent practitioner during a disaster

A 6. Primary source verification of licensure begins as soon as the immediate situation is under control and is completed within 72 hours from the time the volunteer practitioner presents to the organization.

Note: *In the extraordinary circumstance that primary source verification cannot be completed in 72 hours (for example, no means of communication or a lack of resources), it is expected that it be done as soon as possible. In this extraordinary circumstance, there must be documentation of the following: why primary source verification could not be performed in the required time frame; evidence of a demonstrated ability to continue to provide adequate care, treatment, and services; and an attempt to rectify the situation as soon as possible. Primary source verification of licensure would not be required if the volunteer practitioner has not provided care, treatment, and services under the disaster privileges.*

B 7. The organization oversees the professional practice of volunteer licensed independent practitioners.

A 8. The organization makes a decision (based on information obtained regarding the professional practice of the volunteer) within 72 hours related to the continuation of the disaster privileges initially granted.

Standard HR.4.40

There are mechanisms, including a fair hearing and appeal process, for addressing adverse decisions regarding reappointment denial, reduction, suspension, or revocation of clinical privileges that may relate to quality of care, treatment, and service issues.

Rationale for HR.4.40

Mechanisms for fair hearing and appeals processes are designed to allow the affected individual a fair opportunity to defend herself or himself regarding the adverse decision to an unbiased hearing committee, and an opportunity to appeal the decision of the committee to the governance function. The purpose of a fair hearing and appeal is to assure full consideration and reconsideration of quality

* **DMAT** A group of medical and support personnel designed to provide emergency medical care during a disaster or other unusual event. The DMAT is a component of the National Disaster Medical System (NDMS).

and safety issues and, under the current structure of reporting to the NPDB, to allow practitioners an opportunity to defend themselves.

Elements of Performance for HR.4.40

The organization has developed a fair hearing and appeals process that does the following:

B 1. Is designed to provide a uniform and fair process

B 2. Has a mechanism to schedule a hearing of such requests

B 3. Has identified the procedures for the hearings to follow

B 4. Identifies or defines the composition of the hearing committee

B 5. Provides for a mechanism to appeal an adverse decision through the governance function

Standard HR.4.50

Clinical privileges and appointments/reappointments are reviewed and revised at least every two years.

Elements of Performance for HR.4.50

A 1. Policies and procedures or rules and regulations specify a period of no more than two years between appointments and reappointments and between granting, renewing, and revising clinical privileges.

C Ⓜ 2. Credential files for licensed independent practitioners contain substantive information and indicate that clinical privileges are reviewed or revised at least every two years and are revised as needed; in addition, appointments and reappointments are made for a period of no more than two years.

A 3. A reappraisal is conducted at the time of reappointment or renewal or revision of clinical privileges.

A 4. The reappraisal addresses current competence and includes the following:
- Confirmation of adherence to organization policies and procedures, rules, or regulations
- Relevant information from organization performance improvement activities when evaluating professional performance, judgment, and clinical or technical skills
- Any results of review of the individual's clinical performance
- Clinical performance in the organization that is outside acceptable standards

B 5. Credentials files contain clear evidence that the full range of privileges has been included in the reappraisal.

HR

Standards HR.4.60 Through HR.5.40
Not applicable

Management of Information

Overview

The **goal** of the information management function is to support decision making to improve patient outcomes, improve health care documentation, improve patient safety, and improve performance in patient care, treatment, and services; governance; management; and support processes. While efficiency, effectiveness, patient safety, and the quality of patient care can be improved by computerization and other technologies, the principles of good information management apply to paper-based or electronic methods. The standards in this chapter are designed to be equally compatible with paper-based systems, electronic systems, or hybrid systems.

An organization's provision of care, treatment, and services is a complex endeavor that is highly dependent on information. Furthermore, when many individuals and areas throughout the organization are involved in the provision of care, treatment, and services, their work is coordinated and integrated. As a result, organizations treat information as an important resource to be managed effectively and efficiently. Managing information is an active, planned activity. The organization's leaders have overall responsibility for managing information, just as they do for managing the organization's human, material, and financial resources.

The quality of care, treatment, and services is affected by the many transitions in information management that are currently in progress in health care, such as the transition from handwriting and traditional paper-based documentation to electronic information management, as well as the transition from free text* to structured† and interactive text.‡

To achieve the goals of this function, the following processes are performed:

- Identifying information needs
- Designing the structure of the information management system
- Capturing,§ organizing, storing, retrieving, processing,|| and analyzing# data and information

---

* **Free text** Free-flowing, nonstructured type of speaking, writing, or inputting of information.

† **Structured text** Process that requires authors to put specific information into specific fields with passive guidance by the information system. In paper-based systems, a form encourages a practitioner to fill in fields or boxes. Electronic systems use the same principle for templates or macros, which are guides used to create standardized information documentation. The purpose is to produce data of more consistent quality, make information more usable for decision support, make information more complete and more easily retrievable, and save documentation time.

‡ **Interactive text** A more complex version of structured text, as it interactively prompts and provides feedback to the person using it. Typically, it uses a higher level of computer intelligence that interacts with the person who records information.

§ **Capture** The process of recording representations of human thought, perceptions, or actions, as well as device-generated data or information that is gathered and/or computed about a patient as part of a health care encounter or about other matters in an organization.

|| **Processing** The process that manipulates data and information by editing and updating.

\# **Analyzing** The process that interprets the data and transforms it into information.

IM

- Transmitting,* reporting, displaying, integrating, and using data and information
- Safeguarding data† and information

The standards in this chapter focus on organizationwide information planning and management processes to meet the organization's internal and external information needs. The standards describe a vision for effectively and continuously improving information management in health care organizations. Achieving this vision involves the following:

- Providing for timely and easy access to complete information throughout the organization
- Providing for data accuracy
- Balancing requirements of security‡ and ease of access
- Producing and using aggregate data to pursue opportunities for improvement
- Providing for data comparability within and among organizations, where possible, by following national, state, and other recognized standards and guidelines on form and content
- Accessing and using external knowledge bases and comparative data to pursue opportunities for improvement
- Redesigning information-related processes to improve efficiency and effectiveness, as well as patient safety and quality of patient care, treatment, and services
- Increasing collaboration and information sharing to enhance patient care

* **Transmission** The sending of data and information from one location to another.

† **Data** Uninterpreted observations or facts.

‡ **Security** The protection of data from intentional or unintentional destruction, modification, or disclosure.

Standards

The following is a list of all standards for this chapter. They are presented here for your convenience without footnotes or other explanatory text. If you have a question about a term used here, please check the Glossary.

Note: *A revised standard numbering system is being used with the reformatted standards. This revised numbering system will allow for more flexibility to add standards while maintaining the current label for each standard.*

Information Management Planning

IM.1.10 The organization plans and designs information management processes to meet internal and external information needs.

Confidentiality and Security

IM.2.10 Information privacy and confidentiality are maintained.

IM.2.20 Information security, including data integrity, is maintained.

IM.2.30 Continuity of information is maintained.

Information Management Processes

IM.3.10 The organization has processes in place to effectively manage information, including the capturing, reporting, processing, storing, retrieving, disseminating, and displaying of clinical/service and nonclinical data and information.

Information-Based Decision Making

IM.4.10 The information management system provides information for use in decision making.

Knowledge-Based Information

IM.5.10 Knowledge-based information resources are readily available, current, and authoritative.

Patient-Specific Information

IM.6.10 The organization has a complete and accurate medical record for patients assessed, cared for, treated, or served.

IM.6.20 Records contain patient-specific information, as appropriate to the care, treatment, and services provided.

IM.6.30 The medical record thoroughly documents operative or other high-risk procedures and the use of moderate or deep sedation or anesthesia. (*See also* standards PC.13.30 and PC.13.40.)

IM.6.40 For patients receiving continuing ambulatory care services, the medical record contains a summary list(s) of significant diagnoses, procedures, drug allergies, and medications.

IM.6.50 Designated qualified staff accept and transcribe verbal or telephone orders from authorized individuals.

IM.6.60 The organization provides access to relevant information from a patient's record as needed for use in patient care, treatment, and services.

IM.6.70 Through IM.6.280 Not applicable

Standards, Rationales, Elements of Performance, and Scoring

Information Management Planning

Standard IM.1.10

The organization plans and designs information management processes to meet internal and external information needs.

Rationale for IM.1.10

Organizations vary in size, complexity, governance, structure, decision-making processes, and resources. Information management systems and processes vary accordingly. Only by first identifying the information needs can one then evaluate the extent to which they are planned for and at what performance level the needs are being met. Planning for the management of information does not require a formal written information plan but does require evidence of a planned approach that identifies the organization's information needs and supports its goals and objectives.

Elements of Performance for IM.1.10

B 1. The organization bases its information management processes on an assessment of internal and external information needs:
- The assessment identifies the flow of information throughout an organization, including information storage and feedback mechanisms
- The assessment identifies the data and information needed: within and among departments, services, or programs; within and among the staff, the leadership, and the governance for supporting relationships with outside services and contractors; with licensing, accrediting, and regulatory bodies; with purchasers, payers, and employers; for supporting informational needs between the organization and the patients; and for participating in research and databases

B 2. To guide development of processes for managing information used internally and externally, the organization assesses its information management needs based on the following:
- Its mission
- Its goals
- Its services
- Staff
- Patient safety considerations
- Quality of care, treatment, and services
- Mode(s) of service delivery
- Resources

IM

- Access to affordable technology
- Identification of barriers to effective communication among caregivers

B 3. The organization bases its management, staffing, and material resource allocations for information management on the scope and complexity of care, treatment, and services provided.

B 4. Identified staff participates in assessment, selection, integration, and use of information management systems for clinical/service and organization information.

B 5. The organization has an ongoing process to assess the needs of the organization, departments, and individuals for knowledge-based information.

B 6. The organization uses the assessment for knowledge-based information as a basis for planning.

Confidentiality and Security

Standard IM.2.10

Information privacy and confidentiality are maintained.

Rationale for IM.2.10

Confidentiality of data and information applies across all systems and to automated, paper, and verbal communications, as well as to clinical/service, financial, and business records and employee-specific information. The capture, storage, and retrieval processes for data and information are performed on a timely* basis without compromising the data and information's confidentiality. Protecting privacy and confidentiality of information is the responsibility of the whole organization. In achieving this responsibility, the organization provides safeguards for patient privacy and information confidentiality. These safeguards are consistent with available technology and legitimate needs for accessibility of the information by authorized individuals for the delivery of care, treatment, and services; effective functioning of the organization; research; and education.

Elements of Performance for IM.2.10

A 1. The organization has a written policy(ies) for addressing the privacy† and confidentiality‡ of information that is based on and consistent with law or regulation.

* Defined by organization policy and based on the intended use of the information.

† **Privacy** An individual's right to limit the disclosure of personal information.

‡ **Confidentiality** The safekeeping of data/information so as to restrict access to individuals who have need, reason, and permission for such access.

B 2. The organization's policy, including changes to the policy, has been communicated to staff.

B 3. The organization implements the policy.

B 4. The organization monitors compliance with the policy.

B 5. The organization improves privacy and confidentiality of information by monitoring information and developments in technology.

C Ⓜ 6. Individuals for whom identifiable health data and information are maintained or collected are made aware of how the data will be used and whether it will be disclosed.

B 7. Personal identifiers are removed to the extent possible for uses and disclosures of health information, consistent with maintaining the usefulness of the information.

C Ⓜ 8. Protected health information* is used for the purposes identified or as required by law or regulation and not further disclosed without patient authorization.

B 9. The organization preserves the privacy and confidentiality of data and information identified as sensitive.

Standard IM.2.20

Information security, including data integrity, is maintained.

Rationale for IM.2.20

Policies and procedures address security procedures that allow only authorized staff to gain access to data and information. These policies range from access to the paper chart to the various security levels and distribution of passwords in an electronic system. The basic premise of the policies is to provide the security and protection for sensitive patient, staff, and other information, while facilitating access to data by those who have a legitimate need. The capture, storage, and retrieval processes for data and information are designed to provide for timely access without compromising the data and information's security and integrity.

Elements of Performance for IM.2.20

A 1. The organization has a written policy(ies) for addressing information security, including data integrity* that is based on and consistent with law or regulation.

B 2. The organization's policy, including changes to the policy, has been communicated to staff.

---

* **Protected health information** Health information that contains information such that an individual person can be identified as the subject of that information.

† **Integrity** In the context of data security, data integrity means the protection of data from accidental or unauthorized intentional change.

B 3. The organization implements the policy.

B 4. The organization monitors compliance with the policy.

B 5. The organization improves information security, including data integrity, by monitoring information and developments in technology.

B 6. The organization develops and implements controls to safeguard data and information, including the patient record, against loss, destruction, and tampering.

B 7. Controls to safeguard data and information include the following:
- Policies indicating when the removal of records is permitted
- Protection against unauthorized intrusion, corruption, or damage
- Minimization of the risk of falsification of data and information
- Guidelines for preventing the loss and destruction of records
- Guidelines for destroying copies of records
- Protection of records in a manner that minimizes the possibility of damage from fire and water

B 8. Policies and procedures, including plans for implementation, for electronic information systems address the following: data integrity, authentication,* nonrepudiation,† encryption‡ as warranted, and auditability§ as appropriate to the system and types of information, for example, patient information and billing information.

Standard IM.2.30

Continuity of information is maintained.

Rationale for IM.2.30

The purpose of the business continuity/disaster recovery plan is to identify the most critical information needs for patient care, treatment, and services and business processes, and the impact on the organization if these information systems were severely interrupted. The plan identifies alternative means for processing data, providing for recovery of data, and returning to normal operations as soon as possible.

Elements of Performance for IM.2.30

IM

B 1. The organization has a business continuity/disaster recovery plan for its information systems.

---

* **Authentication** The validation of correctness for both the information itself and the person who is the author or user of information.

† **Nonrepudiation** The inability to dispute a document's content or authorship.

‡ **Encryption** The process of transforming plain text (readable) into cipher text that is unreadable without a special software key.

§ **Auditability** The ability to do a methodical examination and verification of all information activities such as entering and accessing.

B 2. For electronic systems, the business continuity/disaster recovery plan includes the following:
- Plans for scheduled and unscheduled interruptions, which includes end-user training with the downtime procedures
- Contingency plans for operational interruptions (hardware, software, or other systems failure)
- Plans for minimal interruptions as a result of scheduled downtime
- An emergency service plan
- A back-up system (electronic or manual)
- Data retrieval, including retrieval from storage and information presently in the operating system, retrieval of data in the event of system interruption, and backup of data

B 3. The plan is tested periodically as defined by the organization (or in accordance with law or regulation) to ensure that the business interruption backup techniques are effective.

B 4. The business continuity/disaster recovery plan is implemented when information systems are interrupted.

Introduction to Managing Information for Clinical/Service and Organization Decision Making

An organization's ability to make decisions depends on having ready access to reliable and accurate information. To support the decision-making process, the organization captures, processes, stores, and retrieves the needed information. It then supplies the information to management and others involved in the decision-making process.

Standards IM.3.10 and IM.4.10 address the procedures involved in information management in support of clinical/service and organization decision making. These procedures are critical to patient care and safety and the organization's efficient management. The procedures also apply in paper-based, electronic, or a hybrid information management environment.

The standards are relevant to organizations transitioning from a paper-based environment to an electronic environment. The first standard addresses the tasks of collecting, processing, storing, retrieving, reporting, and disseminating data and information. The second standard addresses the use of the information.

Information Management Processes

Standard IM.3.10

The organization has processes in place to effectively manage information, including the capturing, reporting, processing, storing, retrieving, disseminating, and displaying of clinical/service and nonclinical data and information.

Rationale for IM.3.10

Records resulting from data capture and report generation* are used for communication and continuity of the patient's care or financial and business operations over time. Records are also used for other purposes, including litigation and risk management activities, reimbursement, and statistics. Improved data capture and report generation systems enhance the value of the records. Potential benefits include improved patient care, quality and safety, improved efficiency, effectiveness and reduced costs in patient care, and financial and business operations. To maximize the benefits of data capture and report generation, these processes exhibit the following characteristics: unique ID, accuracy, completeness, timeliness,† interoperability,‡ retrievability,§ authentication and accountability,‖ auditability, confidentiality, and security.

The processing, storing, and retrieving functions are integral to electronic, computerized, and paper-based information systems in organizations. Important considerations for these functions include data elements, data accuracy, data confidentiality, data security, data integrity, permanence of storage (the time a medium safely stores information), ease of retrievability, aggregation of information, interoperability, clinical/service practice considerations, performance improvement, and decision support processing.

A goal for information storage is to be linked or centrally organized and accessible. This could include the organization having an index identifying where the information is stored and how to access it; or, as the organization moves to electronic systems, the organization creates information systems to be interoperable within the enterprise. As more organizations automate various processes and activities, it is important to share critical data among systems. As challenges of interoperability have arisen, standards organizations for the information technology field have stepped in to develop industry standards. It is important that the organization is aware of the standards development organizations and their recommendations.

* **Report generation** The process of analyzing, organizing, and presenting recorded information for authentication and inclusion in the patient's health care record or in financial or business records.

† **Timeliness** The time between the occurrence of an event and the availability of data about the event. Timeliness is related to the use of the data.

‡ **Interoperability** Enables authorized users to capture, share, and report information from any system, whether paper- or electronic-based.

§ **Retrievability** The capability of efficiently finding relevant information.

‖ **Accountability** All information is attributable to its source (person or device).

Internally and externally generated data and information are accurately disseminated to users. Access to accurate information is required to deliver, improve, analyze, and advance patient care and the systems that support health care delivery. Information is accessed and disseminated through electronic information systems or paper-based records and reports. The use of information is considered in developing forms, screen displays, and standard or ad hoc reports.

Elements of Performance for IM.3.10

B 1. Information technology industry standards or organization policies are used and address the following:
- Uniform data definitions
- Data capture
- Data display
- Data transmission

2. Standardize a list of abbreviations, acronyms, symbols, and dose designations that are not to be used throughout the organization.

Note: *The preceding requirement is not scored here. It is scored at Goal 2, Requirement 2B.*

B 3. Minimum data sets, terminology, definitions, classifications, vocabulary, and nomenclature, including abbreviations, acronyms, symbols, and dose designations are standardized throughout the organization.

B 4. Quality control systems are used to monitor data content and collection activities:
- The method used provides for timely and economical data collection with the degree of accuracy, completeness, and discrimination necessary for their intended use
- The method used minimizes bias in the data and regularly assesses the data's reliability, validity, and accuracy
- Those responsible for collecting and reviewing the data are accountable for information accuracy and completeness

B 5. Storage and retrieval systems are designed to support organization needs for clinical/service and organization-specific information:
- Storage and retrieval systems are designed to balance the ability to retrieve data and information with the intended use for the data and information
- Storage and retrieval systems are designed to balance security and confidentiality issues with accessibility
- Systems for paper and electronic records are designed to reduce disruption or inaccessibility during such times as diminished staffing and scheduled and unscheduled downtimes of electronic information systems

A 6. Data and information are retained for sufficient time to comply with law or regulation.

B 7. Knowledgeable staff and tools are available for collecting, retrieving, and analyzing data and their transformation into information.

B 8. Data are organized and transformed into information in formats useful to decision makers.

B 9. Dissemination of data and information is timely* and accurate.

B 10. Data and information are disseminated in standard formats and methods to meet user needs and provide for retrievability and interpretation.

Information-Based Decision Making

Standard IM.4.10

The information management system provides information for use in decision making.

Rationale for IM.4.10

Information management supports timely and effective decision making at all organization levels. The information management processes support managerial and operational decisions; performance improvement activities; and patient care, treatment, and service decisions. Clinical and strategic decision making depends on information from multiple sources, including the patient record, knowledge-based information, comparative data/information, and aggregate data/information.

Elements of Performance for IM.4.10

B 1. The organization has the ability to collect and aggregate data and information to support care, treatment, and service delivery and operations, including the following:
- Individual care, treatment, and services and care, treatment, and service delivery
- Decision making
- Management and operations
- Analysis of trends
- Performance comparisons over time throughout the organization and with other organizations
- Performance improvement
- Infection control
- Patient safety

B 2. To support clinical decision making, information found in the patient record is
- Readily accessible
- Accurate

---

* Defined by organization policy and based on the intended use of the information.

- Complete
- Organized for retrieval of data
- Timely*

B 3. Comparative performance data and information are used for decision making, when available.

Knowledge-Based Information

Standard IM.5.10

Knowledge-based information resources are readily available, current, and authoritative.

Rationale for IM.5.10

Organization practitioners and staff have access to knowledge-based information† to do the following:

- Acquire and maintain the knowledge and skills needed to maintain and improve competence
- Assist with clinical/service and management decision making
- Provide appropriate information and education to patients and families
- Support performance improvement and patient safety activities
- Support the institution's educational and research needs

Elements of Performance for IM.5.10

1. Not applicable

B 2. The organization provides access to knowledge-based information resources‡ needed by staff in any of the following forms: print, electronic, Internet, or audio.

B 3. Knowledge-based information resources are available to clinical/service staff through electronic means, after-hours access to an in-house collection, or other methods.

B 4. The organization has a process for providing access to knowledge-based information resources when electronic systems are unavailable.

IM

* Defined by organization policy and based on the intended use of the information.

† **Knowledge-based information** A collection of stored facts, models, and information that can be used for designing and redesigning processes and for problem solving. In the context of this manual, knowledge-based information is found in the clinical, scientific, and management literature.

‡ Examples of knowledge-based information resources include current texts, periodicals, indexes, abstracts, reports, documents, databases, directories, discussion lists, successful practices, equipment and maintenance user manuals, standards, protocols, practice guidelines, clinical trials, and other resources.

Patient-Specific Information

Standard IM.6.10

The organization has a complete and accurate medical record for patients assessed, cared for, treated, or served.

Rationale for IM.6.10

Patient-specific data and information are contained in the medical record to facilitate patient care, treatment, and services; serve as a financial and legal record; aid in research; support decision analysis; and guide professional and organization performance improvement. This information is maintained as a paper record or as electronic health information.*

Elements of Performance for IM.6.10

A 1. Only authorized individuals make entries in the medical record.

A 2. The organization defines which entries made by nonindependent practitioners require countersigning consistent with law or regulation.

A 3. Standardized formats are used for documenting all care, treatment, and services provided to patients.

C Ⓜ 4. Medical record entries† are dated, the author identified and, when necessary according to law or regulation or organization policy, authenticated, either by written signature, electronic signature, or computer key or rubber stamp.‡

C Ⓜ 5. The author authenticates either by written signature, electronic signature, or computer key or rubber stamp the following:
- The history and physical examination
- Operative reports
- Consultations
- Diagnostic and therapeutic procedures
- Follow-up or discharge orders

C Ⓜ 6. The medical record contains sufficient information to identify the patient; support the diagnosis/condition; justify the care, treatment, and

* **Electronic health information** A computerized format of the health care information in paper records that is used for the same range of purposes as paper records, namely to familiarize readers with the patient's status; document care, treatment, and services; plan for discharge; document the need for care, treatment, and services; assess the quality of care, treatment, and services; determine reimbursement rates; justify reimbursement claims; pursue clinical or epidemiological research; and measure outcomes of the care, treatment, and service process.

† For paper-based records, countersignatures entered for purposes of authentication after transcription or for verbal orders are dated when required by law or regulations or organization policy. For electronic records, electronic signatures will be date-stamped.

‡ Authentication is shown by written signatures or initials, rubber-stamp signatures, or computer key. Authorized users of signature stamps or computer keys sign a statement assuring that they alone will use the stamp or key.

services; document the course and results of care, treatment, and services; and promote continuity of care among providers.

7. Not applicable

B 8. The organization has a policy on the timely entry of information into the patient's medical record.

A 9. The organization defines a complete record and the time frame within which the record is completed.

10. Not applicable

11. Not applicable

B 12. Medical records are reviewed on an ongoing basis.

B 13. The review of medical records is based on organization-defined indicators that address the presence, timeliness, readability (whether handwritten or printed), quality, consistency, clarity, accuracy, completeness, and authentication of data and information contained within the record.

B 14. The retention time of medical record information is determined by the organization based on law or regulation and on its use for patient care, treatment, and services; legal, research, and operational purposes; and educational activities.

15. Not applicable

16. Not applicable

A 17. Original medical records are not released unless the organization is responding appropriately to laws or regulations, court orders, or subpoenas.

C Ⓜ 18. Medical records of patients who have received urgent or immediate care, treatment, and services contain the following information:
- Times and means of arrival
- Whether the patient left against medical advice
- The conclusions at termination of treatment, including final disposition, condition, and instructions for follow-up care, treatment, and services
- A copy of the record that is available to the practitioner or medical organization providing follow-up care, treatment, and services

Standard IM.6.20

Records contain patient-specific information, as appropriate to the care, treatment, and services provided.

Elements of Performance for IM.6.20

C Ⓜ 1. Medical records contain, as applicable, the following clinical/case information:
- Documentation and findings of assessments*
- Conclusions or impressions drawn from medical history and physical examination
- Diagnosis, diagnostic impression, or conditions
- Diagnostic and therapeutic orders
- Diagnostic and therapeutic procedures, tests, and results
- Operative and other invasive procedures
- Progress notes made by authorized individuals, including the date; staff person; and care, treatment, and service provided
- Reassessments and plan of care revisions
- Consultation reports
- Allergies to foods and medicines
- Medications ordered or prescribed
- Dosages of medications administered (including the strength, dose, or rate of administration; administration devices used; access site or route; known drug allergies; patient's response to medication; and adverse drug reactions)
- Relevant diagnoses/conditions established during the course of care, treatment, and services

C Ⓜ 2. Medical records contain, as applicable, the following demographic information:
- Patient's name, gender, address, phone number, date of birth, height, and weight and the name and phone number of any legally authorized representative
- Legal status of patients receiving behavioral health care services
- The patient's language and communication needs

C Ⓜ 3. Medical records contain, as applicable, the following information:
- Evidence of known advance directives when indicated
- Evidence of informed consent when required by organization policy
- Referrals or communications made to external or internal care providers and community agencies
- Treatment summaries and other pertinent documents to promote continuity of care
- Documentation of clinical research interventions that is distinct from entries related to regular patient care
- Records of communication with the patient regarding care, treatment, and services (for example, telephone calls or e-mail)
- Patient-generated information (for example, information entered into the record over the Web or in previsit computer systems)

C Ⓜ 4. When appropriate, summaries of treatment and other documents provided by the organization are forwarded to other care providers.

---

* *See* the "Provision of Care, Treatment, and Services" chapter in this book.

For Medicare-Certified Ambulatory Surgical Centers

A Ⓜ 5. Medical records must contain the discharge diagnosis.

Standard IM.6.30

The medical record thoroughly documents operative or other high-risk procedures and the use of moderate or deep sedation or anesthesia. (*See also* standards PC.13.30 and PC.13.40.)

Elements of Performance for IM.6.30

C Ⓜ 1. The licensed independent practitioner (responsible for the patient) records the provisional diagnosis before the operative or other high-risk procedures.*

C Ⓜ 2. Operative or other high-risk procedure reports dictated or written immediately† after an operative or other high-risk procedure record the name of the licensed independent practitioner and assistants; procedure(s) performed and description of the procedure; findings; estimated blood loss; specimens removed; and postoperative diagnosis.

Note: *The exception to the requirement is when an operative or other high-risk procedure progress note is written immediately after the procedure* (see *EP 3*)*, in which case the full operative or other high-risk procedure report can be written or dictated within a time frame defined by the organization.*

C Ⓜ 3. An operative or other high-risk procedure progress note is entered in the medical record immediately after the procedure, if the full operative or other high-risk procedure report cannot be entered into the record immediately after the operation or procedure.

C Ⓜ 4. The completed operative or other high-risk procedure report is authenticated by the licensed independent practitioner and made available in the medical record as soon as possible after the procedure.

C Ⓜ 5. Postoperative documentation records the patient's vital signs and level of consciousness; medications (including intravenous fluids) and blood and blood components administered; unusual events or complications, including blood transfusion reactions; and the management of those events.

---

* **Operative and other high-risk procedures** Procedures including operative, other invasive, and noninvasive procedures that place the patient at risk. The focus is on procedures and therefore is not meant to include use of medications that place patients at risk.

† **Immediately after a procedure** Defined as "upon completion of the operation or procedure, before the patient is transferred to the next level of care." This is to ensure that pertinent information is available to the next caregiver. In addition, if the surgeon accompanies the patient from the operating room to the next unit or area of care, the operative note or progress note can be written in that unit or area of care.

C Ⓜ 6. Postoperative documentation records the patient's discharge from the postsedation or postanesthesia care area by the responsible licensed independent practitioner or according to discharge criteria.

C Ⓜ 7. The use of approved discharge criteria to determine the patient's readiness for discharge is documented in the medical record.

C Ⓜ 8. Postoperative documentation records the name of the licensed independent practitioner responsible for discharge.

For Medicare-Certified Ambulatory Surgical Centers

C Ⓜ 9. Medical records must contain the results of preoperative diagnostic studies before surgery, if performed.

Standard IM.6.40

For patients receiving continuing ambulatory care services, the medical record contains a summary list(s) of significant diagnoses, procedures, drug allergies, and medications.

Rationale for IM.6.40

Summary lists facilitate continuity of care over time for a single provider or among several providers. To support quality and safe patient care, it is important that this information be easily and quickly available to staff. As a large variety and variation of record keeping currently exist, any system that achieves this goal, either paper-based or electronic, is acceptable.

Elements of Performance for IM.6.40

C Ⓜ 1. The summary list(s) is initiated for the patient by the third visit and maintained thereafter.

C Ⓜ 2. The summary list(s) contains the following information:
- Known* significant medical diagnoses and conditions
- Known significant operative and invasive procedures
- Known adverse and allergic drug reactions
- Known long-term medications, including current medications, over-the-counter drugs, and herbal preparations

C Ⓜ 3. The summary list(s) is quickly and easily available for practitioners to access needed information.

IM

Standard IM.6.50

Designated qualified staff accept and transcribe verbal or telephone orders from authorized individuals.

* "Known" refers to information gathered during ambulatory care assessment and treatment.

Rationale for IM.6.50

Processes for receiving, transcribing, and authenticating verbal or telephone orders are established to protect the quality of patient care, treatment, and services.

Elements of Performance for IM.6.50

A 1. Qualified personnel are identified, as defined by organization policy and in accordance with law or regulation, and authorized to receive and record verbal or telephone orders.

C Ⓜ 2. Verbal or telephone orders are dated and identify the names of the individuals who gave, received, and implemented the order.

A 3. When required by law or regulation, verbal or telephone orders are authenticated within the specified time frame.

4. For verbal or telephone orders or for telephonic reporting of critical test results, verify the complete order or test result by having the person receiving the information record and "read back" the complete order or test result.

Note: *The preceding requirement is not scored here. It is scored at Goal 2, Requirement 2A.*

Standard IM.6.60

The organization provides access to relevant information from a patient's record as needed for use in patient care, treatment, and services.

Rationale for IM.6.60

To facilitate continuity of care, providers have access to information about all previous care, treatment, and services provided to a patient by the organization.

Elements of Performance for IM.6.60

B 1. The organization has a process to track the location of all components of the medical record.

B 2. The organization uses a system to assemble required information or make available a summary of information relative to the patient care, treatment, and services provided.

Standards IM.6.70 Through IM.6.280

Not applicable

Glossary

abuse Intentional maltreatment of an individual which may cause injury, either physical or psychological. *See also* neglect.

mental abuse Includes humiliation, harassment, and threats of punishment or deprivation.

physical abuse Includes hitting, slapping, pinching, or kicking. Also includes controlling behavior through corporal punishment.

sexual abuse Includes sexual harassment, sexual coercion, and sexual assault.

accountability *See* information management.

accreditation Determination by the Joint Commission's accrediting body that an eligible health care organization complies with applicable Joint Commission standards. *See also* accreditation decisions.

accreditation cycle A period of accreditation at the conclusion of which, accreditation expires unless a full survey is performed.

accreditation decisions Categories of accreditation that an organization can achieve based on a Joint Commission survey. These decision categories are:

- **Accredited** The organization is in compliance with all standards at the time of the on-site survey or has successfully addressed all requirements for improvement (*see* definition), via submission of an Evidence of Standards Compliance (ESC) report (*see* definition), within 45 days following the posting of the Accreditation Survey Findings Report.
- **Provisional Accreditation** The organization fails to successfully address all requirements for improvement in an ESC report within 45 days following the posting of the Accreditation Survey Findings Report.
- **Conditional Accreditation** The organization is not in substantial compliance with the standards, as usually evidenced by a count of the number of not compliant standards at the time of survey which is between 1½ and 3 standard deviations above the mean number of not compliant standards for organizations in that accreditation program. The organization must remedy identified problem areas through preparation and submission of an ESC report and subsequently undergo an on-site, follow-up survey.
- **Preliminary Denial of Accreditation** There is justification to deny accreditation to the organization, as usually evidenced by a count of the number of not compliant standards at the time of survey which is 3 or more standard deviations above the mean number of standards identified as not compliant for organizations in that accreditation program. The decision is subject to review and appeal prior to the determination to deny accreditation; the appeal process may also result in a decision other than Denial of Accreditation.
- **Denial of Accreditation** The organization has been denied accreditation. All review and appeal opportunities have been exhausted.
- **Preliminary Accreditation** The organization demonstrates compliance with selected standards in the first of two surveys conducted under the Early Survey Policy Option 1 (*see* definition).

accreditation process A continuous process whereby health care organizations are required to demonstrate to the Joint Commission that they are providing safe, high-quality care, as determined by compliance with Joint Commission standards, National Patient Safety Goals recommendations, and performance measurement requirements. Key components of this process are an on-site evaluation of an organization by Joint Commission surveyors, a Periodic Performance Review, and quarterly submission of performance measurement data to the Joint Commission, as applicable.

accreditation survey findings Findings from an on-site evaluation conducted by Joint Commission's surveyors that results in an organization's accreditation decision.

Accreditation Survey Findings Report A report of an organization's survey findings; the report includes Requirements for Improvement (*see* definition) and supplemental findings (*see* definition), as appropriate.

administration 1. The fiscal and general management of an organization, as distinct from the direct provision of services. 2. *See* medication management/administration.

admitting Acceptance of a patient to the healthcare setting or service.

admitting privileges Authority issued to admit individuals to a health care organization. Individuals with admitting privileges may practice only within the scope of the clinical privileges granted by the organization's governing body.

advance directive A document or documentation allowing a person to give directions about future medical care or to designate another person(s) to make medical decisions if the individual loses decision-making capacity. Advance directives may include living wills, durable powers of attorney, do-not-resuscitate orders (DNRs), right to die, or similar documents listed in the Patient Self-Determination Act which express the patient's preferences.

advanced practice registered nurse A registered nurse who has gained additional knowledge and skills through successful completion of an organized program of nursing education that prepares nurses for advanced practice roles and who has been certified by the board of nursing to engage in the practice of advanced practice nursing.

When standards reference the term "licensed independent practitioner," this language is not to be construed to limit the authority of a licensed independent practitioner to delegate tasks to other qualified health care personnel (for example, physician assistants and advanced practice registered nurses) to the extent authorized by state law or a state's regulatory mechanism or federal guidelines and organizational policy.

adverse drug event A patient injury resulting from a medication, either because of a pharmacological reaction to a normal dose, or because of a preventable adverse reaction to a drug resulting from an error.

adverse drug reaction (ADR) Unintended, undesirable, or unexpected effects of prescribed medications or of medication errors that require discontinuing a medication or modifying the dose; require initial or prolonged hospitalization; result in disability; require treatment with a prescription medication; result in cognitive deterioration or impairment; are life threatening; result in death; or result in congenital anomalies.

ambulatory health care All types of health services provided to individuals on an outpatient basis. Ambulatory care services are provided in many settings ranging from freestanding ambulatory surgical facilities, to primary care settings, to diagnostic radiology.

ambulatory health care occupancy *See* occupancy.

analyzing *See* information management.

anesthesia and sedation The administration to an individual, in any setting, for any purpose, by any route, medication to induce a partial or total loss of sensation for the purpose of conducting an operative or other procedure. Definitions of four levels of sedation and anesthesia include the following:

minimal sedation (anxiolysis) A drug-induced state during which patients respond normally to verbal commands. Although cognitive function and coordination may be impaired, ventilatory and cardiovascular functions are unaffected.

moderate sedation/analgesia ("conscious sedation") A drug-induced depression of consciousness during which patients respond purposefully to verbal commands, either alone or accompanied by light tactile stimulation. Reflex withdrawal from a painful stimulus is *not* considered a purposeful response. No interventions are required to maintain a patent airway, and spontaneous ventilation is adequate. Cardiovascular function is usually maintained.

deep sedation/analgesia A drug-induced depression of consciousness during which patients cannot be easily aroused, but respond purposefully following repeated or painful stimulation. The ability to independently maintain ventilatory function may be impaired. Patients may require assistance in maintaining a patent airway and spontaneous ventilation may be inadequate. Cardiovascular function is usually maintained.

anesthesia Consists of general anesthesia and spinal or major regional anesthesia. It does *not* include local anesthesia. General anesthesia is a drug-induced loss of consciousness during which patients are not arousable, even by painful stimulation. The ability to independently maintain ventilatory function is often impaired. Patients often require assistance in maintaining a patent airway, and positive pressure ventilation may be required because of depressed spontaneous ventilation or drug-induced depression of neuromuscular function. Cardiovascular function may be impaired.

anesthetic gases Any gas delivered through the respiratory system as a component of general anesthesia or sedation. This may include inhalation anesthetics distributed in liquid form that when vaporized produce an anesthetic gas (for example, isoflurane, sevoflurane) or nonliquid compressed gases (for example, nitrous oxide). Oxygen is not included in this definition.

anesthetizing location Any area used for the administration of anesthetic agents.

appeal process The process afforded to an organization that receives a Preliminary Denial of Accreditation (*see* accreditation decisions), which includes the organization having a right to make a presentation to a Review Hearing Panel (*see* definition) before the Accreditation Committee takes final action to deny accreditation.

assessment **1.** For purposes of patient assessment, the process established by an organization for obtaining appropriate and necessary information about each individual seeking entry into a health care setting or service. The information is used to match an individual's need with the appropriate setting, care level, and intervention. **2.** For purposes of performance improvement, the systematic collection and review of patient-specific data.

auditability *See* information management.

authenticate To verify that an entry is complete, accurate, and final.

authentication *See* information management.

behavioral health A broad array of mental health, chemical dependency, habilitation, and rehabilitation services provided in settings such as inpatient, residential, and outpatient.

best practices Clinical, scientific, or professional practices that are recognized by a majority of professionals in a particular field. These practices are typically evidence based and consensus driven.

biologicals Medicines made from living organisms and their products, including serums, vaccines, antigens, and antitoxins.

blood component A fraction of separated whole blood, for example, red blood cell, plasma, platelets, and granulocytes.

blood derivative A pooled blood product, such as albumin, gamma globulin, or Rh immune globulin whose use is considered significantly lower in risk than that of blood or blood components.

blood transfusion services Services relating to transfusing and infusing individuals with blood, blood components, or blood derivatives.

blood usage measurement An activity that entails measuring, assessing, and improving the ordering, distributing, handling, dispensing, administering, and monitoring of blood and blood components.

business occupancy *See* occupancy.

bylaws A governance framework that establishes the roles and responsibilities of a body and its members.

capture *See* information management.

care planning (or planning of care) Individualized planning and provision of services that address the needs, safety, and well-being of the patient. The plan, which formulates strategies, goals, and objectives, may include narratives, policies and procedures, protocols, practice guidelines, clinical paths, care maps, or a combination of these.

chemical dependency services Services of a health care organization that are designed to address environmental, interpersonal, and intrapersonal factors for individuals with alcohol and/or drug dependencies in either a designated program or track (that is, the organization is advertising and/or presenting to the public, has policies and procedures in place, and has trained staff to address the individual needs).

chemical restraint *See* restraint.

CLIA '88 The Clinical Laboratory Improvement Amendments of 1988.

clinical laboratory A facility that is equipped to examine material derived from the human body to provide information for use in the diagnosis, prevention, or treatment of disease; also called medical laboratory.

clinical privileges Authorization granted by the appropriate authority (for example, the governing body) to a practitioner to provide specific care, treatment, or services in an organization within well-defined limits, based on the following factors, as applicable: license, education, training, experience, competence, health status, and judgment.

clinical practice guidelines *See* practice guidelines.

clinical/service groups Groups of patients in distinct, clinical populations for which data are collected. Tracer patients are selected according to clinical service groups.

community The individuals, families, groups, agencies, facilities, or institutions within the geographic area served by a health care organization.

competence or competency A determination of an individual's skills, knowledge, and capability to meet defined expectations.

complex organization An organization that provides or provides for more than one level of care (for example, acute, subacute, chronic) and type (for example, pediatric, dental, behavioral health) of health care service, usually in more than one type of setting (for example, hospital, behavioral, home). An example is an organization that provides acute care, long term care, and home care services.

complex organization survey A Joint Commission survey in which standards from more than one accreditation manual are used in assessing compliance. This type of survey may include using specialist surveyors appropriate to the standards selected for survey.

compliance with a standard (see definition) Meeting the requirements of a standard through compliance with its element(s) of performance.

component A health care delivery entity (for example, service, program, related entity) that meets survey eligibility criteria under one of the Joint Commission accreditation programs. Multiple components comprise a complex organization.

confidentiality An individual's right, within the law, to personal and informational privacy, including his or her health care records. *See also* information management.

GL

consultation **1.** Provision of professional advice or services. **2.** For purposes of Joint Commission accreditation, advice that is given to staff members of surveyed organizations relating to compliance with standards that are the subject of the survey.

consultation report **1.** A written opinion by a consultant that reflects, when appropriate, an examination of the individual and the individual's medical record(s). **2.** Information given verbally by a consultant to a care provider that reflects, when appropriate, an examination of the individual. The individual's care provider usually documents those opinions in the clinical/case record.

continuing care Care provided over time; in various settings, programs, or services; spanning the illness-to-wellness continuum.

continuing education Education beyond initial professional preparation that is relevant to the type of care delivered in an organization, that provides current knowledge relevant to an individual's field of practice or service responsibilities, and that may be related to findings from performance-improvement activities.

continuity The degree to which the care of individuals is coordinated among practitioners, among organizations, and over time.

continuum of care Matching the individual's ongoing needs with the appropriate level and type of care, treatment, or service within an organization or across multiple organizations.

contract A formal agreement for care, treatment, or services with any organization, agency, or individual that specifies the services, personnel, products, or space provided by, to, or on behalf of the organization and specifies the consideration to be expended in exchange. The agreement is approved by the governing body or comparable entity.

contracted services Services provided through a written agreement with another organization, agency, or individual. The agreement specifies the services or personnel to be provided on behalf of the applicant organization and the fees to provide these services or personnel.

control chart A graphic display of data in the order they occur with statistically determined upper and lower limits of expected common-cause variation. A control chart is used to identify special causes of variation, to monitor a process for maintenance, and to determine if process changes have had the desired effect.

control limit In statistics, an expected limit of common-cause variation, sometimes referred to as either an upper or a lower limit. Variation beyond a control limit is evidence that special causes are affecting a process. Control limits are calculated from process data and are not to be confused with engineering specifications or tolerance limits. Control limits are typically plotted on a control chart.

coordination of care The process of coordinating care, treatment, or services provided by a health care organization, including referral to appropriate community resources and liaison with others (such as the individual's physician, other health care organizations, or community services involved in care or services) to meet the ongoing identified needs of individuals, to ensure implementation of the plan of care, and to avoid unnecessary duplication of services.

credentialing The process of obtaining, verifying, and assessing the qualifications of a health care practitioner to provide patient care services in or for a health care organization.

credentials Documented evidence of licensure, education, training, experience, or other qualifications.

Credentials Verification Organization (CVO) Any ambulatory care organization that bases its decision in part on information obtained from a CVO should have confidence in the completeness, accuracy, and timeliness of information. To achieve this level of confidence, the organization should evaluate the agency providing the information initially and then periodically as appropriate. The principles that guide such an evaluation include the following:

- The agency makes known to the user the data and information it can provide.
- The agency provides documentation to the user describing how its data collection, information development, and verification process(es) are performed.
- The user is given sufficient, clear information on database functions, including any limitations of information available from the agency (practitioners not included in the database), the time frame for agency responses to requests for information, and a summary overview of quality control processes related to data integrity, security, transmission accuracy, and technical specifications.
- The user and agency agree on the format for transmitting credentials information about an individual from the CVO.
- The user can easily discern what information transmitted by the CVO is from a primary source and what is not.
- For information transmitted by the agency that can go out of date (licensure, board certification), the CVO provides the date the information was last updated from the primary source.
- The CVO certifies that the information transmitted to the user accurately represents the information obtained by it.
- The user can discern whether the information transmitted by the CVO from a primary source is all the primary source information in the CVO's possession pertinent to a given item or, if not, where additional information can be obtained.
- The user can engage the CVO's quality control processes when necessary to resolve concerns about transmission errors, inconsistencies, or other data issues that may be identified from time to time.
- The user has a formal arrangement with the CVO for communicating changes in credentialing information.

criteria **1.** Expected level(s) of achievement, or specifications against which performance or quality may be compared. **2.** For purposes of eligibility for a Joint Commission survey, the conditions necessary for health care organizations and networks to be surveyed for accreditation by the Joint Commission.

data *See* information management.

decentralized laboratory testing *See* point-of-care testing.

decentralized pharmaceutical services *See* pharmaceutical care and services.

deemed status Status conferred by the Centers for Medicare & Medicaid Services (CMS) on a health care organization accredited by an organization whose standards and survey process are determined by CMS to be equivalent to those of the Medicare program or other federal laws, such as the Clinical Laboratory Improvement Amendments of 1988 (CLIA '88). Accreditation is voluntary and seeking deemed status through accreditation is an option, not a requirement.

delineation of clinical privileges The listing of the specific clinical privileges an organization's staff member is permitted to perform in the organization.

dental services Services provided by a dentist, or a qualified individual under the supervision of a dentist, to improve or maintain the health of an individual's teeth, oral cavity, and associated structures.

dentist An individual who has received the degree of either doctor of dental surgery or doctor of dental medicine and who is licensed to practice dentistry.

designated equivalent sources Selected agencies that have been determined to maintain a specific item(s) of credential(s) information that is identical to the information at the primary source. Designated equivalent sources include but are not limited to the following:

- The American Medical Association (AMA) Physician Masterfile for verification of a physician's United States and Puerto Rican medical school graduation and residency completion
- The American Board of Medical Specialities (ABMS) for verification of a physician's board certification
- The Educational Commission for Foreign Medical Graduates (ECFMG) for verification of a physician's graduation from a foreign medical school
- The American Osteopathic Association (AOA) Physician Database for pre-doctoral education accredited by the AOA Bureau of Professional Education; postdoctoral education approved by the AOA Council on Postdoctoral Training; and Osteopathic Specialty Board Certification
- The Federation of State Medical Boards (FSMB) for all actions against a physician's medical license
- The American Academy of Physician Assistants (AAPA) Profile for physician assistant education and National Certification Commission (NCCPA) certification

dietetic services The delivery of care pertaining to the provision of nutrition and food service to individuals.

disaster *See* emergency.

discharge The point at which an individual's active involvement with an organization or program is terminated and the organization or program no longer maintains active responsibility for the care of the individual.

GL

discharge planning A formalized process in a health care organization through which the need for a program of continuing and follow-up care is ascertained and, if warranted, initiated for each patient.

disinfection The use of a chemical procedure that eliminates virtually all recognized pathogenic microorganisms but not necessarily all microbial forms (for example, bacterial endospores) on inanimate objects.

dispensing *See* medication management; pharmacy services.

drug *See* medication.

drug administration *See* medication management.

drug allergies A state of hypersensitivity induced by exposure to a particular drug antigen resulting in harmful immunologic reactions on subsequent drug exposures, such as a penicillin drug allergy. *See* medication.

drug dispensing *See* medication management.

e-App The electronic version of an organization's application for accreditation.

Early Survey Policy A policy that provides two options to organizations undergoing their initial Joint Commission survey. Under both options, the organization undergoes two surveys. Under option 1, the first survey is limited and successful completion results in Preliminary Accreditation (*see* accreditation decisions). Under option 2, the first survey is a full survey, and successful completion can lead to the organization being Accredited (*see* accreditation decisions). The second survey in both options is a full survey.

effectiveness The degree to which care is provided in the correct manner, given the current state of knowledge, to achieve the desired or projected outcome(s) for the individual.

efficacy The degree to which the care of the individual has been shown to accomplish the desired or projected outcome(s).

efficiency The relationship between the outcomes (results of care) and the resources used to deliver care.

electronic health information *See* information management.

elements of performance (EPs) The specific performance expectations and/or structures or processes that must be in place in order for an organization to provide safe, high-quality care, treatment, and services.

emergency **1.** An unexpected or sudden occasion, as in emergency surgery needed to prevent death or serious disability. **2.** A natural or man-made event that significantly disrupts the environment of care (for example, damage to the organization's building(s) and grounds due to severe winds, storms, or earthquakes); that significantly disrupts care and treatment (for example, loss of utilities such as power, water, or telephones due to floods, civil disturbances, accidents, or emergencies in the organization or its community); or that results in sudden, significantly changed or increased demands for the organization's services (for example, bioterrorist attack, building collapse, or plane crash in the organization's community). Some emergencies are called "disasters" or "potential injury creating events" (PICEs).

emergency, life-threatening A situation (for example, major trauma, neck injury) in which an individual may require resuscitation or other support to sustain life.

emergency management plan The organization's written document describing the process it would implement for managing the consequences of natural disasters or other emergencies that could disrupt the organization's ability to provide care, treatment, and services. The plan identifies specific procedures that describe mitigation, preparedness, response, and recovery strategies, actions, and responsibilities. *See also* emergency, mitigation activities, preparedness activities.

encryption *See* information management.

endemic infection *See* infection, endemic.

entry The process by which an individual comes into a setting, including screening and/or assessment by the organization or the practitioner in order to determine the capacity of the organization or practitioner to provide the care, treatment, or services required to meet the individual's needs.

environmental tours Activities routinely used by the organization to determine the presence of unsafe conditions and whether the organization's current processes for managing environmental safety risks are practiced correctly and are effective.

epidemic infection *See* infection, epidemic.

epidemiologically significant infection *See* infection, epidemiologically significant.

equipment management Activities selected and implemented by the organization to assess and control the clinical and physical risks of fixed and portable equipment used for diagnosis, treatment, monitoring, and care.

evidenced-based Based on empirical evidence or in the absence of empirical evidence, expert consensus (such as consensus statements promoted by professional societies).

evidence-based guidelines Guidelines that have been scientifically developed based on current literature and are consensus driven. These are also referred to as National Guidelines or Professional Guidelines.

Evidence of Standards Compliance (ESC) report A report submitted by a surveyed organization within 45 days of its survey, which details the action(s) that it took to bring itself into compliance with a standard or clarifies why the organization believes that it was in compliance with the standard for which it received a requirement for improvement. An ESC must address compliance at the element of performance (EP) level and include a measure of success (MOS) (*see* definition) for all appropriate EP corrections.

failure modes and effect analysis *See* risk assessment, proactive.

family The person(s) who plays a significant role in an individual's life. This may include a person(s) not legally related to the individual. This person(s) is often referred to as a surrogate decision maker if authorized to make care decisions for the individual should he or she lose decision-making capacity. *See also* guardian; surrogate decision maker.

fire-safety management Activities selected and implemented by the organization to assess and control the risks of fire, smoke, and other byproducts of combustion that could occur during the organization's provision of care, treatment, or services.

free text *See* information management.

governance The individual(s), group, or agency that has ultimate authority and responsibility for establishing policy, maintaining quality of care, and providing for organization management and planning. The governance may be a separate entity or it may fall within the medical advisory or executive committee. Other names for this group include the board, board of trustees, board of governors, board of commissioners, and partnership.

guardian A parent, trustee, conservator, committee, or other individual or agency empowered by law to act on behalf of or be responsible for an individual. *See also* family; surrogate decision maker.

hazard vulnerability analysis The identification of potential emergencies and the direct and indirect effects these emergencies may have on the health care organization's operations and the demand for its services.

hazardous condition Any set of circumstances (exclusive of the disease, disorder, or condition for which the patient is undergoing care, treatment, or services) defined by the organization that significantly increases the likelihood of a serious adverse outcome.

hazardous materials and waste Materials whose handling, use, and storage are guided or defined by local, state, or federal regulation (for example, the Occupational Safety and Health Administration's Regulations for Bloodborne Pathogens regarding the disposal of blood and blood-soaked items; the Nuclear Regulatory Commission's regulations for the handling and disposal of radioactive waste), hazardous vapors (for example, gluteraldehyde, ethylene oxide, nitrous oxide), and hazardous energy sources (for example, ionizing or nonionizing radiation, lasers, microwave, ultrasound). Although the Joint Commission considers infectious waste as falling into this category of materials, federal regulations do not define infectious or medical waste as hazardous waste.

hazardous materials and waste management Activities selected and implemented by the organization to assess and control occupational and environmental hazards of materials and waste that require special handling. *See* hazardous materials and waste.

health care occupancy *See* occupancy.

human subject research The use of individuals in the systematic study, observation, or evaluation of factors on preventing, assessing, treating, and understanding an illness. The term applies to all behavioral and medical experimental research that involves human beings as experimental subjects.

infection The transmission of a pathogenic microorganism to a host, with subsequent invasion and multiplication, with or without resulting symptoms of disease.

GL

endemic infection The usual level or presence of an agent or disease in a defined population during a defined period.

epidemic infection A higher than expected level of infection by a common agent in a defined population during a defined period.

health care–associated infection An infection acquired while receiving care, treatment, or services in the health care organization.

infection control program Organized system of services designed to meet the needs of the organization or individual in relation to the surveillance, prevention, and control of infection.

information management Terms applicable to information management functions:

- **accountability** All information is attributable to its source (person or device).
- **analyzing** The process that interprets data and transforms it into information.
- **auditability** The ability to do a methodical examination and verification of all information activities such as entering and accessing.
- **authentication** The validation of correctness for both the information itself and the person who is the author or user of information.
- **capture** The process of recording representations of human thought, perceptions, or actions, as well as device-generated data or information that is gathered and/or computed about a patient as part of a health care encounter or about other matters in a health care organization.
- **confidentiality** The safekeeping of data/information so as to restrict access to individuals who have need, reason, and permission for such access.
- **data** Uninterpreted observations or facts.
- **electronic health information** A computerized format of the health care information in paper records that is used for the same range of purposes as paper records, namely to familiarize readers with the patient's status; to document care, treatment, and services; to plan for discharge; to document the need for care, treatment, and services; to assess the quality of care, treatment, and services; to determine reimbursement rates; to justify reimbursement claims; to pursue clinical or epidemiological research; and to measure outcomes of the care, treatment, and service process.
- **encryption** The process of transforming plain text (readable) into cipher text that is unreadable without a special software key.

- **free text** Free-flowing, nonstructured type of speaking, writing, or inputting information.
- **integrity** In the context of data security, *data integrity* means the protection of data from accidental or unauthorized intentional change.
- **interactive text** A more complex version of structured text, as it interactively prompts and provides feedback to the person using it. Typically, it uses a higher level of computer intelligence that interacts with the person who records information.
- **interoperability** Enables authorized users to capture, share, and report information from any system, whether paper based or electronic based.
- **knowledge-based information** A collection of stored facts, models, and information that can be used for designing and redesigning processes and for problem solving. In the context of the manual, knowledge-based information is found in the clinical, scientific, and management literature.
- **nonrepudiation** The inability to dispute a document's content or authorship.
- **privacy** An individual's right to limit the disclosure of personal information.
- **processing** The manipulation of data and information by editing and updating.
- **protected health information** Health information that contains information such that an individual person can be identified as the subject of that information.
- **report generation** The process of analyzing, organizing, and presenting recorded information for authentication and inclusion in the patient's health care record or in financial or business records.
- **retrievability** The capability of efficiently finding relevant information.
- **security** The protection of data from intentional or unintentional destruction, modification, or disclosure.
- **structured text** Process that requires authors to put specific information into specific fields with passive guidance by the information system. In paper-based systems, a form encourages a practitioner to fill in fields or boxes. Electronic systems use the same principle for templates or macros, which are guides used to create standardized information documentation. The purpose is to produce data of more consistent quality, make information more usable for decision support, make information complete and more easily retrievable, and save documentation time.
- **timeliness** The time between the occurrence of an event and the availability of data about the event. Timeliness is related to the use of the data.
- **transmission** The sending of data and information from one location to another.

informed consent Agreement or permission accompanied by full notice about what is being consented to. A patient must be apprised of the nature, risks, and alternatives of a medical procedure or treatment before the physician or other health care professional begins any such course. After receiving this information, the patient then either consents to or refuses such a procedure or treatment.

initial survey An accreditation survey of a health care organization not previously accredited by the Joint Commission, or an accreditation survey of an organization performed without reference to any prior survey findings.

integrity *See* information management.

interactive text *See* information management.

interim life safety measures (ILSM) A series of 11 administrative actions intended to temporarily compensate for significant hazards posed by existing National Fire Protection Association 101® 2000 *Life Safety Code®* (*LSC*) deficiencies or construction activities. *See also* *Life Safety Code®*; fire safety management.

interoperability *See* information management.

interpretation services Interpretation services provide for the communication needs of patients who have limited English proficiency or are deaf/hard of hearing. An interpreter is a person who renders a message spoken or signed in one language into one or more languages. Unlike translation, which works only with written text, interpretation works only with spoken/signed language.

intravenous (IV) admixture The preparation of pharmaceutical product that requires the measured addition of a medication to a 50 ml or greater bag or bottle of IV fluid (for example, IV, IM, IT, SC). It does not include the draw-ing-up of medications into a syringe for immediate use (that is, reconstitution), or the assembly and activation of an IV system that does not involve the measurement of the additive.

invasive procedure A procedure involving puncture or incision of the skin, or insertion of an instrument or foreign material into the body.

investigational medication A medication or placebo used as part of a research protocol or clinical trial.

Joint Commission on Accreditation of Healthcare Organizations (Joint Commission) An independent, not-for-profit organization dedicated to improving the quality of care in organized health care settings. Founded in 1951, its members represent the American College of Physicians-American Society of Internal Medicine, the American College of Surgeons, the American Dental Association, the American Hospital Association, the American Medical Association, the public, and the nursing profession. The Joint Commission engages in issues and activities concerning the advancement of health care safety and quality, including public policy initiatives, standards development, and accreditation and certification programs.

knowledge-based information *See* information management.

laboratory *See* pathology and clinical laboratory services.

leader An individual who sets expectations, develops plans, and implements procedures to assess and improve the quality of the organization's governance, management, clinical, and support functions and processes. Leaders include, when applicable to the organization's structure, the owners, members of the governing body, the chief executive officer, director of nursing, medical director, and other senior managers and the leaders of the licensed independent practitioners.

licensed independent practitioner Any individual permitted by law and by the organization to provide care and services, without direction or supervision, within the scope of the individual's license and consistent with individually granted clinical privileges.

When standards reference the term "licensed independent practitioner," this language is not to be construed to limit the authority of a licensed independent practitioner to delegate tasks to other qualified health care personnel (for example, physician assistants and advanced practice registered nurses) to the extent authorized by state law or a state's regulatory mechanism or federal guidelines and organizational policy.

licensure A legal right that is granted by a government agency in compliance with a statute governing an occupation (such as medicine, nursing, psychiatry, or clinical social work) or the operation of an activity (such as in a long term care or residential treatment center).

***Life Safety Code*® (*LSC*)** A set of standards for the construction and operation of buildings, intended to provide a reasonable degree of safety to life during fires and prepared, published, and periodically revised by the National Fire Protection Association and adopted by the Joint Commission to evaluate health care organizations under its life-safety management program. *See also* interim life safety measures; fire-safety management; occupancy.

life-support equipment Any device used for the purpose of sustaining life and whose failure to perform its primary function, when used according to manufacturer's instructions and clinical protocol, will lead to patient death in the absence of immediate intervention (examples include ventilators, anesthesia machines, and heart-lung bypass machines).

loss of protective reflexes An inability to handle secretions without aspiration or to maintain a patent airway independently.

management of information *See* information management.

measure of success (MOS) A numerical or quantifiable measure usually related to an audit that determines if an action was effective and sustained; due four months after Evidence of Standards Compliance (*see* definition) approval.

measurement The systematic process of data collection, repeated over time or at a single point in time.

medical equipment Fixed and portable equipment used for the diagnosis, treatment, monitoring, and direct care of individuals. *See also* equipment management.

medical history A component of the medical record consisting of an account of an individual's history, obtained whenever possible from the individual, and including at least the following information: chief complaint, details of the

GL

present illness or care needs, relevant past history, and relevant inventory by body systems.

medical record *See* record.

medical record review The process of measuring, assessing, and improving the quality of medical record documentation—that is, the degree to which medical record documentation is accurate, complete, and performed in a timely manner. This process is carried out with the cooperation of relevant departments or services.

medication Any prescription medications; sample medications; herbal remedies; vitamins; nutriceuticals; over-the-counter drugs; vaccines; diagnostic and contrast agents used on or administered to persons to diagnose, treat, or prevent disease or other abnormal conditions; radioactive medications; respiratory therapy treatments; parenteral nutrition; blood derivatives; intravenous solutions (plain, with electrolytes and/or drugs); and any product designated by the Food and Drug Administration (FDA) as a drug. This definition of medication does not include enteral nutrition solutions (which are considered food products), oxygen, and other medical gases.

medication error Any preventable event that may cause inappropriate medication use or jeopardize patient safety. *See also* adverse drug reaction; sentinel event.

medication history A delineation of the drugs used by an individual (both past and present), including prescribed and unprescribed drugs and alcohol, along with any unusual reactions to those drugs. *See* medication.

medication management The process an organization uses to provide medication therapy to patients receiving care, treatment, and services from the organization. The steps in the medication management process include:

- **selection** Safe and appropriate selection of medications available for prescribing, storage, and/or use in the organization.
- **procurement** The task of obtaining selected medications from a source outside the organization. It does not include obtaining a medication from the organization's own pharmacy, which is considered as part of the ordering and dispensing processes.
- **storage** The task of appropriately maintaining a supply of medications on the organization's premises.
- **secure** In locked containers, in a locked room, or under constant surveillance.
- **prescribing or ordering** Synonymous terms for when a licensed independent practitioner transmits a legal order or prescription to the organization directing the preparing, dispensing, and administering of a specific medication to a specific patient. It does not include requisitions for medication supplies.
- **transcribing** The process by which an order from a licensed independent practitioner is documented either in writing or electronically.
- **preparing** The compounding, manipulation, or other activity needed to get a medication ready for administration exactly as ordered by the licensed independent practitioner.
- **dispensing** Providing, furnishing, or otherwise making available a supply of medications to the individual for whom it was ordered or their representative by a licensed pharmacy according to a specific prescription or medication order, or by a licensed independent practitioner authorized by law to dispense. Dispensing does not involve providing an individual a dose of medication previously dispensed by the pharmacy.
- **administration** The provision of a prescribed and prepared dose of an identified medication to the individual for whom it was ordered to achieve its pharmacological effect. This includes directly introducing the medication into or onto the individual's body.
- **self-administration** Independent use by a patient of a medication, including medications that may be held by the organization for independent use by the patient.
- **monitoring** The ongoing evaluation of an individual to whom a medication was administered, to ascertain the effectiveness and efficacy of the medication therapy and prevent the occurrence of any serious adverse outcomes.
- **medication-management measurement** The measurement, assessment, and improvement of the prescribing or ordering, preparing and dispensing, administering, and monitoring of medications.

mental abuse *See* abuse.

minimum data set An agreed-on and accepted set of terms and definitions constituting a core of data; a collection of related data items.

mission statement A written expression that sets forth the purpose of an organization or one of its components. The generation of a mission statement usually precedes the formation of goals and objectives.

mitigation activities Those activities an organization undertakes in attempting to lessen the severity and impact of a potential emergency. *See* emergency.

multidisciplinary team A group of clinical staff members composed of representatives of a range of professions, disciplines, or service areas.

near miss Used to describe any process variation which did not affect an outcome, but for which a recurrence carries a significant chance of a serious adverse outcome. Such a "near miss" falls within the scope of the definition of a sentinel event, but outside the scope of those sentinel events that are subject to review by the Joint Commission under its Sentinel Event Policy.

neglect The absence of minimal services or resources to meet basic needs. Neglect includes withholding or inadequately providing food and hydration (without physician, patient, or surrogate approval), clothing, medical care, and good hygiene. It may also include placing the individual in unsafe or unsupervised conditions. *See also* abuse.

network An entity offering comprehensive or specialty services that provides, or provides for, integrated health care services to a defined population of individuals. Networks are characterized by a centralized structure that coordinates and integrates services provided by components and practitioners participating in the network.

nonrepudiation *See* information management.

GL

nursing The health profession dealing with nursing care and services as (1) defined by the Code of Ethics for Nurses with Interpretive Statements, Nursing's Social Policy Statement, Nurses' Bill of Rights, Scope and Standards of Nursing Practice of the American Nurses Association and specialty nursing organizations; and (2) defined by relevant state, commonwealth, or territory nurse practice acts and other applicable laws and regulations.

nursing care Professional processes of assessment, diagnosis, planning, implementation, and evaluation based on the art and science of nursing to promote health, its recovery, or a peaceful and dignified death. This includes, but is not limited to, assisting individuals, families, communities, and/or populations in understanding health needs and carrying out therapeutic plans and activities.

nursing services One or more defined units or departments within a health care organization with accountability for the delivery of quality nursing care to individuals, families, communities, and/or populations. Personnel, fiscal, capital, and intellectual resources focus on patient safety via interdisciplinary collaboration, integrated data and information management, and communication within all planning, implementation, and evaluation activities.

nursing staff Personnel within a health care organization who are accountable for providing and assisting in the provision of nursing care. Such personnel must include Registered Nurses (RNs), and may include others such as Advanced Practice Registered Nurses (APRNs), Licensed Practical or Vocational Nurses (LPNs/LVNs), and nursing assistants or other designated unlicensed assistive personnel.

nutriceuticals Nutritional supplements formulated in a pharmaceutical dosage form and used with the intention of deriving medical or health benefits, including preventing and treating disease. Such products may range from isolated nutrients, dietary supplements, and diets to genetically engineered "designer" foods, herbal products, and processed foods such as cereals, soups, and beverages.

nutrition The sum of the processes by which one takes in and uses nutrients.

nutrition assessment A comprehensive process for defining an individual's nutrition and hydration status using medical, nutrition, and medication intake histories; physical examination; anthropomorphic measurements; and laboratory data.

nutrition care Interventions and counseling to promote appropriate nutrition and fluid intake, based on nutrition and hydration assessment and information about food, other sources of nutrients, and meal preparation consistent with the individual's cultural background and socioeconomic status. Nutrition therapy, a component of medical treatment, includes enteral and parenteral nutrition.

nutrition screening A process used to indicate the need for a nutritional assessment to determine whether a patient is malnourished or at risk for malnourishment.

occupancy

ambulatory health care occupancy An occupancy used to provide, care, treatment, or services to four or more patients at the same time that either (1) renders them incapable of providing their own means of self-preservation in an emergency, or (2) provides outpatient surgical treatment requiring general anesthesia.

business occupancy An occupancy used to provide outpatient care, treatment, or services that does not meet the criteria in the ambulatory health care occupancy definition (for example, three or fewer patients at the same time who are either rendered incapable of self-preservation in an emergency or are undergoing general anesthesia).

health care occupancy An occupancy used for purposes such as medical or other treatment or care of persons suffering from physical or mental illness, disease or infirmity; and for the care of infants, convalescents, or infirm aged persons. Health care occupancies provide sleeping facilities for four or more occupants and are occupied by persons who are mostly incapable of self-preservation because of age, physical or mental disability, or because of security measures not under the occupant's control. Health care occupancies include hospitals, nursing homes, and limited care facilities.

residential occupancy An occupancy in which sleeping accommodations are provided for normal residential purposes and include all buildings designed to provide sleeping accommodations.

operative and other high-risk procedures Surgical or other procedures that put the patient at risk of death or disability. This does not include use of medications that place patients at risk.

oral and maxillofacial surgeon An individual who has successfully completed a postgraduate program in oral and maxillofacial surgery accredited by a nationally recognized accrediting body approved by the United States Department of Education. As determined by the medical staff, the individual is also currently competent to perform a complete history and physical examination in order to assess the medical, surgical, and anesthetic risks of the proposed operative and other procedure(s).

organization's strengths Areas in which an organization's performance is exemplary, as evidenced by the implementation of innovative approaches to meeting Joint Commission standards. An organization will not be cited for having a strength if the organization has a related noncompliant standard and/or partially compliant EP.

pathology and clinical laboratory services The services that provide information on diagnosis, prevention, or treatment of disease or the assessment of health, through the examination of the structural and functional changes in tissues and organs of the body that cause or are caused by disease. It also includes the biological, microbiological, serological, chemical, immunohematological, hematological, or other examination of materials derived from the human body.

patient An individual who receives care, treatment, or services. For hospice providers, the patient and family are considered a single unit of care. Synonyms used by various health care fields include client, resident, customer, patient and family unit, consumer, and health care consumer.

patient tracer The process used by the Joint Commission of evaluating a patient's total care experience within a health care organization.

peer recommendation Information submitted by an individual(s) in the same professional discipline as the applicant reflecting their perception of the practitioner's clinical practice, ability to work as part of a team, and ethical behavior or the documented peer evaluation of practitioner-specific data collected from various sources for the purpose of evaluating current competence.

performance improvement The continuous study and adaptation of a health care organization's functions and processes to increase the probability of achieving desired outcomes and to better meet the needs of individuals and other users of services.

Periodic Performance Review (PPR) An additional requirement of the accreditation process whereby an organization reviews its compliance with all applicable Joint Commission standards; completes and submits to the Joint Commission a Plan of Action (*see* definition) for any standard not in full compliance, including the identification of a Measure of Success (MOS) (*see* definition); and chooses to engage in a telephone discussion with a member of the Standards Interpretation Group staff to determine the acceptability of the Plan of Action. The PPR will encourage organizations to be in continuous compliance with Joint Commission standards. At the time of the next full survey, surveyors will validate that the MOS were implemented and effective.

pharmaceutical care and services Services provided directly or through written contract with another organization that include procuring, preparing, dispensing, and/or distributing pharmaceutical products and the ongoing monitoring of the recipient to identify, prevent, and resolve medication-related problems.

pharmaceutical equivalence The degree to which two formulations of the same medication are identical in strength, concentration, and dosage form.

pharmacist An individual who has a degree in pharmacy and is licensed and registered to prepare, preserve, compound, and dispense drugs and chemicals.

pharmacy A licensed location where drugs are stored and dispensed.

pharmacy services The provision of pharmaceutical care and services involving the preparation and dispensing of medications, and medication-related devices and supplies by a licensed pharmacy, with or without the provision of clinical or consultant pharmacist services.

physical abuse *See* abuse.

physical restraint *See* restraint.

physician A doctor of medicine or doctor of osteopathy who, by virtue of education, training, and demonstrated competence, is granted clinical privileges by the organization to perform a specific diagnostic or therapeutic procedure(s) and who is fully licensed to practice medicine.

physician assistant An individual who practices medicine with supervision by licensed physicians, providing patients with services ranging from primary medicine to specialized surgical care. The scope of practice is determined by state law, the supervising physician's delegation of responsibilities, the individual's education and experience, and the specialty and setting in which the individual works.

When standards reference the term "licensed independent practitioner," this language is not to be construed to limit the authority of a licensed independent practitioner to delegate tasks to other qualified health care personnel (for example, physician assistants and advanced practice registered nurses) to the extent authorized by state law or a state's regulatory mechanism or federal guidelines and organizational policy.

physician licensure The process by which a legal jurisdiction, such as a state, grants permission to a physician to practice medicine after finding that he or she has met acceptable qualification standards. Licensure also involves ongoing regulation of physicians by the legal jurisdiction, including the authority to revoke or otherwise restrict a physician's license to practice.

plan A detailed method, formulated beforehand, that identifies needs, lists strategies to meet those needs, and sets goals and objectives. The format of the plan may include narratives, policies and procedures, protocols, practice guidelines, clinical paths, care maps, or a combination of these.

plan of action A plan detailing the action(s) that an organization will take in order to come into compliance with a Joint Commission standard. A plan of action must be completed for each element of performance (EP) (*see* definition) associated with a not compliant standard. A measure of success (MOS) (*see* definition) must also be included in the plan of action as indicated in the accreditation manual.

plan for improvement For purposes of Joint Commission accreditation, an organization's written statement that details the procedures to be taken and time frames to correct existing *Life Safety Code*® deficiencies. *See also* Statement of Conditions (SOC); interim life safety measures; *Life Safety Code*®.

podiatrist An individual who has received the degree of doctor of podiatric medicine and who is licensed to practice podiatry.

point-of-care testing Analytical testing performed at sites outside the traditional laboratory environment, usually at or near the site where care is delivered to individuals. Testing may range from simple waived procedures, such as fecal occult blood, to more sophisticated chemical analyzers. The testing may be under the control of the main laboratory, the direction of another specialized laboratory (such as for arterial blood gas), or under the nursing service. Testing may be categorized as waived, moderate, or high complexity under CLIA '88. Also called alternate site testing, decentralized laboratory testing, and distributed site testing.

policies and procedures The formal, approved description of how a governance, management, or clinical care process is defined, organized, and carried out.

practice guidelines Tools that describe processes found by clinical trials or by consensus opinion of experts to be the most effective in evaluating and/or treating a patient who has a specific symptom, condition, or diagnosis or that describe a specific procedure. Synonyms include clinical practice guideline, practice parameter, protocol, preferred practice pattern, and guideline.

Preliminary Denial of Accreditation *See* accreditation decisions.

preparedness activities Those activities an organization undertakes to build capacity and identify resources that may be used if an emergency occurs. *See* emergency.

prescribing or ordering *See* medication management.

primary source The original source or an approved agent of that source of a specific credential that can verify the accuracy of a qualification reported by an individual health care practitioner. Examples include medical school, graduate education, and state medical board and federal and state licensing boards.

primary source verification Verification of an individual health care practitioner's reported qualifications by the original source or an approved agent of that source. Methods for conducting primary source verification of credentials include direct correspondence, documented telephone verification or secure electronic verification from the original qualification source, or reports from credentials verification organizations that meet the 10 Joint Commission requirements (see the note for Standard HR.1.20, EP 3.

priority focus areas Processes, systems, or structures in a health care organization that significantly impact the quality and safety of care. The priority focus areas are

- Assessment and Care/Services
- Communication
- Credentialed Practitioners
- Equipment Use
- Infection Control
- Information Management
- Medication Management
- Organizational Structure
- Orientation and Training
- Patient Safety
- Physical Environment
- Quality Improvement Expertise and Activities
- Rights and Ethics
- Staffing

primary priority focus area Every standard is linked to one or more priority focus areas. When a surveyor has findings under a standard, he or she determines which of the linked priority focus areas is most related to the specific finding; this becomes the *primary* priority focus area. For example, a finding under standard HR.1.10 may be linked to the primary priority focus area of Staffing.

secondary priority focus areas These are priority focus areas that, in addition to the primary priority focus area, are related to a specific finding. For example, a finding under standard HR.1.10 may be linked to a secondary priority focus area of Orientation and Training. The organization's Accreditation Report lists the secondary priority focus area(s).

Priority Focus Process (PFP) The process for standardizing the priorities for sampling during an organization's survey based on information collected about the organization prior to survey. The process also helps to focus the survey on areas that are critical to that organization's client safety and quality-of-care processes. Examples of such information may include, but are not limited to, data from the organization's e-App (see definition); past survey finding data; complaint and sentinel event information; and data collected from external sources.

Priority Focus Tool (PFT) An automated tool that supports the Priority Focus Process through the use of algorithms, or sets of rules, to transform a health care organization's data into information that guides the survey process.

privacy *See* information management.

privileging The process whereby a specific scope and content of patient care services (that is, clinical privileges) are authorized for a health care practitioner by a health care organization, based on evaluation of the individual's credentials and performance. *See* licensed independent practitioner.

processing *See* information management.

program An organized system of services designed to address the needs of the organization or individual.

protected health information *See* information management.

Provisional Accreditation *See* accreditation decisions.

Public Information Policy A Joint Commission policy governing the disclosure of specific information about the performance of a health care organization or network, as well as accreditation-related information that will remain confidential. This policy covers the Joint Commission's Quality Reports, information publicly disclosed on request, complaint information, aggregate performance data, data released to government agencies, and the Joint Commission's right to clarify information an accredited organization releases about its accreditation status.

qualified individual An individual or staff member who is qualified to provide care, treatment, or services by virtue of the following: education; training; experience; competence; registration, certification, or applicable licensure; and law or regulation. Examples of qualified individuals can include: activities coordinator, administrator, audiologist, child psychiatrist, clinical chaplain, creative arts therapist, dietetic services supervisor, dietitian, registered dietitian, health information administrator, health information technician, licensed practical nurse (LPN), medical radiation physician, medical technologist, music therapist, occupational therapist, occupational therapy assistant, physiatrist, physical therapist assistant, physical therapist, psychiatric nurse, psychologist, radiologic technologist, recreational therapist, recreational therapist assistant or technician, respiratory care technician, respiratory therapist, respiratory therapy technician, social work assistant, social worker, and speech-language pathologist.

quality control A process that consists of measuring performance, comparing performance against goals, and acting on the differences when performance falls short of defined goals.

quality of care The degree to which health services for individuals and populations increase the likelihood of desired health outcomes and are consistent with current professional knowledge. Dimensions of performance include the following: patient perspective issues; safety of the care environment; and accessibility, appropriateness, continuity, effectiveness, efficacy, efficiency, and timeliness of care.

Quality Report A report that is available to the public that provides information about an organization's accreditation decision and the effective date for the decision, any special quality awards the organization received, the accreditation services included in the organization's accreditation award, any disease-specific care certification(s) and the effective date of each certification received by the organization, the implementation of National Patient Safety Goals by the organization, the organization's performance against National Quality Goals, and the organization's performance in relation to Patient Experience of Care measures.

range orders Orders in which the dose or dosing interval varies over a prescribed range, depending on the situation or individual's status.

rationale for a standard Background, justification, or additional information about a standard. A rationale is *not* scored. Not every standard has a rationale.

reassessment Ongoing data collection, which begins on initial assessment, comparing the most recent data with the data collected at earlier assessments.

record **1.** The account compiled by physicians and other health care professionals of a variety of patient health information, such as assessment findings, treatment details, and progress notes. **2.** (data source) Data obtained from the records or documentation maintained on a patient in any health care setting (for example, hospital, home care, long term care, practitioner office). Includes automated and paper medical record systems.

referral The sending of an individual (1) from one clinician to another clinician or specialist, (2) from one setting or service to another, or (3) by one physician (the referring physician) to another physician(s) or other resource, either for consultation or care.

registered nurse An individual who is qualified by an approved postsecondary program or baccalaureate or higher degree in nursing and licensed by the state, commonwealth, or territory to practice professional nursing.

report generation *See* information management.

reprocessing All operations performed to render a contaminated reusable or single-use device patient-ready. The steps may include cleaning and disinfection/sterilization. The manufacturer of reusable devices and single use devices that are marketed as nonsterile should provide validated reprocessing instructions in the labeling.

requirement for improvement A recommendation that is required to be addressed in an organization's Evidence of Standards Compliance (*see* definition), and needs to be addressed in order for the organization to retain its accreditation decision. Failure to adequately address a requirement for improvement after two opportunities will result in a recommendation to place the organization in Conditional Accreditation (*see* definition).

residential occupancy *See* occupancy.

respiratory care services Delivery of care to provide ventilatory support and associated services for individuals.

restraint Any method (chemical or physical) of restricting a patient's freedom of movement, including seclusion, physical activity, or normal access to his or her body that (1) is not a usual and customary part of a medical diagnostic or treatment procedure to which the patient or his or her legal representative has consented; (2) is not indicated to treat the patient's medical condition or symptoms; or (3) does not promote the patient's independent functioning.

- **chemical restraint** The inappropriate use of a sedating psychotropic drug to manage or control behavior.
- **physical restraint** Any method of physically restricting a person's freedom of movement, physical activity, or normal access to his or her body.

resuscitative services Personnel, supplies, and processes used to resuscitate an individual.

retrievability *See* information management.

Review Hearing Panel A panel of three individuals, including one member of the Joint Commission Accreditation Committee, which hears a presentation on the facts of the case by an organization in Preliminary Denial of Accreditation, should the organization desire such a presentation.

risk assessment, proactive An assessment that examines a process in detail, including sequencing of events; assesses actual and potential risk, failure, or points of vulnerability; and, through a logical process, prioritizes areas for improvement based on the actual or potential patient care impact (criticality).

risk-management activities Clinical and administrative activities that organizations undertake to identify, evaluate, and reduce the risk of injury to patients, staff, and visitors and the risk of loss to the organization itself.

root cause analysis A process for identifying the basic or causal factor(s) that underlie variation in performance, including the occurrence or possible occurrence of a sentinel event.

safety The degree to which the risk of an intervention (for example, use of a drug or a procedure) and risk in the care environment are reduced for a patient and other persons, including health care practitioners.

safety management Activities selected and implemented by the organization to assess and control the impact of environmental risk and to improve general environmental safety.

scope of care or services The activities performed by governance, managerial, clinical, or support staff.

security *See* information management.

security management A component of an organization's management of the environment of care program that maintains and improves the general security of the care environment.

sedation *See* anesthesia and sedation.

self-admimistration *See* medication management, administration.

sentinel event An unexpected occurrence involving death or serious physical or psychological injury, or the risk thereof. Serious injury specifically includes loss of limb or function. The phrase "or the risk thereof" includes any process variation for which a recurrence would carry a significant chance of a serious adverse outcome.

sexual abuse *See* abuse.

Shared Visions–New Pathways® An initiative to progressively sharpen the focus of the accreditation process on care systems critical to the safety and quality of patient care.

staff As appropriate to their roles and responsibilities, all people who provide care, treatment, and services in the organization, including those receiving pay (for example, permanent, temporary, and part-time personnel, as well as contract employees), volunteers and health profession students. The definition of staff does not include licensed independent practitioners who are not paid staff or who are not contract employees.

staffing effectiveness The number, competence, and skill mix of staff as related to the provision of needed services.

standard A statement that defines the performance expectations, structures, or processes that must be in place for an organization to provide safe and high-quality care, treatment, and service.

Statement of Conditions™ (SOC) A proactive document that helps an organization do a critical self-assessment of its current level of compliance and describe how to resolve any *Life Safety Code®* (*LSC*) deficiencies. The SOC was created to be a "living, ongoing" management tool that should be used in a management process that continually identifies, assesses, and resolves *LSC* deficiencies.

sterilization The use of a physical or chemical procedure to destroy all microbial life, including highly resistant bacterial endospores.

structured text *See* information management.

supplemental finding A recommendation that is not required to be addressed in an organization's Evidence of Standards Compliance (*see* definition) but should be addressed by the organization internally. A supplemental finding will also be factored into an organization's Priority Focus Process at its next survey.

surrogate decision maker Someone appointed to act on behalf of another. Surrogates make decisions only when an individual is without capacity or has given permission to involve others. *See also* family.

survey A key component in the accreditation process, whereby a surveyor(s) conducts an on-site evaluation of an organization's compliance with Joint Commission standards.

full survey A survey that assesses an organization's compliance with all applicable Joint Commission standards.

initial survey A survey of a health care organization not previously accredited by the Joint Commission, or a survey of an organization performed without reference to any prior survey findings.

surveyor For purposes of Joint Commission accreditation, a licensed physician, surgeon, podiatrist, dentist, nurse, physician assistant or administrator, or any other health care professional who meets the Joint Commission's surveyor selection criteria, evaluates standards compliance, and provides education and consultation regarding standards compliance to surveyed organizations or networks and systems.

system A set of interrelated parts that work together toward a common goal.

system tracer A session during the on-site survey devoted to evaluating high-priority safety and quality-of-care issues on a systemwide basis throughout the organization. Examples of such issues may include infection control, medication management, staffing effectiveness, and the use of data.

systems analysis The evaluation of how well a health care organization's systems function.

telemedicine The use of health care information exchanged from one site to another via electronic communications for the health and education of the patient or health care provider and for the purpose of improving patient care, treatment, and services.

threshold for Conditional Accreditation At least two but not more than three standard deviations above the mean number of Not Compliant standards; the threshold for Conditional Accreditation is one rule for receiving Conditional Accreditation.

threshold for Preliminary Denial of Accreditation At least three standard deviations above the mean number of Not Compliant standards; the threshold for Preliminary Denial of Accreditation is one rule for receiving Preliminary Denial of Accreditation.

timeliness *See* information management.

tracer methodology A process surveyors use during the on-site survey to analyze an organization's systems, with particular attention to identified priority focus areas, by following individual patients through the organization's health care process in the sequence experienced by the patients. Depending on the health care setting, this may require surveyors to visit multiple care units, departments, or areas within an organization or a single care unit to "trace" the care, treatment, or services rendered to a patient.

transfer The formal shifting of responsibility for the care of an individual (1) from one care unit to another, (2) from one clinical service to another, (3) from one licensed independent practitioner to another, or (4) from one organization to another organization.

translation services Translation services provide *translation* of written documents into other languages. A translator is a person who converts the written text of one language into the written text of one or more languages. Unlike interpretation, which works with spoken/signed language, translation works only with written text.

transmission *See* information management.

urgent A degree of severity of illness or injury that is less severe than immediately life-threatening (emergency), but requiring care more quickly than elective care.

urgent/immediate care services Those services sought for conditions that are considered less critical than those that need to be seen in an emergency center but are not scheduled with the individual's primary care provider or the provider's designee.

utilities management Activities selected and implemented by the organization to assess and control the risks of utility systems of buildings that support the provision of care, treatment, or services. Included are those activities that ensure the operational reliability of such systems and those activities for responding to a failure of such systems.

utility systems Building systems for life support; surveillance, prevention, and control of infection; environment support; and equipment support. May include electrical distribution; emergency power; vertical and horizontal transport; heating, ventilating, and air-conditioning; plumbing, boiler, and steam; piped gases; vacuum systems; or communication systems, including data-exchange systems.

utilization management The examination and evaluation of the appropriateness of the utilization of an organization's resources. Also referred to as a utilization review.

waived testing Tests that meet the Clinical Laboratory Improvement Act of 1988 (CLIA '88) requirements for waived tests; are cleared by the Food and Drug Administration for home use; employ methodologies that are so simple and accurate as to render the likelihood of erroneous results negligible; or pose no risk of harm to the patient if the test is performed incorrectly. *See also* CLIA '88.

written Information that is documented in hard copy or electronic formats.

Index

IX

IX

IX

IX

E

IX

IX

IX

IX

N

IX

O

Q

IX

GWUMC
P1877A